Atlas of Gastrointestinal Pathology as seen on biopsy

For Margaret

Nec desiderio minus est praemium

Current Histopathology

Consultant Editor
Professor G. Austin Gresham, TD, ScD, MD, FRC Path.
Professor of Morbid Anatomy and Histology, University of Cambridge

Volume Six

ATLAS OF GASTROINTESTINAL PATHOLOGY
AS SEEN ON BIOPSY

BY I. M. P. DAWSON

Emeritus Professor of Pathology and Honorary Consultant Pathologist
University Hospital
Nottingham

1983 **MTP PRESS LIMITED**
a member of the KLUWER ACADEMIC PUBLISHERS GROUP
BOSTON / THE HAGUE / DORDRECHT / LANCASTER

Published by
MTP Press Limited
Falcon House
Cable Street
Lancaster, England

British Library Cataloguing in Publication Data

Dawson, Ian M. P.
    Atlas of gastrointestinal pathology—(Current
histopathology; v. 6)
    1. Gastroenterology
    I. Title   II. Series
    616.3'307   RC803

ISBN-13:978-94-009-6585-0   e-ISBN-13:978-94-009-6583-6
DOI: 10.1007/978-94-009-6583-6

Phototypesetting by Georgia Origination, Liverpool.
Colour origination by Replica Photo-Litho
Reproducers Limited, Stockport.

Manchester.

Contents

Current Histopathology Series

Consultant Editor's Note

At the present time books on morbid anatomy and histology can be divided into two broad groups: extensive textbooks often written primarily for students and monographs on research topics.

This takes no account of the fact that the vast majority of pathologists are involved in an essentially practical field of general Diagnostic Pathology providing an important service to their clinical colleagues. Many of these pathologists are expected to cover a broad range of disciplines and even those who remain solely within the field of histopathology usually have single and sole responsibility within the hospital for all this work. They may often have no chance for direct discussion on problem cases with colleagues in the same department. In the field of histopathology, no less than in other medical fields, there have been extensive and recent advances, not only in new histochemical techniques but also in the type of specimen provided by new surgical procedures.

There is a great need for the provision of appropriate information for this group. This need has been defined in the following terms.

(1) It should be aimed at the general clinical pathologist or histopathologist with existing practical training, but should also have value for the trainee pathologist.
(2) It should concentrate on the practical aspects of histopathology taking account of the new techniques which should be within the compass of the worker in a unit with reasonable facilities.
(3) New types of material, e.g. those derived from endoscopic biopsy should be covered fully.
(4) There should be an adequate number of illustrations on each subject to demonstrate the variation in appearance that is encountered.
(5) Colour illustrations should be used wherever they aid recognition.

The present concept stemmed from this definition but it was immediately realized that these aims could only be achieved within the compass of a series, of which this volume is one. Since histopathology is, by its very nature, systemized, the individual volumes deal with one system or where this appears more appropriate with a single organ.

Gastrointestinal Pathology is a further addition to this series of atlases for the histopathologist. The approach is concise, comprehensive and to the point which makes it a valuable volume for the bench worker. Biopsy material gets smaller as the years go by and gastrointestinal samples are amongst the smallest. This atlas begins with an introduction on handling and processing of such specimens which is the key to diagnostic accuracy. The application of new methods to the study of this material is also included.

The author has managed to cover a vast field with remarkable brevity and attention to detail.

G. Austin Gresham
Cambridge

Foreword

Biopsy of the gastrointestinal tract has been revolutionized by the introduction of fibreoptics; the proximal reaches, as far as the second part of the duodenum, and the whole large bowel back to the caecum can now be sampled under direct vision and multiple small biopsies can be obtained. Only in the jejunum and ileum are there still limitations on the sampling of localized as opposed to generalized conditions. The sheer volume of gastrointestinal material passing through our own laboratories has risen steeply over the last years to form some 25% of the total current work load and the rise continues; nearly all of it is in biopsy form rather than as resected specimens.

This great increase has led to other interesting and stimulating developments. First, and to me by far the most important, is the growing co-operation between pathologists and clinicians which has resulted in regular (for us weekly) meetings to discuss interesting patients with their biopsy material, better clinical histories for the pathologist with a greater awareness on his part of endoscopic appearances, and more soundly-based attempts to reason out what has happened when the clinical and pathological findings fail to correlate as they not infrequently do.

Second comes an informed appreciation of the value or otherwise of special techniques, including electron microscopy, plastic embedding with thin sectioning, histochemistry, immunocytochemistry and morphometry in particular suspected conditions. This necessarily includes an appreciation of when they are *not* likely to be helpful and which of them can reasonably be used in a busy district general hospital laboratory as opposed to a more *recherché* (though not necessarily less busy) teaching hospital. These sort of techniques, which I confess interest me greatly because of the additional information which they can yield when rightly chosen, are naturally linked with improved methods of tissue preservation in general, bearing in mind that the need for special techniques often becomes apparent only when the biopsy has been conventionally processed and examined. However, I have firmly stabled this hobbyhorse and have included little that cannot be done in a district general hospital and nothing that I am not prepared to do myself. I have tried to stress, particularly, common lesions which can cause real difficulty in interpretation, such as epithelial dysplasias, rather than rarities, since I still find them the most difficult of all to report; it is nice to talk about one's triumphs in making obscure diagnoses but it is the wrong decisions on reasonably common conditions that haunt one in the small hours.

A word is perhaps necessary about the arrangement of photomicrographs and the selection of references. The former are all arranged so that the luminal surface lies either at the top or to the right (I have inserted some photographs of resected specimens when these are helpful in illustrating a point or in suggesting what the endoscopic appearances look like in the surgically removed specimen); the latter have been selected particularly to give access to the rarer conditions or because they themselves give extensive reference lists which the reader can explore at greater leisure. My hope is that this Atlas may prove a practical working bench book for those interpreting biopsies; conditions which are not normally biopsied receive scant attention and it is in no sense a textbook in picture form.

Acknowledgements

I am deeply indebted to the many clinicians, particularly in the Westminster Hospital Group in London and in the Nottingham hospitals, who have supplied much of the biopsy material here described and photographed and taken part in many stimulating and sometimes uncomfortable discussions. I am equally indebted to fellow pathologists in the same hospitals and elsewhere both in Britain and abroad who have sent me interesting material and may recognize it in print. It is not possible to acknowledge them all individually but my particular thanks are due to Basil Morson at St Marks Hospital, London, who has given me much good advice and counsel during a friendship which has outlasted 25 years, to David Ansell at the City Hospital, Nottingham, Professor R. O. C. Kaschula of Capetown, Dr M. Al-Jafari, formerly of Baghdad, and Dr D. Jenkins of Lincoln, all of whom have given me much interesting material, and to members of our slide club in London and 'Black Box' in Nottingham from whose contributions some material has also been drawn. Virtually all of the photomicrographs were taken on my own microscope at the time of reporting, but the macroscopic photographs and a few photomicrographs are the work of our departmental photographer, Bill Brackenbury, while the electron micrographs are gifts from Graham Robinson and Stan Terras. The histochemical and immunocytochemical preparations were lovingly made by Mrs Janet Palmer, and my personal secretary, Mrs Joy Nice, patiently reduced my handwriting to legible typescript. I am also indebted to my successor, Professor D. R. Turner, who has allowed me continued use of departmental facilities.

Phil Johnstone of MTP Press has been a helpful editor, leaning heavily upon me in the later stages. To all of these and to other colleagues, medical, technical and secretarial, who have helped me at different times and in various ways I am grateful. Finally, as the dedication indicates, I owe to Margaret, my wife, for her practical help, encouragement and caring, very much more than it is possible to put into words.

Pathologists reporting on gastrointestinal biopsies in a routine laboratory normally rely on formaldehyde fixation, paraffin embedding and haematoxylin and eosin staining, supplemented by a limited number of special stains. For most biopsies this routine is satisfactory and other techniques, apart from step or serial sectioning, are unnecessary; in a few biopsies special procedures would be valuable if used and in a few others they are essential[1]. Attention to orientation, fixation and sectioning is, by contrast, vitally important, and it seems worthwhile to begin this book with a section on the handling of biopsies in general. More specific details which apply only to biopsies from particular conditions or sites are given in individual chapters.

Consideration of how to handle an individual biopsy should begin before rather than after the biopsy has been taken. Some biopsies provide less information than they should, either because the clinician has failed to tell the pathologist what he wants to know or because the pathologist has failed to make clear to the clinician exactly how much information he can give. For example, if disaccharidase deficiency is suspected in a child, ordinary histology is likely to be valueless, histochemistry on unembedded material may give some help, while biochemical analysis of unfixed material is the investigation of choice. Ideally every patient should be discussed by clinician and pathologist before biopsy. This is clearly impracticable but for each provisional clinical diagnosis a standard line of procedure can be agreed beforehand and no patient with an unusual or undetermined provisional diagnosis should be biopsied without discussion. Table 1.1 provides a summary of those special investigations which in my view are worthwhile for particular suspected diagnoses and which should be within the range of all laboratories which possess a cryostat, a competent MLSO who can cut good sections and an interested pathologist; I have not included any which I have not found of value or which I am not prepared to do myself. Table 1.2 lists those investigations which can be helpful in particular circumstances but which require specialized equipment. It should be emphasized that conventional processing, appropriately modified if facilities exist for plastic embedding and thin sectioning, is satisfactory for almost all biopsies.

Preservation of Material

For standard paraffin embedding and sectioning, neutral or buffered formaldehyde or 10% formol calcium are the fixatives of choice. I remain unconvinced of the need for mercurial fixation for this type of work. Consideration should be given to the use of modern techniques of plastic embedding, particularly in methacrylate resins which allow reasonable sized blocks to be handled, followed by $0.5-1.5 \mu m$ sections which provide excellent detail and often obviate any need for elec-

Table 1.1 Worthwhile special investigations practicable in a routine laboratory

Suspected diagnosis	Investigation	Preservation	Technique
Intestinal metaplasia	Studies on mucins	Routine fixation	PAS, Alcian Blue at pH 2.5 and 1.0
Malabsorption states in children (selected cases). See text	Enzyme histochemistry IgA in plasma cells Quantitation	Unfixed Consult lab* Routine	Alkaline phosphatase PAP or fluorescent antibody Eye piece graticle counts
Disaccharidase defects	Biochemical enzyme study Histochemical study**	Unfixed Unfixed	Consult biochemists Consult pathologist
Endocrine cell screening	Histochemical study	Routine formalin	Formaldehyde-induced fluorescence Argentaffin technique for 5-HT Argyrophil technique Lead haematoxylin
Hirschsprung's disease	Enzyme histochemistry	Unfixed	Acetylcholinesterase technique
Neuropathological diseases (gangliosidoses)	Lipid histochemistry	Unfixed	Autofluorescence, Sudan black, Oil Red O, Luxol fast blue, Feyrter's thionin, Acid phosphatase

* Different preservatives are called for as to whether a peroxidase or a fluorescent antibody technique are used.
** Only a few laboratories are equipped to do histochemical techniques on disaccharidases.

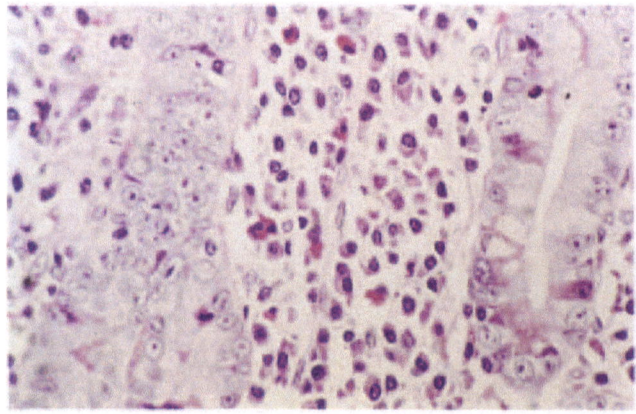

Figure 1.1 Stomach; gastritis. The clarity of detail of intracellular structures is obvious. Methacrylate embedding, 1.0 μm sectioning, toluidine blue stain   ×320

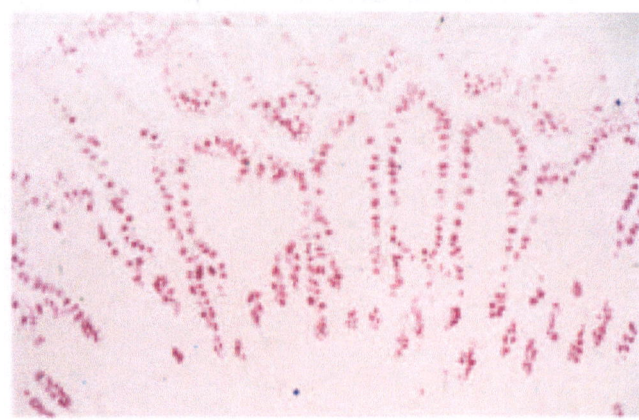

Figure 1.2 Normal small intestine. Neutral mucin demonstrated using a periodic acid-Schiff (PAS) technique.   ×100

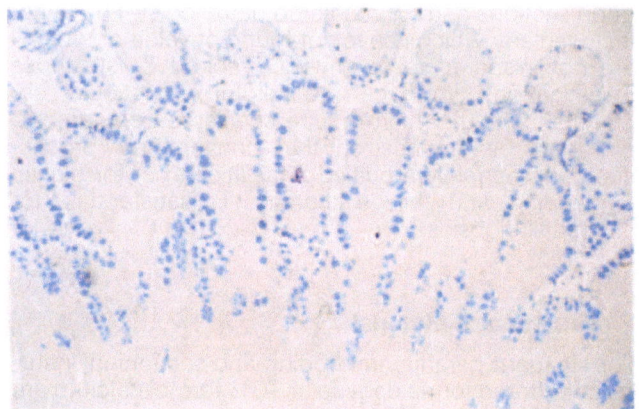

Figure 1.3 Normal small intestine. Sialomucin demonstrated using Alcian blue at pH 2.5.   ×100

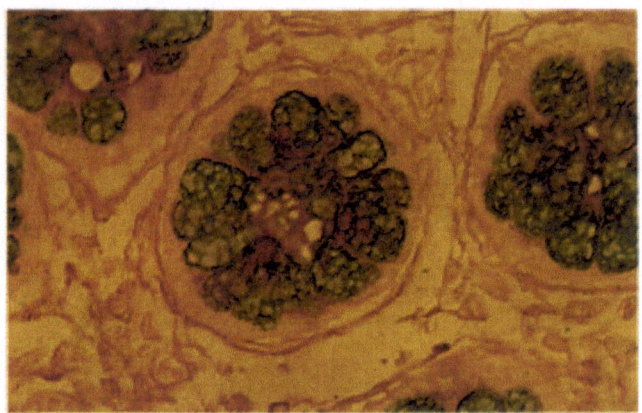

Figure 1.4 Normal rectum. Sialomucin (blue) and sulphomucin (brown) demonstrated simultaneously using an Alcian blue–high iron diamine technique   ×320

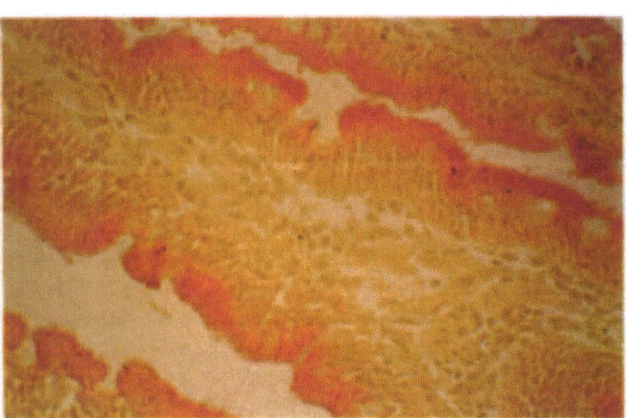

Figure 1.5 Normal small intestine. Shows the normal brush-border distribution of alkaline phosphatase.   Diazonium salt technique ×250

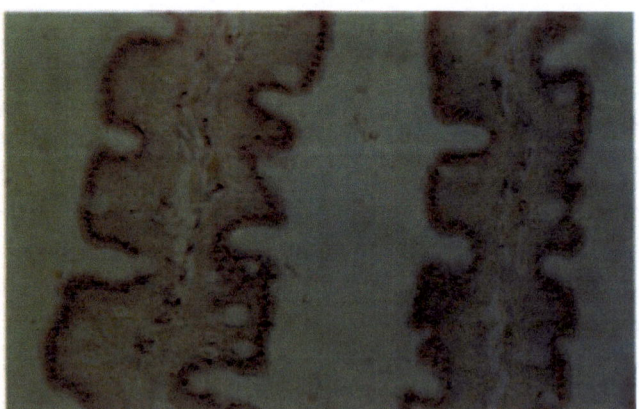

Figure 1.6 Normal small intestine. Shows the distribution of acid phosphatase in phagolysosomes within enterocytes and also within macrophages in the lamina propria.   Diazonium salt technique ×125

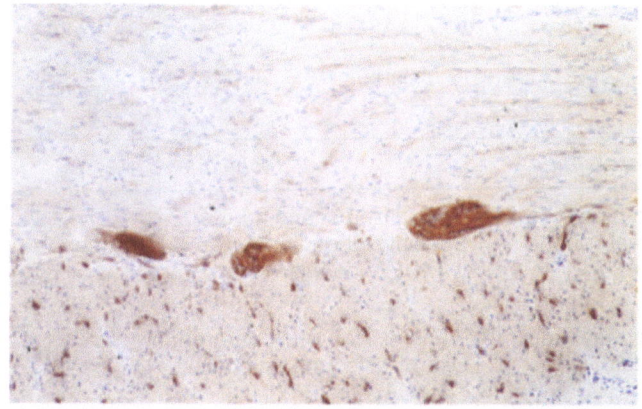

Figure 1.7 Normal rectum. Myenteric plexus showing the clear delineation of ganglion cells. Cholinesterase technique × 100

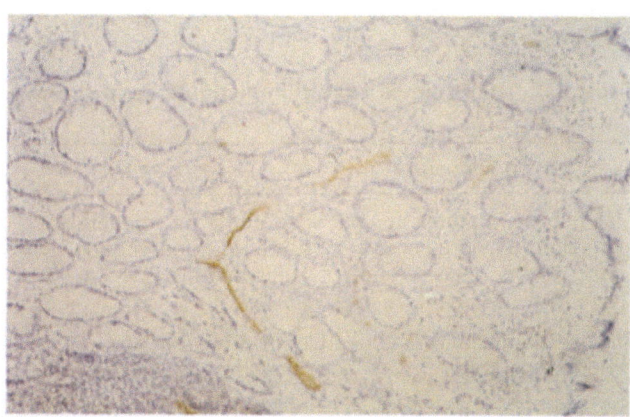

Figure 1.8 Normal rectum. Small nerve fibres are present normally in the mucosa. Cholinesterase technique × 125

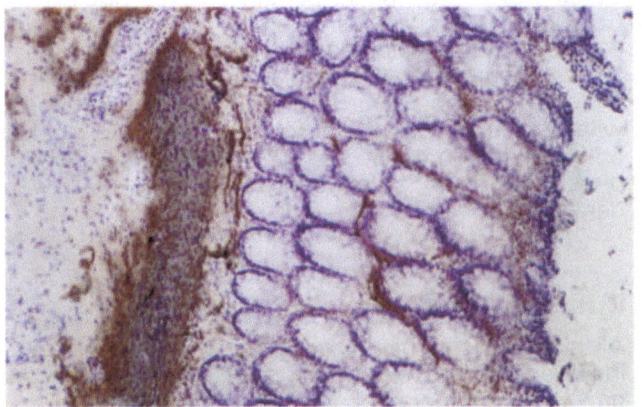

Figure 1.9 Rectum, Hirschsprung's disease. The fibres in the lamina propria are more numerous and thicker, especially in the region of the muscularis mucosae. This finding, which many consider diagnostic, can only be shown by the use of a cholinesterase technique. × 125

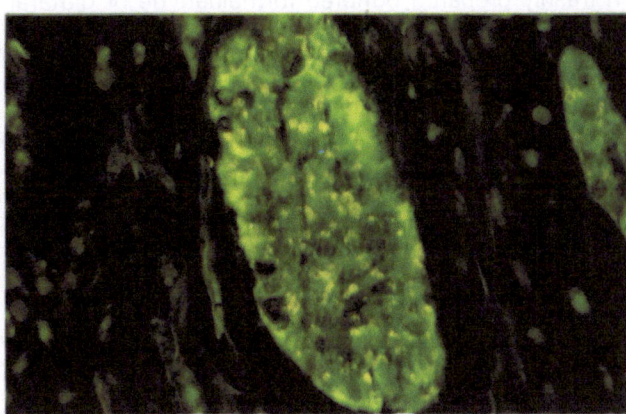

Figure 1.10 Appendix, carcinoid tumour. An island of carcinoid shows green autofluorescence with a specific yellow granular formaldehyde-induced fluorescence indicating the presence of β-carboline. Formaldehyde fixed, unstained section, blue-violet excitation × 250

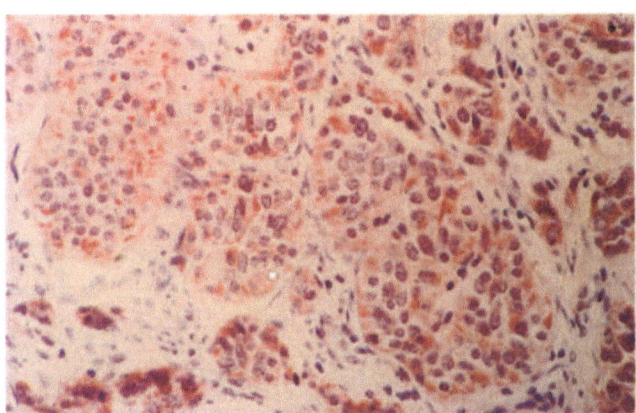

Figure 1.11 Appendix, carcinoid tumour. Islands of tumour showing red granular staining. Diazo reaction × 250

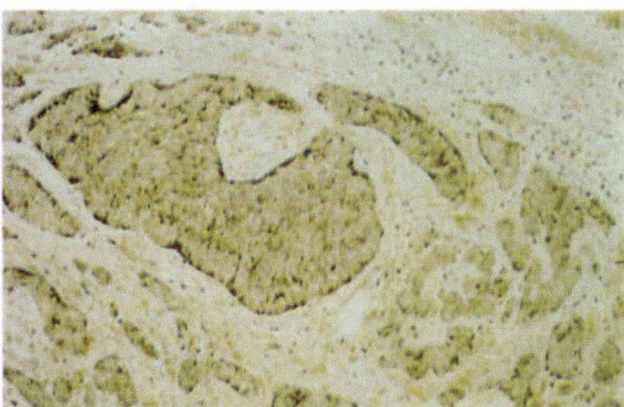

Figure 1.12 Appendix, carcinoid tumour. Islands of tumour showing argentaffin granules, most conspicuous at the edges of the tumour islets. Singh's technique × 125

Table 1.2 Worthwhile special investigations in specialist laboratory

Suspected diagnosis	Investigation	Preservation	Technique
Malabsorption states in children (selected cases)	Scanning e.m. appearance Specialized quantitation of cells and areas	Glutaraldehyde Normal routine	Specialized scanning e.m. Specialized equipment, e.g. Quantimet or MOP Videoplan
Further identification of endocrine cells	Electron microscopy Specialized antibodies	Glutaraldehyde Consult lab*	Transmission e.m. on granules Use of selected antibodies
Whipple's disease	Electron microscopy	Glutaraldehyde	Identification of organisms on e.m.

* Some antibodies (e.g. those to glucagon, gastrin and insulin) can be used on conventionally processed material. Others require special techniques of fixation and processing. Always consult with the laboratory concerned.

tron microscopy (Figure 1.1). If these are contemplated either for thin (1 μm) section or electron microscopy, fix in freshly prepared buffered formaldehyde or glutaraldehyde. For certain immunocytochemical or enzyme techniques either fix in 10% cold formol calcium and then immerse in cold gum sucrose or quench unfixed material. Both techniques are followed by cryostat sectioning. Details of appropriate preservation are given in Plate 1.1, from which it can be seen that different techniques are not necessarily mutually exclusive. It is not always appreciated that properly prepared cryostat sections can be used routinely for most diagnostic purposes: in practice many of our diagnostic paediatric small intestinal biopsies are fixed in cold formaldehyde, immersed in gum sucrose and cryostat sectioned to allow the subsequent use of enzyme techniques.

Quenching is the rapid cooling of biopsy material in a chemically inert liquid which does not vaporize. We use isopentane prechilled in liquid nitrogen. About 30 ml of isopentane placed in a small beaker which can be suspended in a wide-mouthed thermos containing liquid nitrogen is ideal. The isopentane is semisolid at this temperature but soon liquefies on removal from the liquid nitrogen. Tissues are orientated on a cork block or

a chuck (see below) using OCT both to secure tissue to cork and cork to chuck, and the whole is inserted upside-down into the isopentane. It will not fall off. Complete quenching of a small block takes about 10–15 s: do not prolong quenching beyond this time as blocks become brittle. If liquid nitrogen is unavailable, precool the isopentane by packing the beaker round with cardice, and allow 20 s for quenching. Store blocks on chucks or on the cork block in the cooling chamber of a cryostat in sealed cellophane bags to prevent dehydration.

Orientation, Transport and Sectioning

All biopsies less than 3 mm in greatest diameter and intended for fixation, whether single or multiple, should be wrapped in porous paper, immersed in fixative and orientated in the laboratory at the embedding stage. If a special technique is required which precludes fixation, wrap them in porous paper, soak a swab in sterile normal saline, wring out to damp-dry, wrap the porous paper in the swab and send to the laboratory immediately in a sealed container.

Plate 1.1

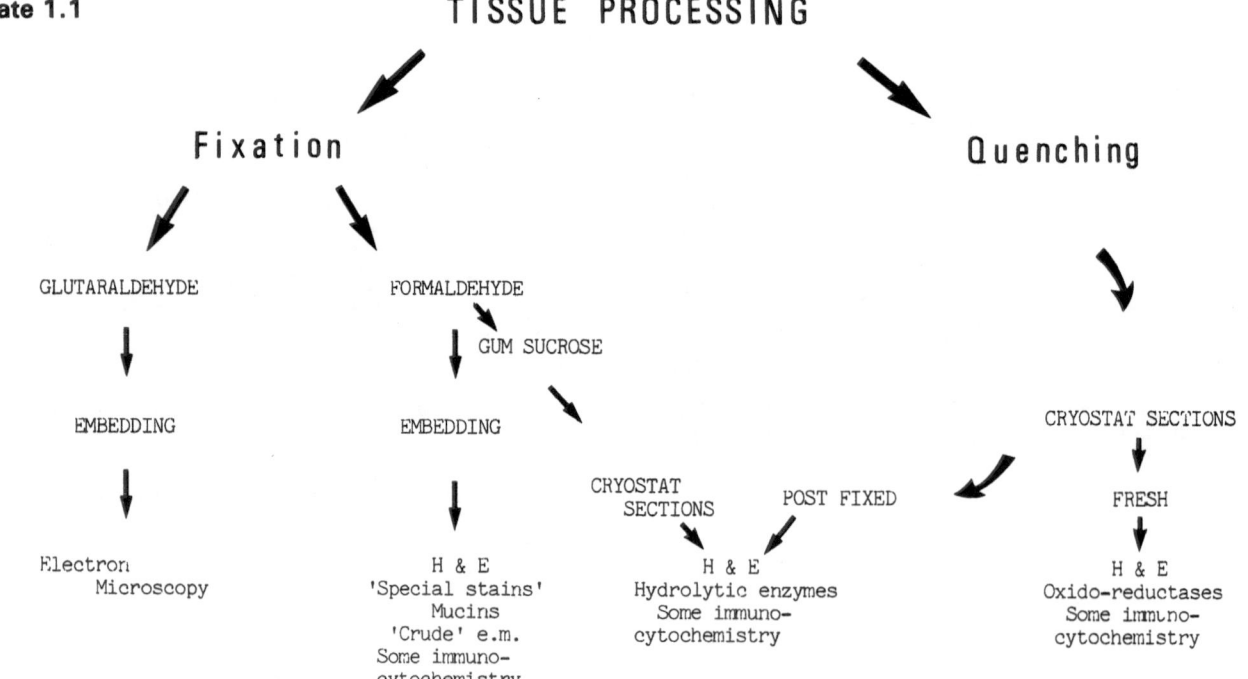

TISSUE PROCESSING

Whether or not the clinician orientates larger biopsies is a matter for discussion, which centres on whether a biopsy placed initially mucosal surface upwards on a firm surface and then immersed in fixative distorts less and is easier to orientate at paraffin wax or plastic embedding than one fixed without orientation or support. My own opinion is that if a clinician is prepared to orientate each biopsy individually using a lens or dissecting microscope, this is preferable; if he is not, fixation without orientation or the use of a support is better than unskilled attempts which can result in the mucosal surface being laid face down on the support with considerable subsequent distortion. I prefer filter paper squares to coverslips, card or plastic mesh as a support material since the fresh biopsy adheres well to it, and fixative penetrates it. Final orientation is always performed or checked on embedding, preferably using a dissecting microscope. This can be difficult with small biopsies, but there is a tendency, especially if the biopsy includes muscularis mucosae, for the mucosal surface to be convex, which is helpful.

If the workload allows, do not block more than two or three fragments from multiple biopsies together: it is difficult to get small biopsies aligned precisely in the same plane and one fragment may well be sectioned almost through before another has been reached.

It is a good working rule, even when 'levels' are likely to be required, to cut a single section first and check the orientation, while realignment is still possible. If 'levels' as opposed to serial sections are needed, keep the intervening sections in case special stains are required.

Special Techniques

The special techniques which I have found of value fall into four categories: histochemical, immunocytochemical, ultrastructural, and morphological or quantitative. There is likely in the future to be a place for scanning electron microscopy in those few departments equipped for it, but I propose here mainly to discuss what can be profitably done in a district hospital laboratory which has at most limited access to electron microscopic facilities.

Histochemistry

A recent review of the value of histochemistry in gastrointestinal studies is available[2]. The most useful techniques are those for mucins in the stomach and colon, for selected enzymes in the small intestine, for cholinesterase to delineate nerve fibres and ganglion cells, semispecific screening methods for endocrine cells, and techniques for investigating storage disorders in children, using histochemical methods for detecting contained substances in ganglion cells.

Mucosubstances

The three most valuable techniques are the use of diastase followed by PAS for neutral mucosubstances, Alcian blue at pH 2.5 for acid non-sulphated mucosubstances (sialomucins) and Alcian blue at pH 1.0 for acid sulphated mucosubstances. PAS and Alcian blue techniques can be combined, and more specialized iron diamine techniques will demonstrate sialomucins and sulphomucins simultaneously but simple single methods are usually preferable (Figures 1.2–1.4). They are readily performed on conventionally processed material.

The normal distribution of mucosubstances and the value of demonstrating them[3-5] are discussed in individual chapters.

Enzymes

Using appropriate techniques with selected substrates it is possible to demonstrate sites of enzymatic activity in mucosal and other cells. The only potential value which such techniques have in mucosal biopsy studies in routine diagnostic work is in the delineation of brush-border (alkaline phosphatase) enzymes in small intestinal biopsies (Figures 1.5 and 1.6) and in the demonstration of altered nerve fibres and absence of ganglion cells in Hirschsprung's disease (Figures 1.7–1.9) using a cholinesterase technique. The value of demonstrating brush-border and phagolysosomal enzymes remains doubtful and is discussed on page 74; the value of cholinesterase studies in Hirschsprung's disease[6] and other ganglion cell disorders is accepted and described on page 146.

Neuroendocrine Cells

A number of semispecific techniques are available for demonstrating neuroendocrine cells in the gut and merit brief comment. These cells may contain a biological amine, a specific polypeptide hormone or both, but the term APUD (Amino Precursor Uptake and Decarboxylation) cell is not always appropriate, as not all the cells can be shown to contain biological amines. They can be provisionally identified as members of the family by semispecific histochemical techniques (see below) and more specifically categorized by the ultrastructural appearance and immunocytochemical reactions of their contained granules[7,8].

Biological amines combine with aldehydes to form compounds which have reducing properties and which fluoresce. Most amines diffuse away in aqueous formalin too rapidly to remain detectable and special techniques such as freeze-drying of tissue and formaldehyde vapour fixation are required to demonstrate them, but 5-hydroxytryptamine (5HT) remains in cell granules in fresh tissue long enough to combine with formaldehyde to form a β-carboline detectable by its fluorescence (Figure 1.10), its ability to couple with diazonium salts (Figure 1.11) and its reducing properties (Figure 1.12) as demonstrated by argentaffin-type reactions.

In practice cell granules which possess these properties after conventional aldehyde fixation can confidently be said to contain 5HT, since other biological amines will have diffused into the aqueous fixative. The side-chains of polypeptide hormones possess ionizable acidic groups and many also contain disulphide bonds. Silver salts will attach to these and can be reduced to visible black metallic silver either by a reducing agent such as a β-carboline already present in the aldehyde-fixed cell (argentaffin reaction, see above) or by adding an external reducing agent (argyrophil reaction) (Figure 1.13). I prefer Singh's modification of the Masson Hamperl technique for argentaffin reactions and Grimelius' technique for argyrophil reactions[8]. The acidic side-chains also combine readily with basic and metachromatic dyes such as lead haematoxylin, toluidine blue or methylene blue, forming insoluble coloured products (Figure 1.14).

Positive staining of intracytoplasmic granules merely indicates the presence of a polypeptide with anionic reactive side-chains; it is reliable for screening but usually does not identify precisely the polypeptide present and a

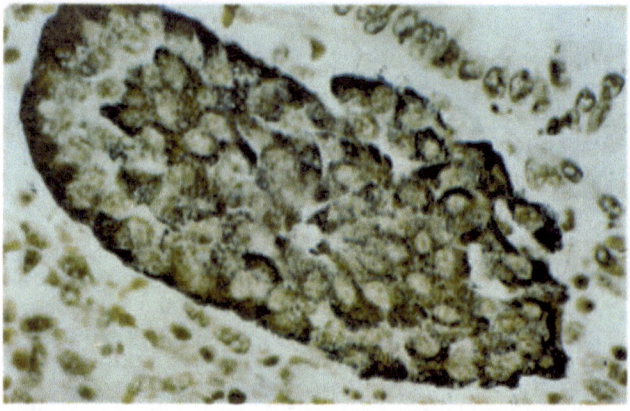

Figure 1.13   Ileum, carcinoid tumour. An islet of tumour showing argyrophil granules; there is also some nuclear staining.   Grimelius technique × 250

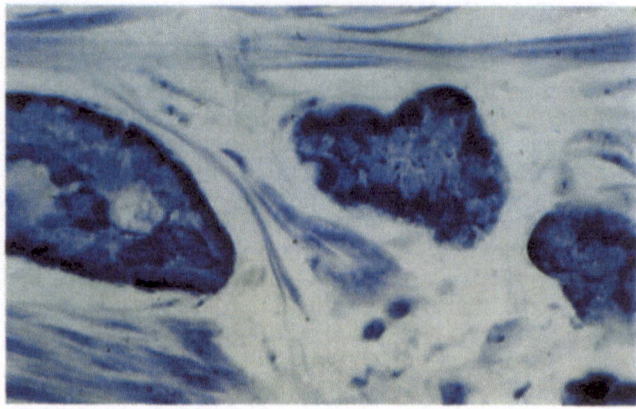

Figure 1.14   Ileum, carcinoid tumour. Two tumour islets contain granules stainable with lead haematoxylin.   × 250

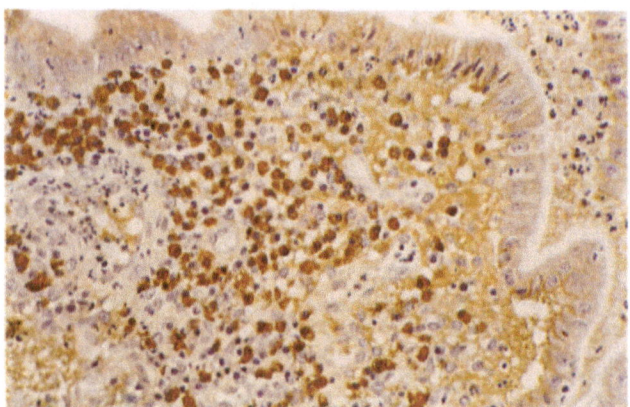

Figure 1.15   Normal rectum. Distribution of plasma cells containing IgA. Peroxidase–antiperoxidase (PAP) technique × 250

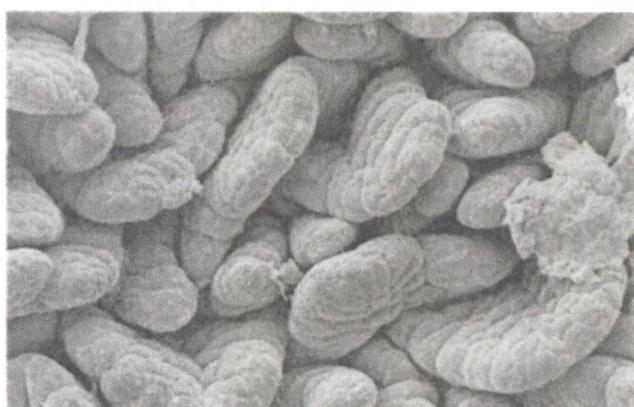

Figure 1.16   Normal small intestine. A scanning electron micrograph shows beautifully the configuration of normal villi.   × 1000

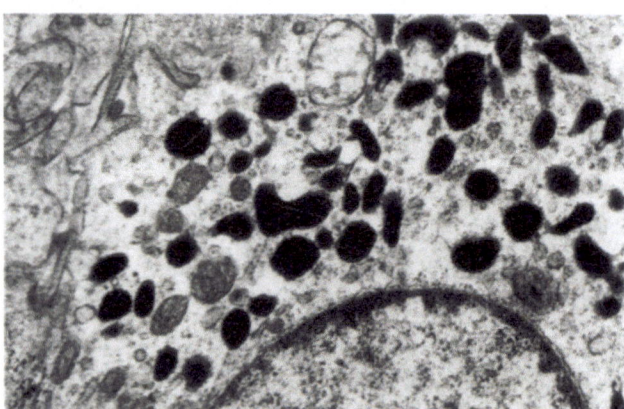

Figure 1.17   Normal small intestine. Transmission electron micrograph of a 5HT-containing cell showing the irregular shape of the granules, some of which are angulated.   × 20 000

negative result does not exclude an endocrine cell, which may have discharged its granule content.

Lipids and Carbohydrates

A number of storage disorders in children, particularly GM1 and GM2 gangliosidoses and Batten's disease, can be diagnosed by applying the appropriate histochemical and ultrastructural techniques to full-thickness biopsy sections of rectum to demonstrate stored material in submucosal and myenteric ganglion cells[9]. The techniques are specialized, and are briefly discussed on page 150.

Immunocytochemistry

There are two separate fields in which immunocytochemistry is becoming increasingly valuable in gastrointestinal pathology.

The first, which is usually allied with simple techniques in quantitation, is in demonstrating the presence of IgA, IgG and IgM in plasma cells within the lamina propria and in estimating the numbers and ratios of each type of plasma cell present; more refined techniques using anti-$\varkappa$, anti-λ and other specific antibodies, including those raised against fractions of complement, can be used to evaluate long and short chain components in monoclonal gammopathies, antigen/antibody reactions in tissues and to identify secretory piece. These techniques can be of value in malabsorption syndromes, in isolated immunoglobulin deficiencies, particulary IgA deficiency, and to some extent in evaluating rectal biopsies in inflammatory bowel disease. Their use is discussed in the appropriate sections.

The second is the use of specific antibodies against polypeptide hormones to identify individual hormones in granules.

Both types of reaction can be performed using fluorochrome-conjugated antibodies and transmission or incident fluorescent illumination or by using peroxidase techniques with conventional light microscopy (Figure 1.15). Full discussions of the relevant merits of each type of technique are available[10]. Fluorescent techniques usually demand the use of quenched unfixed material and cryostat sections; peroxidase techniques can be done on conventionally fixed paraffin embedded material which allow retrospective studies, but trypsinization with its associated disadvantages may be necessary. My preference is for peroxidase techniques but each particular investigation planned must be judged on its merits.

Ultrastructural Techniques

There is increasing evidence that scanning electron microscopy is capable of demonstrating minor defects in the surface mucosa anywhere in the bowel but particularly in the small intestine[11] (Figure 1.16). Scanning electron microscopes, however, are specialized instruments and neither they nor experts in interpreting results obtained by their use are readily available. Transmission electron microscopic facilities are more readily accessible; they are useful in detecting and identifying granules in suspected endocrine cell tumours (Figure 1.17), bacteria in certain diseases such as Whipple's disease, and minor degrees of microvillous damage; material should be preserved in buffered glutaraldehyde and sent to a specialized centre by arrangement.

Quantitation

Simple quantitation is now an accepted part of reporting in many small and large intestinal biopsies, even if the results are not numerically expressed[1]; for example, few pathologists would report a small bowel biopsy as 'flat' without commenting on whether the numbers of intraepithelial lymphocytes were or were not increased relative to absorptive enterocytes or muscularis mucosae, even if the exact counts were not given. Many workers, particulary those in children's units, will measure area and volume of villi relative to basal layer, either using graticules such as Weibel type hexagons or more sophisticated measuring apparatus such as the MOP videoplan or Quantimet[12,13]. Individual cell counts, such as those of IgA, IgG and IgM-containing plasma cells, need to be related to a fixed area, such as that of a given length of muscularis mucosae, which is not likely to vary with the disease under study. My own belief is that measurements of villous and basal layer areas are of value in some patients with partial flattening, that counts of immunoglobulin-containing plasma cells are often helpful in small and large bowel disorders, and that counts of intraepithelial lymphocytes are mandatory. Each is further discussed in the appropriate section.

Reporting Biopsies

There are certain questions which all pathologists must ask themselves whenever they come to report a biopsy. Everyone's list will vary: at the risk of appearing didactic, here is mine.

(1) Is the biopsy adequate for an informed report? This is not simply a matter of size but includes correct orientation, adequacy of depth and a reasonable assurance that it is representative of the organ or lesion. One should not be afraid to say that a biopsy is inadequate if this is genuinely the case.

(2) Has the material been adequately examined? If no obvious lesion is present, all biopsies should be serially or step sectioned before being reported as normal or inadequate. Many pathologists like routinely to serialize or step section every biopsy; I prefer to see a single section first to check orientation, though I like to step section later, unless the diagnosis is obvious.

(3) Are minor changes 'pathological' or within normal limits? This can be one of the most difficult decisions, particularly in deciding whether minor inflammatory changes are significant or can be disregarded (as for example they are usually not significant in cervical biopsies) and whether very mild dysplastic epithelial changes mean anything apart from a mild degree of irritation which is not significant. The problem is further discussed under individual organs.

(4) Have I given all the useful information I can? Pathologists tend to write descriptions: clinicians prefer positive definitive diagnoses. These cannot always be made, but I believe that clinicians have the right to an informed opinion rather than a list of possible differential diagnoses, all of which, from the report, appear equally probable or unlikely. One needs also to consider whether the appropriate special investigations and/or stains have been done. Some pathologists like to

write a report uninfluenced by knowledge of the patient's history: this is a matter of preference but I believe that the full history should always be available and consulted before a final report is issued. Negative statements are often of value in a report if a diagnosis has been suggested on the request form; '?Crohn's disease' on a large bowel biopsy form can be answered by a short statement 'there is no histological evidence to suggest Crohn's disease after serial section in this biopsy', which at least tells the clinician that his clinical supposition has been considered and, while not placed entirely out of court, is not supported by a full examination of the material available.

In my view the ideal report should describe as briefly as possible the material available, any unusual specialized procedure performed on it, and the histological and any other specialized findings. It should end with either a firm diagnosis or, where this is impossible, an opinion on the order of probability of any differential diagnoses made.

References

1. Underwood, J. C. E. (1981). *Introduction to Biopsy Interpretation and Surgical Pathology*. (Berlin: Springer-Verlag)

2. Dawson, I. M. P. (1981). The value of histochemistry in the diagnosis and prognosis of gastrointestinal diseases. In Stoward, P. J. and Polak, J. M. (eds.). *Histochemistry: The Widening Horizons*. pp. 127–162. (Chichester: John Wiley & Sons)

3. Filipe, M. I. and Branfoot, A. C. (1974). Abnormal patterns of mucous secretion in apparently normal mucosa of large intestine with carcinoma. *Cancer*, **34**, 282

4. Filipe, M. I. and Branfoot, A. C. (1976). Mucin histochemistry of the colon. *Curr. Top. Pathol.*, **63**, 143

5. Culling, C. F. A., Reid, P. E. and Dunn, W. L. (1976). A new histochemical method for the identification and visualization of both side chain acylated and non-acylated sialic acids. *J. Histochem. Cytochem.*, **24**, 1225

6. Patrick, W. J. A., Besley, G. T. N. and Smith, I. I. (1980). Histochemical diagnosis of Hirschsprung's disease and a comparison of the histochemical and biochemical activity of acetylcholinesterase in rectal mucosal biopsies. *J. Clin. Pathol.*, **33**, 336

7. Dawson, I. M. P. (1976). The endocrine cells in the gastrointestinal tract and the neoplasms which arise from them *Curr. Top. Pathol.*, **63**, 221

8. Dawson, I. M. P. (1980). Visualisation of the diffuse endocrine system. *J. Clin. Pathol.*, **33**, (Suppl.) (Assoc. Clin. Pathol.) **8**, 7

9. Brett, E. M. and Lake, B. D. (1975). Reassessment of rectal approach to neuropathology in childhood. Review of 307 biopsies over 11 years. *Arch. Dis. Child.*, **50**, 753

10. Robinson, G. (1982). Immunohistochemistry. In Bancroft, J. D. and Stevens, A., (eds.). *Theory and Practice of Histological Techniques*. 2nd edn, pp. 406–427. (Edinburgh and London: Churchill Livingstone)

11. Carr, K. E., Toner, P. G. and Saleh, K. M. (1982). Invited review: Scanning electron microscopy. *Histopathology*, **6**, 3

12. Guix, M., Skinner, J. M. and Whitehead, R. (1979). Measuring intraepithelial lymphocytes, surface area and volume of lamina propria in the jejunal mucosa of coeliac patients. *Gut*, **20**, 275

13. Wright, N. A., Appleton, D. R., Marks, J. and Watson, A. J. (1979). Cytokinetic studies of crypts in convoluted human small intestinal mucosa. *J. Clin. Pathol.*, **32**, 462

Oesophageal biopsies are performed under direct vision and localized lesions can therefore be sampled. Some lesions give rise to strictures which can make sampling below the upper end of the stricture difficult. It is essential to have an adequate history and to know accurately the distance from the incisor teeth at which each separate biopsy was taken. Multiple biopsies must be submitted separately with the level of sampling recorded for each. Only thus can metaplasia to a columnar ('Barrett') type of epithelium in reflux oesophagitis be reliably distinguished from gastric mucosa. In adults the oesophagogastric junction is normally about 40 cm from the incisor teeth; glandular mucosa in biopsies 38 cm or less from the incisors is likely to be metaplastic.

Orientation

Oesophageal biopsies can be difficult to orientate, even using a hand lens or dissecting microscope, since the squamous epithelial surface is often not curved, is not heavily coated with mucus and may not glisten. If sufficient submucosa is included the epithelial surface can appear slightly convex, but this is not as obvious as in gastric or intestinal biopsies and many biopsies consist of epithelium only. I do not think it is helpful for the clinician to do more than lay each biopsy separately on a piece of filter paper in what he judges is the most probable correct orientation before putting it into fixative. Smal biopsies should be wrapped in porous paper without attempts at orientation.

In the laboratory, the pathologist or MLSO should orientate under the dissecting microscope and then cut and stain a single section and re-check the orientation under the light microscope. A provisional assessment and a decision whether to cut serial sections for special stains and/or step sections can then be made, or the orientation can be corrected before further material is cut in an unsuitable plane. It is, in my view, always advisable eventually to serial or step-section all oesophageal material.

Specialized Techniques of Value

With an occasional exception I have not found histochemical, immunocytological or electron microscopic techniques of value in the diagnosis of oesophageal biopsy material and I do not routinely use them. When it is difficult to estimate the thickness of the basal layer, a PAS stain without diastase may help, since it stains glycogen which is present in the stratified squamous zone but not in the basal layer.

The Normal Oesophageal Mucosa

The normal oesophagus is about 25 cm long and is defined as extending from the pharynx to the cardia; for oesophagoscopists with adult patients it begins about 15 cm and ends at about 40 cm from the incisor teeth, and the distance at which any biopsy is taken should always be recorded. It is lined throughout by stratified, non-keratinizing squamous epithelium which contains occasional melanoblasts[1,2] and endocrine cells which are usually argyrophil[2]. Very rarely small islands of columnar epithelium, often ciliated, are seen in adults; they are entirely surrounded by squamous epithelium, are separate from and proximal to the cardia and represent remnants of a normal stage of embryonic development[3]. There is a recognizable proliferating basal layer which forms up to 15% of the total epithelial thickness (Figure 2.1), and connective tissue papillae project surfacewards into the epithelium reaching as far as two-thirds of the way to the lumen[4,5] (Figure 2.2). At the lower end there is an abrupt junction with cardiac mucosa (Figures 2.3 and 2.4). There is a muscularis mucosae of varying thickness, while in the submucosa lie small groups of mucus-secreting acinar and tubular glands which aggregate into small lobules; a number of these lobules are drained by a single duct which is lined by columnar epithelium and possesses a myoepithelial coat (Figures 2.1 and 2.5). A well-formed submucosal lymphatic plexus, important in the assessment of spread of cancer, is present and there are irregularly arranged aggregates of lymphocytes around many gland ducts (Figure 2.5). Polymorphs are not normally present. There is a myenteric nerve plexus between circular and longitudinal muscle coats but no readily identifiable submucosal plexus.

Biopsies often consist of squamous epithelium only and are sometimes orientated obliquely or transversely (Figure 2.6). Provided that the full thickness of mucosa is present a useful report can sometimes be given, though there is little possibility of assessing whether or not inflammatory changes are present.

References

1. de la Pava, S., Nigogosyan, G., Pickren, J. W. and Cabrera, A. (1963). Melanosis of the esophagus. *Cancer*, **16**, 48

2. Tateishi, R., Taniguchi, H., Wada, A., Horai, T. and Taniguchi, K. (1974). Argyrophil cells and melanocytes in oesophageal mucosa. *Arch. Pathol.*, **98**, 87

3. Raeburn, C. (1951). Columnar ciliated epithelium in the adult oesophagus. *J. Pathol. Bacteriol.*, **63**, 157

4. Ismael-Beigi, F. and Pope, C. E. II (1974). Distribution of the histological changes of gastroesophageal reflux in the distal esophagus of man. *Gastroenterology*, **66**, 1109

5. Weinstein, W. M., Bogoch, E. R. and Bowes, K. L. (1975). The normal human esophageal mucosa; a histological reappraisal. *Gastroenterology*, **68**, 40

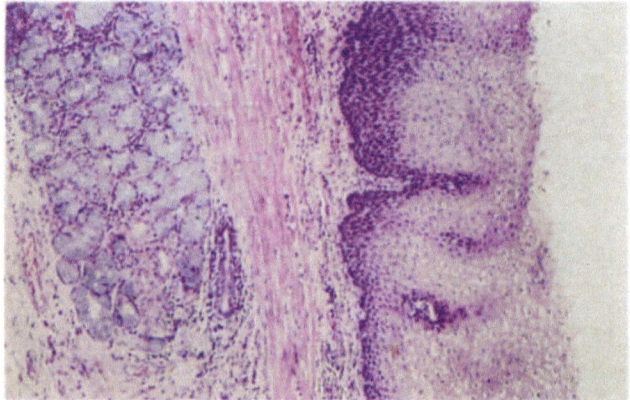

Figure 2.1 Normal oesophageal epithelium, muscularis mucosae, duct and simple mucus glands. The papillae penetrate about two-thirds of the total epithelial thickness, the basal layer forms about 15%. A few round cells lie at the base of the epithelium but there are no polymorphs. An oesophageal gland and duct lie beneath the muscularis mucosae.   H & E × 80

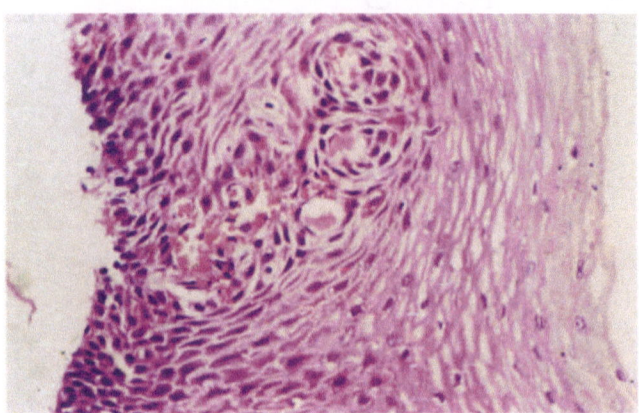

Figure 2.2 Normal papilla; vessels are clearly seen in the connective tissue. The stratification of the superficial epithelium is also well shown.   H & E × 250

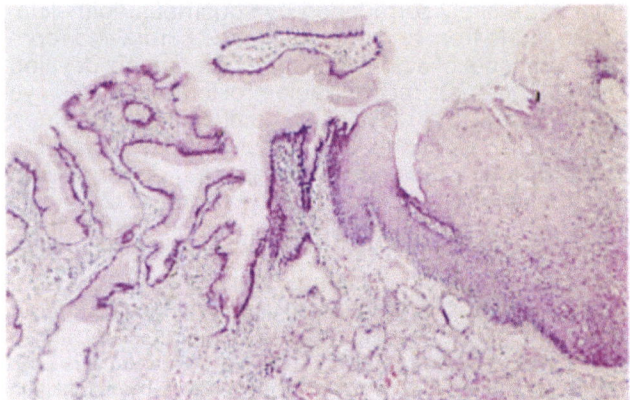

Figure 2.3 Normal cardio-oesophageal junction. Note the abrupt transition to simple cardiac-type glands.   H & E × 125

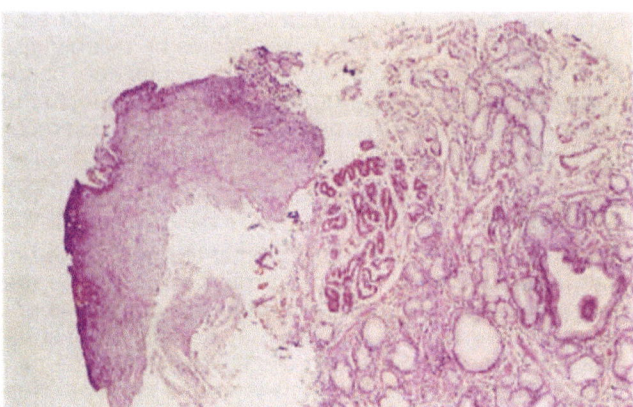

Figure 2.4 Characteristic oesophageal biopsy at 40 cm showing artefactual detachment of oesophageal from cardiac mucosa, which is a common finding.   H & E × 100

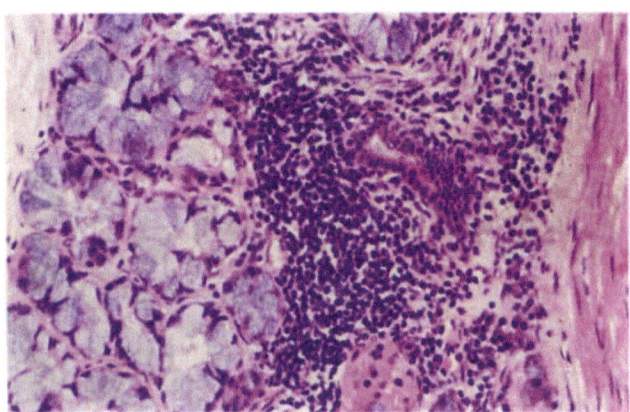

Figure 2.5 Normal oesophageal submucosal glands and duct, surrounded by lymphocytes.   H & E × 250

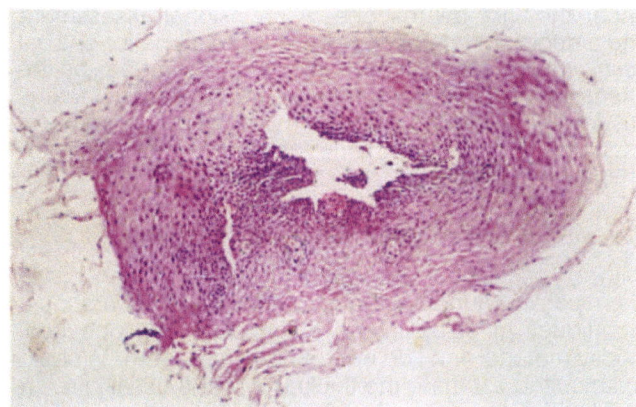

Figure 2.6 Characteristic oesophageal biopsy at less than 40 cm. The biopsy has been cut transversely and only includes epithelium, but is deep enough to examine for squamous epithelial changes. No abnormality is present. H & E × 125

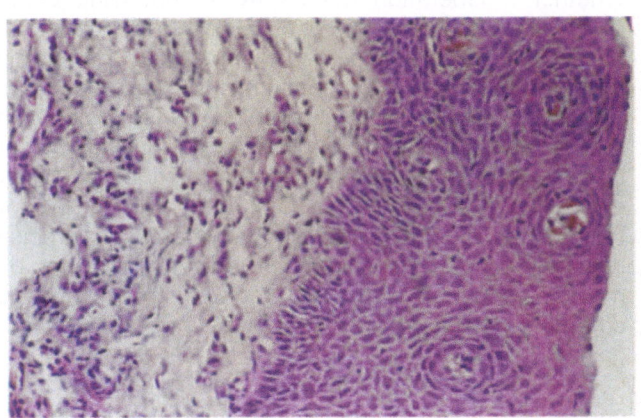

Figure 3.1 Early reflux oesophagitis. There is marked basal hyperplasia involving nearly the full thickness of the epithelium, connective tissue papillae extend almost to the luminal surface and scattered polymorphs are present in the underlying connective tissue. H & E × 125

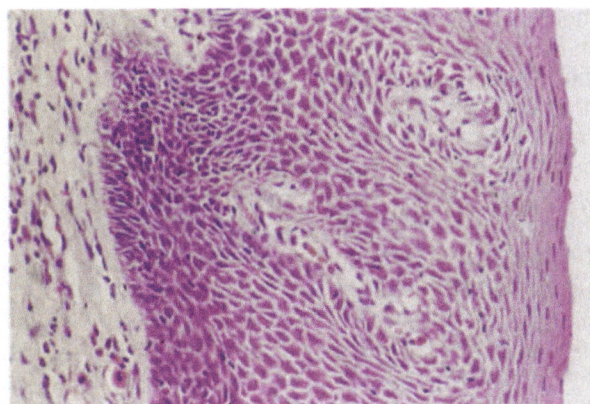

Figure 3.2 Doubtful reflux oesophagitis. There is thickening of the basal layer, papillae extend upwards slightly further than normal and an occasional polymorph is present. Many would regard this as abnormal; I am hesitant as to its significance. H & E × 200

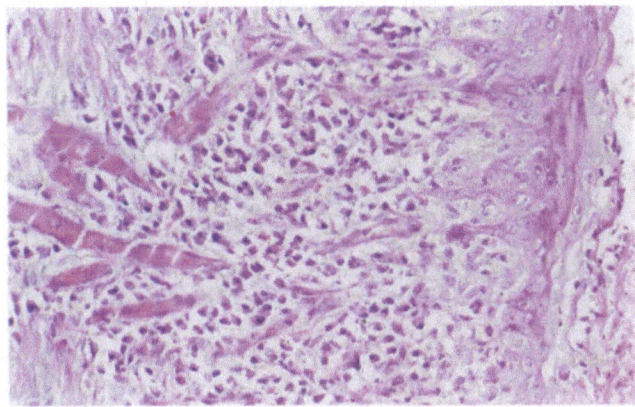

Figure 3.3 Severe reflux oesophagitis. The epithelium is now becoming thinned and eroded. The remains of the lamina propria show increased vascularization and a mixed infiltrate of polymorphs and round cells is present. H & E × 200

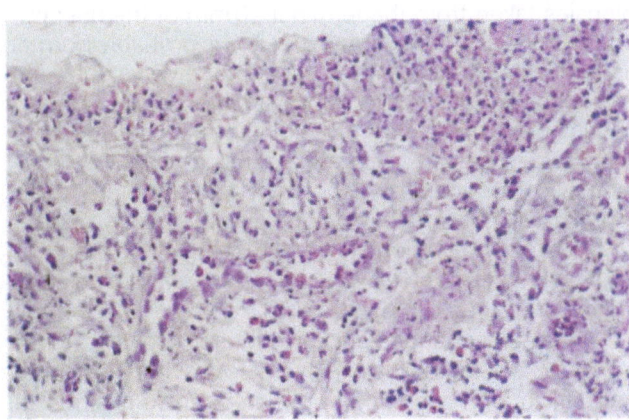

Figure 3.4 Severe reflux oesophagitis. The epithelium is thinned and heavily infiltrated by polymorphs. H & E × 125

Inflammatory Changes

Inflammatory changes in oesophageal biopsies usually result from infections, swallowed extrinsic agents such as lye, or intrinsic irritants such as gastric juice or bile which have been regurgitated or refluxed. They are initially usually acute and the mucosa is often reddened at oesophagoscopy. They may resolve or progress to erosion or ulceration; more chronic changes can also ensue with fibrosis or epithelial metaplasia to a glandular pattern. The most common cause of inflammatory change in the UK is reflux (digestion) oesophagitis, and this is described fully first, followed by comments on less common patterns.

Reflux Oesophagitis

This is a reaction of the normal squamous oesophageal epithelium and submucosa to refluxed gastric juice with, in many patients, associated reflux of bile. Three separate patterns of change are considered to be significant[1-5]. One is hyperplasia of the basal layer beyond its normal 15% of total epithelial thickness, accompanied by a variable but not usually marked degree of nuclear pleomorphism and hyperchromatism; the second is a thinning by erosion of the superficial layers of squamous epithelium so that connective tissue papillae appear to occupy more than two-thirds of the total epithelial thickness; the third is the presence of polymorphonuclear leukocytes in the papillae and around the epithelial rete pegs (Figures 3.1 and 3.2). Pathologists differ as to the diagnostic significance of these three findings. I regard either of the first two alone as insufficient evidence of oesophagitis; together I think they are suggestive but not conclusive. The presence of more than an isolated polymorph in papillae or around rete pegs I regard as more significant and the presence of polymorphs with either basal hyperplasia or upward extension of papillae or both – these two often go together – as reasonable evidence of inflammation. This view needs qualifying in biopsies taken from the terminal 20 mm of the oesophagus where a certain degree of reflux is probably normal and where histological findings do not always correlate well with clinical symptoms or with endoscopic appearances. Care must also be taken to exclude apparent basal hyperplasia and upward extension of papillae artefactually produced by tangential cutting; here polymorphs will not normally be present. It is also proper to say that many pathologists place more reliance than I do on basal hyperplasia alone[3,4] or combined with upward extension of papillae (Figure 3.2).

These early changes appear often to resolve, and on rebiopsy the epithelium appears to have reverted to normal, though sampling errors are hard to exclude. If changes progress the surface epithelium becomes more completely eroded and thinned and can eventually ulcerate (Figures 3.3 and 3.4). The ulcers tend to run longitudinally as troughs, separated by ridges covered by hyperplastic epithelium in which basal hyperplasia, elongated papillae and polymorphs are all usually present. Biopsies from frankly ulcerated areas do not as

a rule present a diagnostic problem since they consist mainly of, or contain within them, inflammatory granulation tissue with a variable amount of fibrosis (Figures 3.5 and 3.6) but it is often impossible to say whether they represent reflux oesophagitis, a reaction to other damaging agents or to carcinoma; step-sectioning is always necessary to exclude an adjacent or underlying neoplasm.

The Lower Oesophagus lined by Columnar Epithelium (Barrett's Oesophagus)

Prolonged exposure to refluxed gastric juice or bile can lead to a metaplasia of the squamous epithelium lining the lower end of the oesophagus to a columnar type. There is considerable argument as to whether this represents an upward extension of gastric mucosa to replace ulcerated or eroded squamous epithelium or whether regeneration occurs from underlying oesophageal mucous glands, but from the standpoint of biopsy interpretation the point is immaterial, though the former supposition is probably correct. The squamous epithelium is replaced for a variable distance proximal to the cardia; the distance of the biopsy from the incisor teeth must be known to allow interpretation. Columnar epithelium at a distance less than 38 cm from the incisor teeth is almost certainly metaplastic whatever its precise histological pattern; between 38 and 40 cm it may be metaplastic or cardiac and its precise histology must be carefully studied; beyond 40 cm it is almost certain to be gastric.

Three patterns of columnar epithelium are described[6], all of which can be associated with inflammatory changes. The most common is an 'intestinal' pattern with a pseudovillous surface, goblet cells which contain sialomucins (Figures 3.7 and 3.8) and sometimes Paneth and endocrine cells, but which differs from small intestine in its enzymic and ultrastructural features[7]. A second resembles simple cardiac epithelium with mucus-secreting surface cells and simple mucous glands (Figure 3.9), while a third resembles normal body epithelium with parietal and pepsinogen-secreting cells (Figure 3.10). These three patterns are found sequentially in the order described, and it is rare to see them transposed in numbered biopsies, though not all patterns are necessarily present in any one patient. Since Barrett-type mucosal metaplasia follows reflux oesophagitis with ulceration, and since metaplasia can be a patchy lesion, biopsy material may also include squamous epithelium showing the inflammatory changes already described. Secondary changes can develop in Barrett-type epithelium. These include goblet cell metaplasia similar to that seen in intestinal metaplasia of gastric epithelium, and peptic ulceration. It is not uncommon also to find chronic inflammatory changes resembling those seen in chronic atrophic gastritis (Figures 3.9 and 3.10). Dysplastic and frank carcinomatous change can also occur in this type of metaplastic mucosa (Figures 3.11 and 3.12, and see page 30) and must be carefully looked for.

Electron microscopic changes in oesophagitis are described which include widening of intercellular spaces, variable mitochondrial damage and an increase in keratohyaline granules[8]. They do not seem to me to offer a more accurate means of diagnosis than conventional light microscopy.

Other Patterns of Oesophagitis

Viral Oesophagitis

Oesophagitis due to herpes simplex or varicella-zoster viruses or to cytomegalovirus is usually seen in immunocompromised patients[9,10] but herpetic infections are also seen in healthy young adults[11]. Shallow ulcers of variable size develop and often become secondarily infected so that evidence of a primary viral origin can be difficult to find. Biopsies from the ulcer floor are generally unhelpful, but biopsies from the ulcer edge often reveal eosinophilic intranuclear inclusions in squamous cells (Figures 3.13 and 3.14).

Candidiasis

Oesophageal candidiasis is also found in immunocompromised patients as well as in association with preexisting oesophagitis and carcinoma[12,13]. Endoscopy reveals white patches or plaques which are not in themselves diagnostic. Histological studies can show features of non-specific oesophagitis including basal hyperplasia, epithelial cell cytoplasmic swelling and the presence of polymorphs, but often all inflammatory changes are inconspicuous. The presence of Candida within the tissues as yeasts or hyphae can be demonstrated by PAS staining (Figure 3.15); one group of authors points out that the demonstration of Candida in surface exudates or slough is not sufficient for diagnosis since the organism is a common mouth commensal[13].

Granulomatous Lesions

Tuberculous ulceration secondary to open pulmonary tuberculosis usually occurs as a terminal event though an occasional primary lesion has been described[14]. There is often caseation and usually a characteristic granulomatous reaction (Figure 3.16). Crohn's disease is also well recognized, not always in association with other clinically obvious gastrointestinal lesions[15]. Characteristic granulomas can be seen and sinus tracks with granulation tissue and fibrosis are described. I have seen one such lesion in 30 years' experience.

Miscellaneous Conditions

Oesophageal inflammation of varying degree, not usually severe enough to ulcerate and indistinguishable histologically from that seen in early reflux oesophagitis, is described in children who receive radiotherapy or antimitotic drugs[16], in nasopharyngeal inflammation, influenza, hypothermia and immediately following ingestion of corrosive fluids. The ingestion of lye is well recognized in the USA as a cause of fibrosis and stricture formation.

Disorders of Ganglion Cells

Ganglion cells are not present in the oesophageal submucosa, but a myenteric plexus is present between the circular and longitudinal smooth muscle coats which surround the middle and lower parts of the oesophagus. There appear to be two types of neurone: a multiaxonal argyrophilic cell which sends out an axon and dendrites to other neurones but not directly to muscle, and a non-argyrophilic cholinesterase-containing neurone which actually supplies muscle[17]. Each is identifiable using appropriate techniques, but as a virtually full-thickness biopsy is needed to include the plexus the question of differentiation does not arise in routine biopsy material. Brief descriptions of conditions affecting ganglion cells are included for completeness.

Achalasia

In this condition the sphincteric mechanism or sling at the cardia fails to relax in coordination with peristalsis and the lower oesophagus becomes dilated, with associated muscle hypertrophy and regurgitation. Careful histochemical studies show that argyrophilic neurones are reduced in number, especially in the upper dilated part of the oesophagus (contrast with Hirschsprung's disease) while cholinesterase-containing cells are normal in number[18,19]. It is always essential to include normal control material to check techniques and to provide a normal ganglion cell count.

Chagas' Disease

Chagas' disease, caused by Trypanosoma cruzi, is found in central and northern South America. The trypanosomes develop in the cone-nosed bug Triatoma megista and enter the bloodstream of man through the skin following a bite and deposition of the bug's faeces on the bitten area. Leishmania forms enter ganglion cells or adjacent histiocytes in smooth muscle and probably release neuro-toxins which directly damage ganglion cells and produce an accompanying inflammatory reaction[20]. The picture differs from that seen in achalasia in that both types of ganglion cell are equally affected and inflammatory cells are present; some ganglion cells usually remain intact.

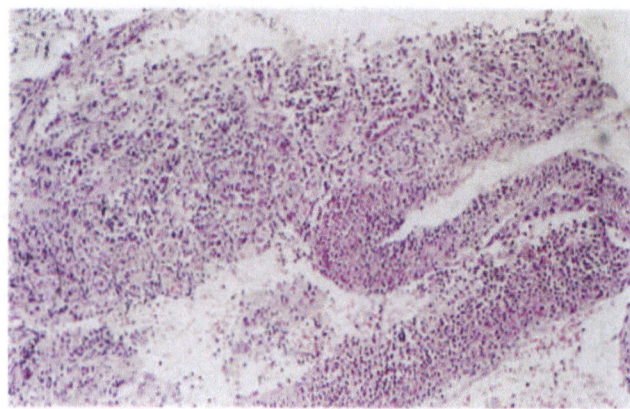

Figure 3.5 Ulceration in reflux oesophagitis. Little squamous epithelium now remains; it is replaced by a fibrinopurulent exudate with underlying purulent granulation tissue.   H & E × 80

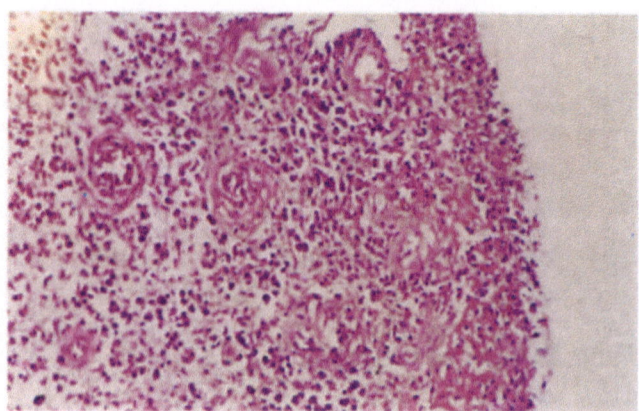

Figure 3.6 Ulceration in reflux oesophagitis. This biopsy consists of granulation and fibrous tissue only, and the inflammatory pattern is non-specific; it could equally well be associated with carcinoma.   H & E × 125

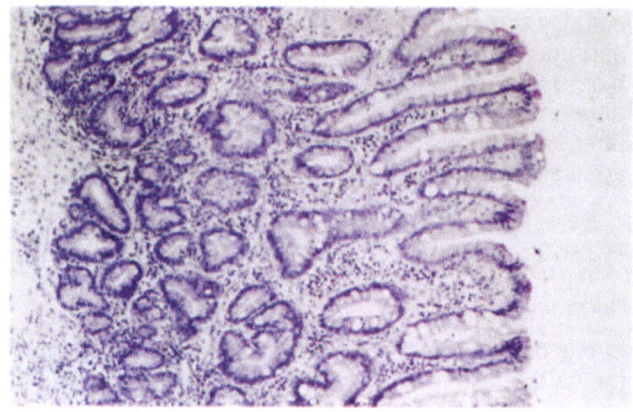

Figure 3.7 Barrett-type epithelium, intestinal pattern. The goblet cells are well shown and there is some pseudovillous formation.   H & E × 250

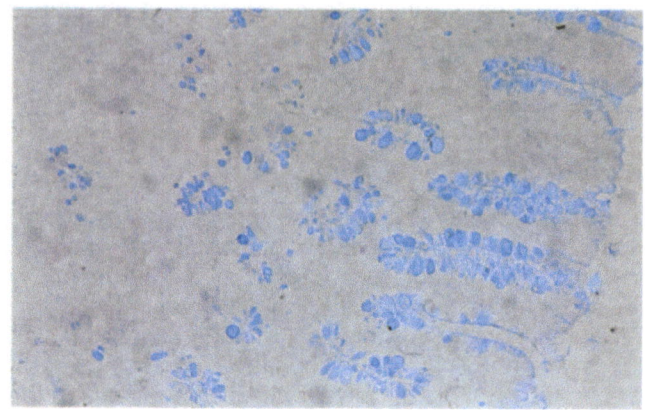

Figure 3.8 Barrett-type epithelium, intestinal pattern. Goblet cells contain sialomucins.   Alcian blue pH 2.5 × 125

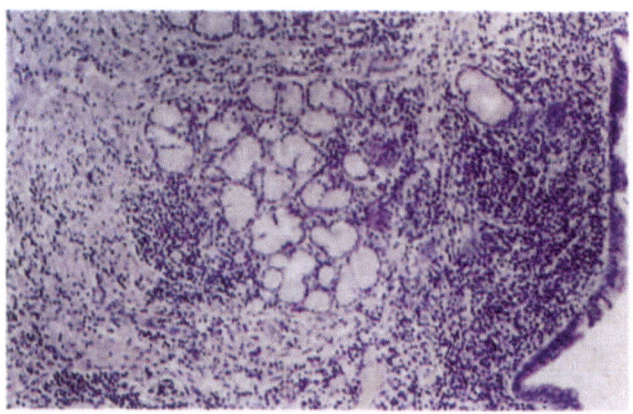

Figure 3.9 Barrett-type epithelium, cardiac pattern. The metaplasia here is accompanied by severe chronic inflammation and surface ulceration but some glands are recognizably simple, mucus-secreting and of cardiac type.   H & E × 100

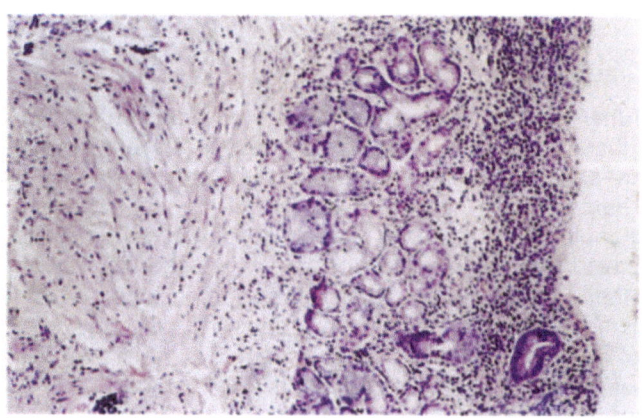

Figure 3.10 Barrett-type epithelium, body pattern. The metaplasia here is also accompanied by severe chronic inflammation and surface ulceration but some specialized cells are recognizable in deeper glands.   H & E × 100

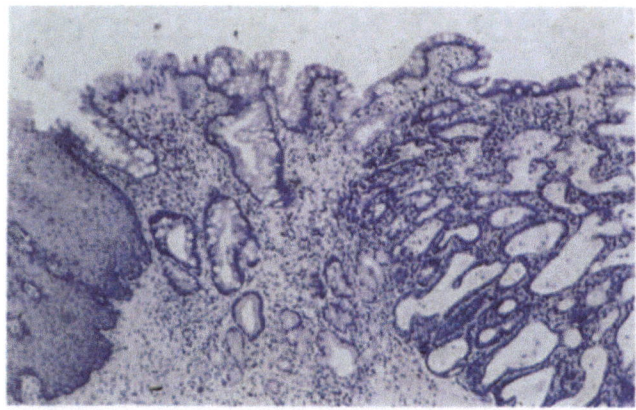

Figure 3.11 Barrett-type epithelium, moderate dysplasia. This interesting biopsy shows normal squamous epithelium (left), a thin zone of intestinal-type epithelium (centre) and a zone of moderately severe glandular dysplasia (right) which is not frankly invasive. Two months later this patient had an oesophagogastrectomy and was found to have widespread dysplasia with early invasive carcinoma. H & E × 100

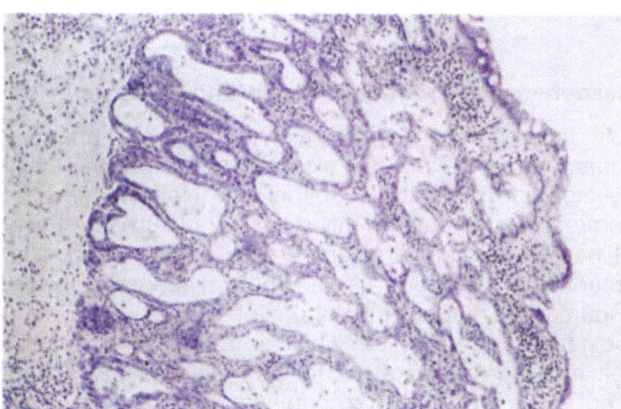

Figure 3.12 Barrett-type epithelium, moderate dysplasia. A slightly higher power view of Figure 3.11 which shows more clearly the well defined lower edge of epithelium without evidence of invasion. H & E × 125

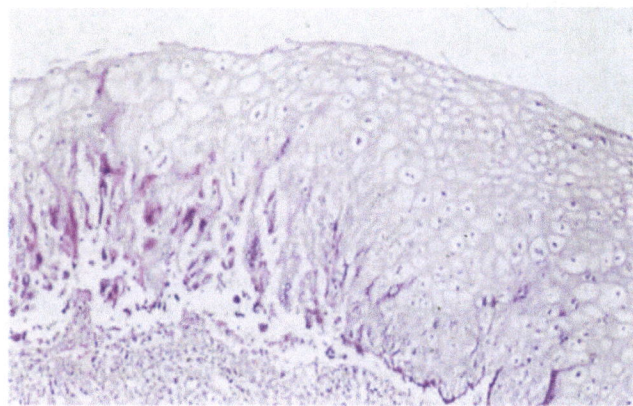

Figure 3.13 Herpetic oesophagitis. The biopsy comes from the edge of an ulcer with much granulation tissue; nuclear inclusions are visible in the frayed rete pegs. H & E × 125

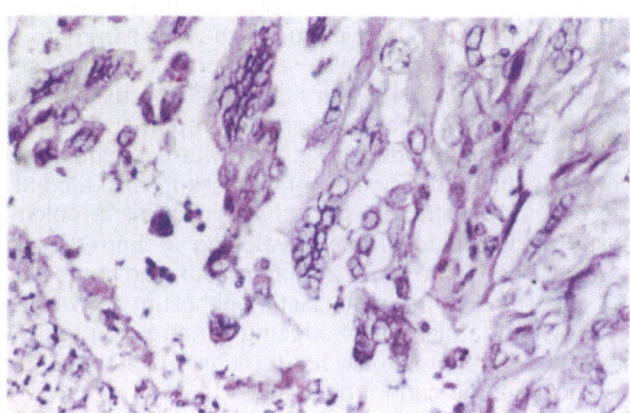

Figure 3.14 Herpetic oesophagitis. Higher-power view to show the intranuclear inclusions. H & E × 250

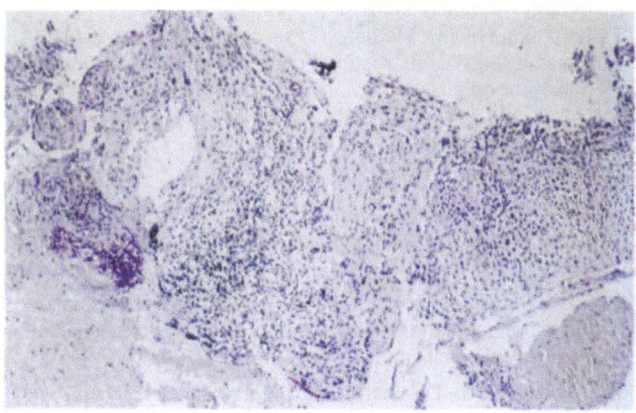

Figure 3.15 Candidiasis of oesophagus. Fungal elements are clearly visible but there is little associated inflammation. PAS × 100

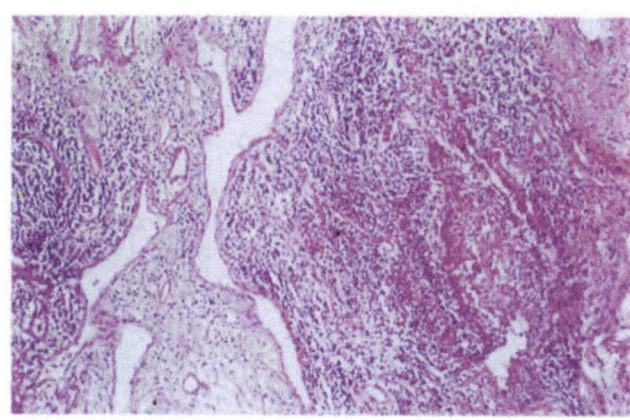

Figure 3.16 Tuberculosis of oesophagus. Ulcerating squamous-epithelium is present (right) with a poorly formed granuloma beneath it. A single giant cell (not shown) was also present but there was no obvious caseation. H & E × 65

Oesophageal Ulceration, Fibrosis and Stricture

Any inflammatory lesion involving the oesophageal squamous epithelium can ulcerate, and ulcers can also develop in Barrett-type epithelium. Neoplasms also commonly ulcerate. An inflammatory ulcer has a base of necrotic slough and granulation tissue when it is recent and of fibrous tissue when of longer duration (Figure 3.6). Biopsy of the edges of the ulcer will define the patterns of epithelium which surround it and may reveal evidence of causation, for example viral inclusions, fungi or the presence of a neoplasm. Biopsy of the base may reveal ulcerated neoplasm but is not usually helpful in primarily inflammatory ulcers.

Biopsies which consist solely or mainly of fibrous tissue (Figures 3.5 and 3.6) can present a real diagnostic problem. Fibrosis occurs in association with ulceration and inflammation from whatever cause, and if severe or extensive can lead to stricture; it also occurs in relation to developing carcinoma and this also can cause stricture. It can be impossible in a biopsy consisting of fibrous tissue with or without inflammatory epithelial change to make a differential diagnosis (Figures 3.17 and 3.18) and such biopsies must always be step or serially sectioned and the report so worded that the clinician understands that when carcinoma is not present in a biopsy it is not necessarily excluded as the cause of a stricture or other lesion. This problem arises also in carcinomas developing in Barrett-type mucosa since there is often inflammation and fibrosis at the upper end of the metaplastic epithelium above the level of the carcinoma, producing a narrowing which can be biopsied proximally but through which the more distal carcinoma cannot be reached.

Miscellaneous Biopsy Findings

Systemic Sclerosis

This can be a generalized systemic disorder or can present in a localized form which only involves the alimentary tract. In either case the appearances in the oesophagus are the same[21]. Since they involve submucosa and muscularis propria but not mucosa, they can only be recognized, if at all, when a considerable depth of submucosa is present in the biopsy. Points to look for are elastosis and intimal fibrosis in small arteries and submucosal fibrosis and collagen formation, with possible atrophy of smooth muscle if any is included. The degree of fibrosis and muscle atrophy varies widely from patient to patient (Figure 3.19).

Glycolytic Acanthosis

This recently described lesion of undetermined aetiology presents as elevated white plaques on the mucosal folds of the lower oesophagus which on biopsy show a picture of basal hyperplasia with large glycogen-containing cells in the stratified layer[22]. There is no dysplasia or cellular atypia and the condition is apparently benign. I have not seen an example.

Eosinophilic Oesophagitis

Eosinophilic gastroenteritis is now well described[23] but I know of no reported examples in the oesophagus. I have, however, seen two patients, both presenting with dysphagia and found to have a 'stricture' on oesophagoscopy, whose biopsies have shown squamous epithelium infiltrated by eosinophils (Figure 3.20). Both responded to steroids but the diagnosis remains unproven.

Inflammatory Fibroid Polyp

These polyps, of undetermined aetiology, are well described in the stomach and small intestine[24] but are extremely rare in the oesophagus. I have seen a single example (Figure 3.21) from a 61-year-old man who had a pedunculated tumour 6.5×3.3 cm in the mid-oesophageal region.

References

1. Ismael-Beigi, F. and Pope, C. E. II (1974). Distribution of the histological changes of gastroesophageal reflux in the distal esophagus of man. *Gastroenterology*, **66**, 1109

2. Weinstein, W. M., Bogoch, E. R. and Bowes, K. L. (1975). The normal human esophageal mucosa; a histological reappraisal. *Gastroenterology*, **68**, 40

3. Behar, J. and Sheahan, D. C. (1975). Histological abnormalities in reflux esophagitis. *Arch. Pathol.*, **99**, 387

4. Thompson, H. (1976). Pathology of reflux oesophagitis. *Clin. Gastroenterol.*, **5**, 143

5. Seefeld, U., Krebs, G. J., Siebermann, R. E. and Blum, A. L. (1977). Esophageal histology in gastroesophageal reflux. Morphometric findings in suction biopsies. *Am. J. Dig. Dis.*, **22**, 956

6. Paull, A., Trier, J. S., Dalton, M. D., Camp, R. C., Loeb, P. and Goyal, R. K. (1976). The histologic spectrum of Barrett's esophagus. *N. Engl. J. Med.*, **295**, 476

7. Berenson, M. M., Herbst, J. J. and Freeston, J. W. (1974). Enzyme and ultrastructural characteristics of esophageal columnar epithelium. *Am. J. Dig. Dis.*, **19**, 895

8. Hopwood, D., Milne, G. and Logan, K. R. (1979). Electron microscopic changes in human oesophageal epithelium in oesophagitis. *J. Pathol.*, **129**, 161

9. Nash, G. and Ross, J. S. (1974). Herpetic esophagitis: a common cause of esophageal ulceration. *Hum. Pathol.* **5**, 339

10. Buss, D. H. and Schlary, M. (1979). Herpes virus infection of the esophagus and other visceral organs in adults: incidence and clinical significance. *Am. J. Med.*, **66**, 457

11. Springer, D. J., Da Costa, L. R. and Beck, I. T. (1979). A syndrome of acute selflimiting ulcerative esophagitis in young adults probably due to herpes simplex virus. *Dig. Dis. Sci.*, **24**, 535

12. Kodsi, B. E., Wickremesinghe, P. C., Kozinn, P. J., Iswara, K. and Goldberg, P. K. (1976). Candida esophagitis – a prospective study of 27 cases. *Gastroenterology*, **71**, 715

13. Scott, B. B. and Jenkins, D. (1982). Gastro-oesophageal candidiasis. *Gut*, **23**, 137

14. Annamalai, A. and Shreekumar, S. (1972). Tuberculosis of the esophagus. *Am. J. Gastroenterol.*, **57**, 166

15. LiVolsi, V. A. and Jaretzki, A. III (1973). Granulomatous esophagitis. A case of Crohn's disease limited to the esophagus. *Gastroenterology*, **64**, 313

16. Newburger, P. E., Cassady, J. R. and Jaffe, N. (1978). Esophagitis due to adriamycin and radiation therapy for childhood malignancy. *Cancer*, **42**, 417

17. Smith, B. (1970). The neurological lesion in achalasia of the cardia. *Gut*, **11**, 388

18. Adams, C. W. M., Marples, E. A. and Trounce, J. R. (1960). Achalasia of the cardia and Hirschsprung's disease. The amount and distribution of cholinesterases. *Clin. Sci.*, **19**, 473

19. Adams, C. W. M., Brain, R. H. F., Ellis, F. G., Kauntz, R. and Trounce, J. R. (1960). Achalasia of the cardia. *Guys Hosp. Rep.*, **110**, 191

20. Betarello, A. and Pinotti, H. W. (1976). Oesophageal involvement in Chagas' disease. *Clin. Gastroenterol.*, **5**, 27

21. Atkinson, M. and Summerling, M. D. (1966). Oesophageal changes in systemic sclerosis. *Gut*, **7**, 402

22. Bender, M. D., Allison, J., Cuartas, F. and Montgomery, C. (1973). Glycolytic acanthosis of the esophagus: a form of benign epithelial hyperplasia. *Gastroenterology*, **65**, 373

23. Johnstone, J. M. and Morson, B. C. (1978). Eosinophilic gastroenteritis. *Histopathology*, **2**, 335

24. Johnstone, J. M. and Morson, B. C. (1978). Inflammatory fibroid polyp of the gastrointestinal tract. *Histopathology*, **2**, 349

Figures 3.17–3.21 will be found overleaf.

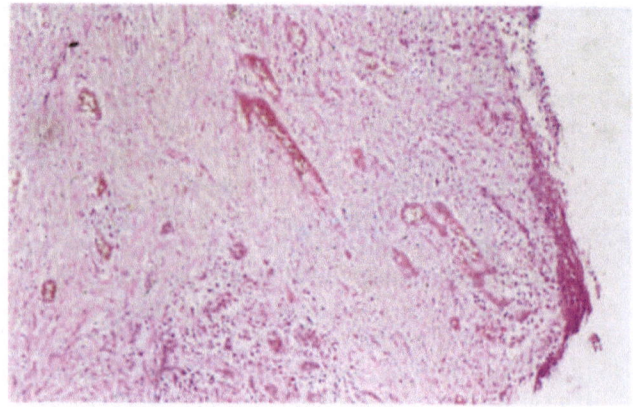

Figure 3.17   Fibrosis of oesophagus. This biopsy from a stricture showed only ulcerated epithelium with chronic inflammation and fibrosis on the initial section.   H & E × 65

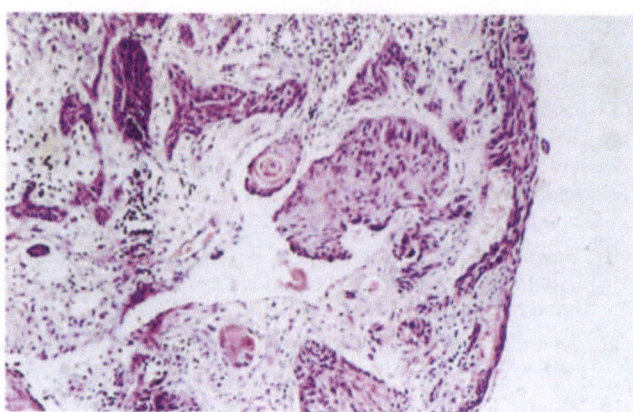

Figure 3.18   Carcinoma with associated fibrosis. Deeper levels cut from the biopsy illustrated in Figure 3.17 revealed islands of squamous cell carcinoma. H & E × 100

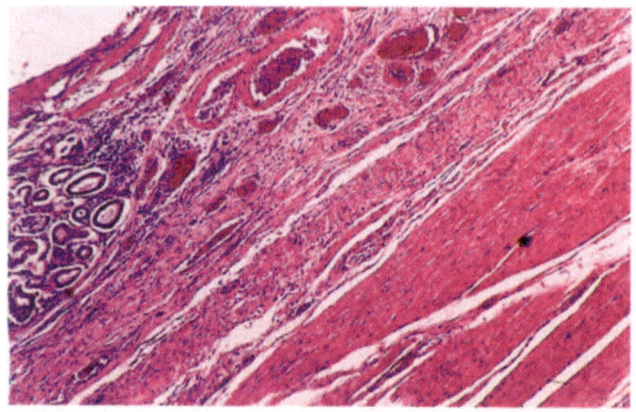

Figure 3.19   Systemic sclerosis. This illustration, from a resected specimen, shows submucosal fibrosis and collagen formation. In none of the four biopsies I have seen in this condition was there sufficient submucosa to make a definitive diagnosis.   H & E × 32

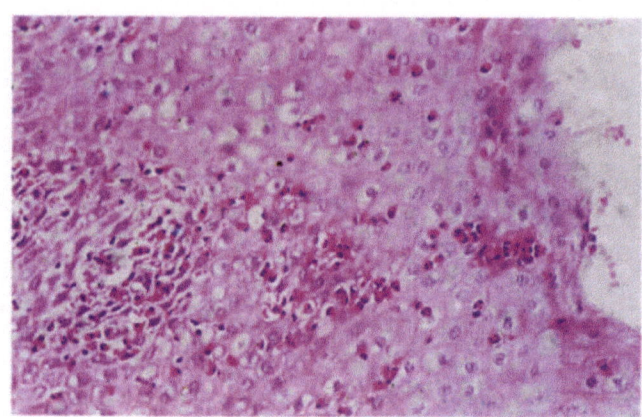

Figure 3.20   Possible eosinophilic oesophagitis. The squamous epithelium is heavily infiltrated with eosinophils but no subepithelial tissue was included in the biopsy.   H & E × 250

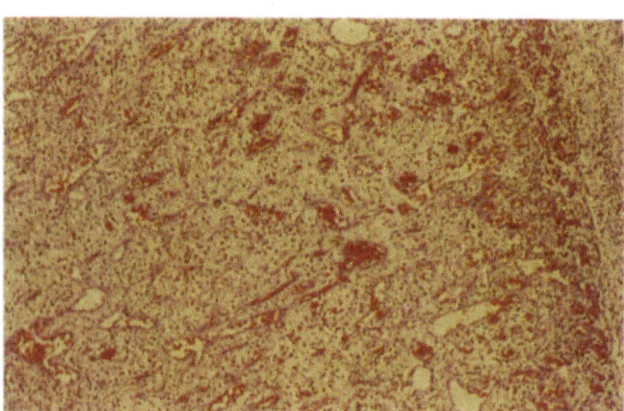

Figure 3.21   Inflammatory fibroid polyp. The polyp is composed of vascular granulation-type tissue with a more fibrous component in places. There is considerable secondary inflammation but many of the infiltrating cells are eosinophils.   H & E × 65

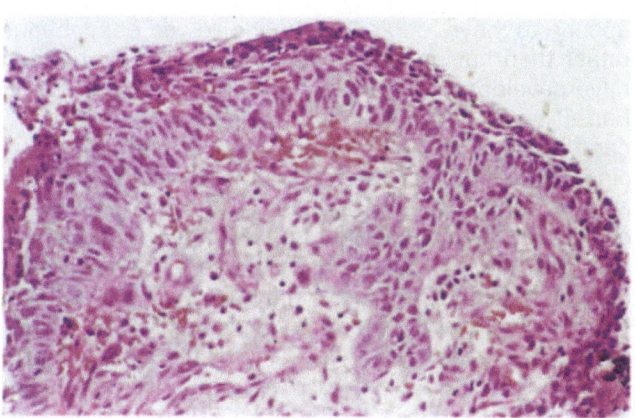

Figure 4.1 Moderate epithelial dysplasia. Cell nuclei in the basal layer are pleomorphic and hyperchromatic but there is no obvious increase in mitoses and some stratification is still present. H & E × 125

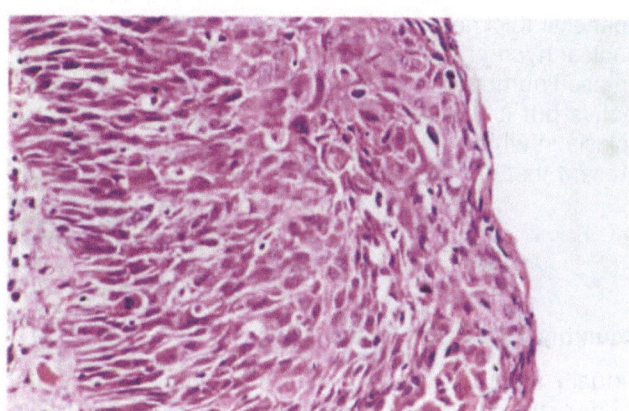

Figure 4.2 Moderate/severe epithelial dysplasia. The basal layer is thickened and the nuclei more pleomorphic and hyperchromatic than in Figure 4.1 with an increased number of mitotic figures. Some attempt at stratification is still present. H & E × 250

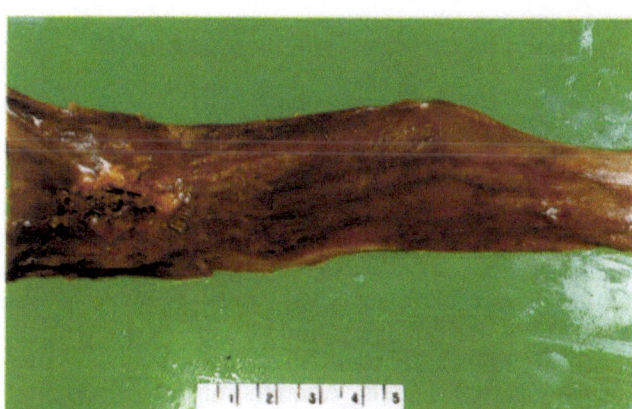

Figure 4.3 Resected early squamous carcinoma beginning as an annular plaque and showing secondary ulceration. The adjacent epithelium was dysplastic.

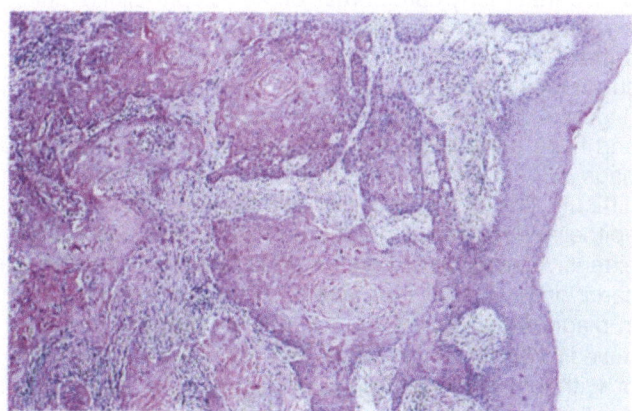

Figure 4.4 Well-differentiated keratinizing squamous carcinoma with cell nest formation. H & E × 65

Squamous Epithelial Dysplasia

In many sites in the body epithelial dysplasia is well recognized as a lesion which commonly precedes carcinoma. Until recently this lesion had not been described in the squamous-lined oesophagus, but careful studies in countries with a high incidence of squamous carcinoma using step section techniques have shown that dysplasia progressing from mild to severe is likely to lead to carcinoma in up to 25% of patients, though reversion of dysplasia to normal can also occur[1]. Dysplastic changes have also been described in association with postcricoid carcinoma in Paterson–Kelly (Plummer–Vinson) syndrome[2] though the webs often seen in this syndrome are not dysplastic. Since dysplastic changes can be found without accompanying carcinoma their neoplastic potential is clearly important.

Moderate and severe dysplasias are not difficult to recognize (Figures 4.1 and 4.2), but milder forms can be difficult to differentiate from basal hyperplasia. Points to look for are a basal layer involving more than 50% of epithelial thickness, a greater than expected degree of nuclear hyperchromatism and pleomorphism and an increased number of mitotic figures. Interpretation is subjective but it is probably only the severe forms of dysplasia in which little or no recognizable stratification is present that are precancerous (Figure 4.2).

Squamous Cell Carcinoma

Virtually all of the carcinomas in the upper and middle thirds of the oesophagus and from 50 to 70% of those in the lower third are squamous-celled. Those in the upper third have a high female incidence, usually associated with Paterson–Kelly syndrome; those in middle and lower thirds predominate in males. There are racial and geographic variations in incidence – the lesion is particularly common in parts of China, Japan and Africa – and a number of predisposing factors including diet and alcohol are postulated. There is now increasing evidence that many carcinomas begin as epithelial dysplasia[1] and that early visible carcinomas consisting of circumscribed or annular plaques confined to mucosa and submucosa arise from adjacent dysplastic epithelium[3] (Figure 4.3). These early lesions may erode and ulcerate and have been likened to early gastric carcinoma (see page 53). In biopsy material, early carcinoma can be difficult to distinguish from severe full-thickness epithelial dysplasia if no submucosa is included. Once extensive invasion has occurred, keratinizing squamous carcinoma with cell nest formation presents no problem in diagnosis (Figure 4.4). It is not uncommon to see a mixed pattern of basal cell and squamous cell types with or without some keratinization (Figure 4.5). Non-keratinizing undifferentiated squamous cell and spindle cell patterns and anaplastic adenocarcinomas can be extremely difficult to categorize (Figure 4.6) and can be mistaken both for so-called 'carcinosarcoma' (see page 31) and for oat cell carcinoma. A search of serial sections will sometimes reveal single cell keratinization in anaplastic squamous carcinoma; PAS staining may reveal isolated mucin-containing cells in adenocarcinoma and electron microscopy, even on material removed from a paraffin section, will usually show endocrine granules if these are present. A major problem, already emphasized, is that carcinomas ulcerate and excite an inflammatory and fibrous reaction and in some instances this type of material only appears in the first section looked at and sometimes forms the entire biopsy (see Figures 3.17 and 3.18); step or serial sectioning must *always* be performed.

Glandular Epithelial Dysplasia

This pattern of dysplasia can be seen in Barrett-type mucosa (see Figures 3.11 and 3.12) and in the mucosa of the stomach proper (see page 51) and in either site it is potentially precancerous. There is increasing evidence that the majority of adenocarcinomas which appear to have originated in the lower oesophagus rather than having spread upwards from the stomach have developed on a basis of pre-existing dysplasia in Barrett-type epithelium[4], and that dysplastic epithelium can be found not only at the edges of these adenocarcinomas but in other parts of the metaplastic epithelium as well, so that its recognition in biopsy material becomes important. Pathologists have tended to grade dysplastic changes into mild, moderate or severe on a basis of nuclear hyperchromatism, crowding and stratification; increased nuclear–cytoplasmic ratio; an increase in numbers of mitoses, which also are found above the proliferative crypt level; and a loss of mucus secretion (see Figures 3.11 and 3.12). It is reported that polymorph infiltration is not a feature of dysplasia as opposed to hyperplasia[4] but I have not found this a distinguishing feature in my own material. Where it is possible to classify the epithelium in which dysplasia has occurred as being of intestinal, cardiac or fundal type (see page 22) dysplasia can apparently occur in all three patterns, but again this is not well commented on in the literature and my own observations are limited.

Adenocarcinoma

Adenocarcinomas form some 30–50% of tumours in the lower third of the oesophagus; some are of primary gastric origin and have spread upwards but there is increasing evidence that many arise from dysplastic change in an acquired Barrett-type of metaplastic columnar epithelium following reflux oesophagitis or ingestion of irritant liquids. When this has happened there is likely to be ulceration and fibrosis with some degree of stricture above the carcinoma, and biopsy may not disclose the presence of malignancy. When differentiated adenocarcinoma is present in a biopsy its recognition is not usually difficult (Figure 4.7); when small fragments only of suspected anaplastic carcinoma are present, a PAS strain for neutral mucin may help.

Adenosquamous Carcinoma

Rarely, a biopsy from the lower end of the oesophagus shows both adenocarcinomatous and squamous carcinomatous elements (Figure 4.8); true mixed patterns do occur and collision tumours have been described, but care must be taken to exclude the possibility of squamous metaplasia in an adenocarcinoma or of a squamous carcinoma infiltrating the upper end of Barrett-type metaplastic columnar epithelium showing dysplastic change.

'Junctional' Change and Primary Malignant Melanoma

Melanoblasts are known to be present in normal oesophageal mucosa, and although statistically a melanomatous tumour in the oesophagus is more likely to be secondary than primary, primary tumours do occur and some are preceded by junctional change (Figures 4.9 and 4.10)[5]. They are usually polypoid and project into the lumen of the middle or lower third of the oesophagus; both the junctional change and the tumour have the typical characteristics of melanomas in the skin, but pigment is usually plentiful.

'Oat Cell' Carcinomas

A number of malignant tumours resembling oat cell carcinoma of bronchus have been described as primary oat cell or small cell carcinoma of the oesophagus[6]; the cells composing them are sometimes argyrophilic and can contain endocrine cell granules on electron microscopy; some secrete ACTH (Figure 4.11). They appear to be a counterpart of oat cell carcinoma of bronchus and probably arise from endocrine cells which are known to be present in oesophageal and tracheobronchial mucosa (see page 19); oesophagus and bronchus have a common embryological origin. Care must be taken to exclude a secondary deposit from a primary bronchial tumour and to differentiate an oat cell carcinoma from an anaplastic squamous carcinoma and from malignant lymphoma or leiomyosarcoma; electron microscopy on material taken from a paraffin section is often adequate to decide whether endocrine-type granules are or are not present, and is of value.

Adenoid Cystic Carcinoma

Rare examples of histologically characteristic primary adenoid cystic carcinoma (Figure 4.12) are reported[7]; they arise either from the submucosal oesophageal mucus glands or their ducts.

'Carcinosarcoma'

A number of so-called carcinosarcomas have been described in the oesophagus. Many pathologists question the existence of such a tumour, which by definition must contain carcinomatous and sarcomatous elements, believing that these tumours are either squamous carcinomas with a large metaplastic spindle cell component which can be mistaken for sarcoma, or that the spindle cell element is reactive and not neoplastic[8]. Most of them are polypoid and the general noncommittal name 'polypoid carcinoma of oesophagus' has been suggested[9]. The example illustrated here (Figures 4.13 and 4.14), one of only two which I have seen, shows undoubted carcinomatous elements with mitotic figures in the 'sarcomatous' element, and I am not fully convinced that the term carcinosarcoma should be unconditionally abandoned.

Leiomyomatous Tumours

Smooth muscle tumours are the commonest benign oesophageal tumour, can arise from the muscularis mucosae or propria and project into the lumen to a variable degree; ulceration of the overlying mucosa is not uncommon[10]. Biopsy appearances can be confusing if this tumour is not borne in mind (Figure 4.15): the smooth muscle elements can be mistaken for fibrous tissue and the whole misdiagnosed as an inflammatory lesion. They can also resemble neural elements or can look so anaplastic as to cause problems in diagnosis. It is not normally possible on biopsy (or indeed after resection) to say whether or not the tumour is malignant: the size of the neoplasm is often a better guide than the histological appearances.

References

1. Studies on relationship between epithelial dysplasia and carcinoma of the esophagus (1975) compiled by coordinating groups for the research of esophageal carcinoma, Horan province and the Chinese Academy of Medical Sciences. *Chin. Med. J.*, **1**, 110

2. Entwhistle, C. C. and Jacobs, A. (1965). Histological findings in the Paterson Kelly syndrome. *J. Clin. Pathol.*, **18**, 408

3. Barge, J., Molas, G., Maillard, J. N., Fekete, F., Bogomoletz, W. V. and Potet, F. (1980). Superficial oesophageal carcinoma: an oesophageal counterpart of early gastric cancer. *Histopathology*, **5**, 499

4. Haggitt, R. C., Tryzelaar, J., Ellis, F. H. and Colcher, H. (1978). Adenocarcinoma complicating columnar epithelium lined (Barrett's) esophagus. *Am. J. Clin. Pathol.*, **70**, 1

5. Raven, R. W. and Dawson, I. (1964). Malignant melanoma of the oesophagus. *Br. J. Surg.*, **51**, 551

6. Horai, T., Kobayashi, A., Tateishi, R., Wada, A., Taniguchi, H., Taniguchi, K., Sano, M. and Tamura, H. (1978). A cytologic study on small cell carcinoma of the esophagus. *Cancer*, **41**, 1890

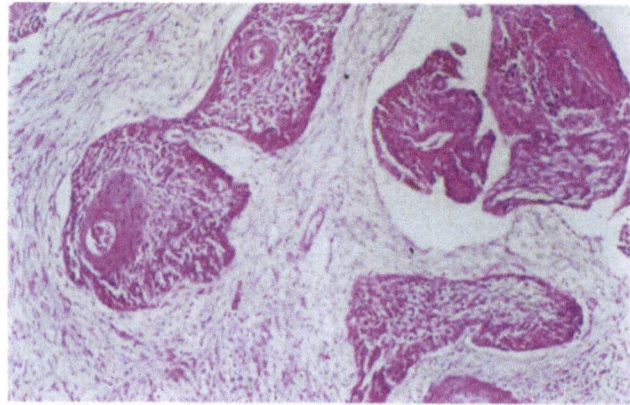

Figure 4.5 Mixed pattern of carcinoma showing squamous and basal cell features.   H & E × 100

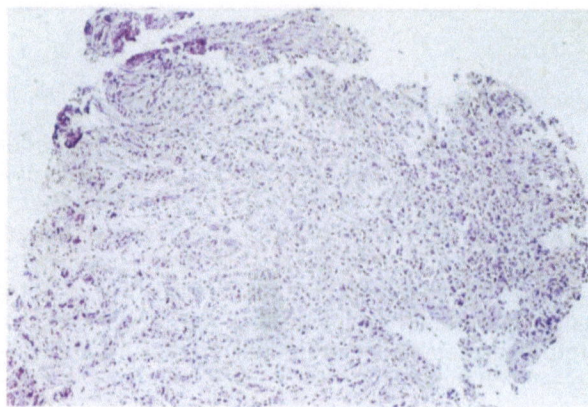

Figure 4.6 Anaplastic carcinoma as seen in biopsy. One can do little more than report that an undifferentiated neoplasm is present: PAS staining can be helpful in trying to exclude anaplastic adenocarcinoma.   H & E × 65

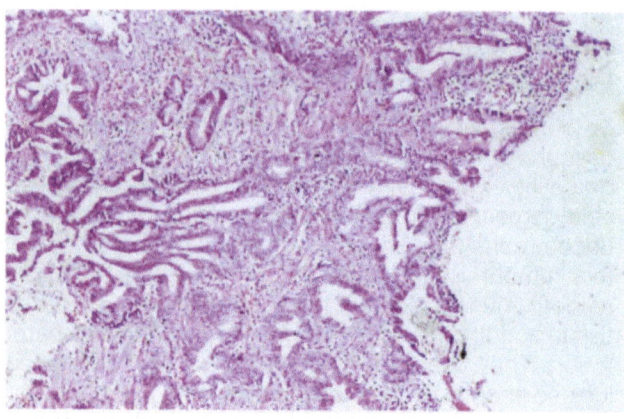

Figure 4.7 Moderately differentiated adenocarcinoma in an oesophageal biopsy at 38 cm. There was no evidence of a Barrett-type epithelium in this patient and subsequent resection revealed an extensive carcinoma at the cardio-oesophageal junction.   H & E × 100

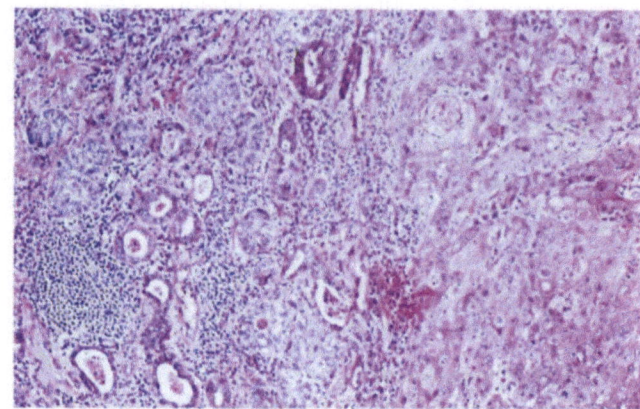

Figure 4.8 Adenosquamous carcinoma. On the right is poorly differentiated squamous carcinoma which more superficially showed keratinization: on the left is well-differentiated adenocarcinoma. In the resected specimen there was little intermingling of the two growths, suggesting collision carcinomas. H & E × 125

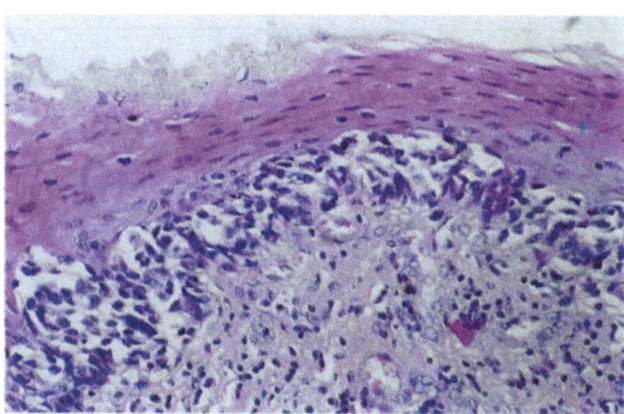

Figure 4.9 Junctional change adjacent to melanoma of oesophagus. This mimics the change seen in skin lesions: note the flattened overlying epithelium and disrupted basal layer.   H & E × 250

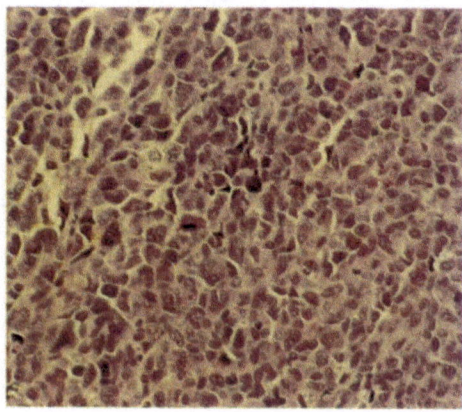

Figure 4.10 Malignant melanoma, showing marked cellular pleomorphism but little or no pigment in this particular example.   H & E × 250

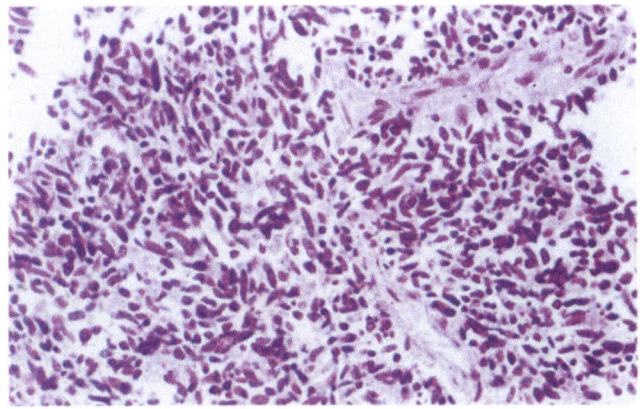

Figure 4.11 Oat cell carcinoma. Cells are scattered in the connective tissue beneath the epithelium and can closely resemble lymphocytes or leiomyoma cells; nuclei are more elongated and there is a slight tendency, seen here, to grouping or clumping which is not usually seen in primary lymphoid tumours. H & E × 250

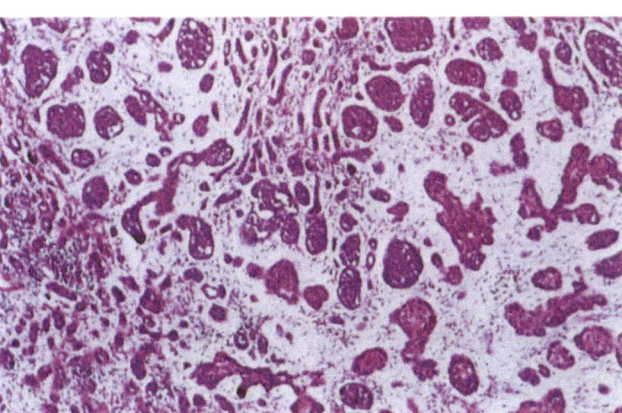

Figure 4.12 Adenoid cystic carcinoma. The resemblance to similar salivary and skin tumours is obvious. H & E × 100

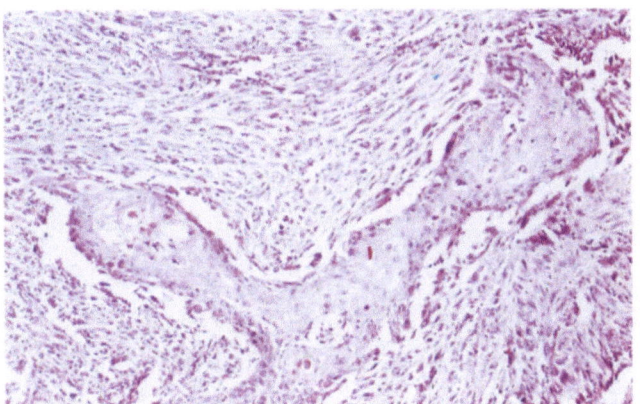

Figure 4.13 'Carcinosarcoma', showing moderately differentiated squamous cell carcinoma in a 'stroma' of anaplastic spindle cells suggestive of fibrosarcoma. H & E × 125

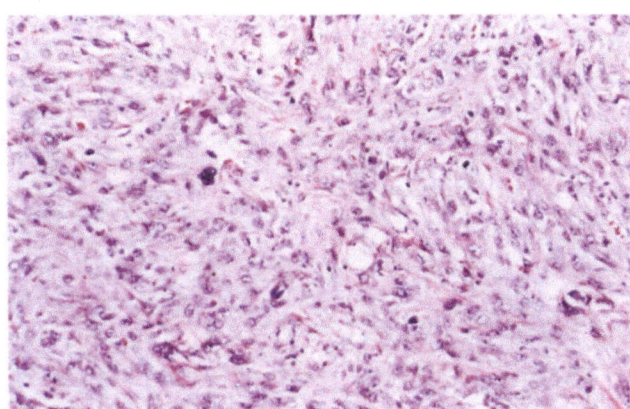

Figure 4.14. Higher-power view of the 'stroma' in Figure 4.13. Seen by itself this suggests sarcoma but many would argue for spindle cell squamous carcinoma. H & E × 250

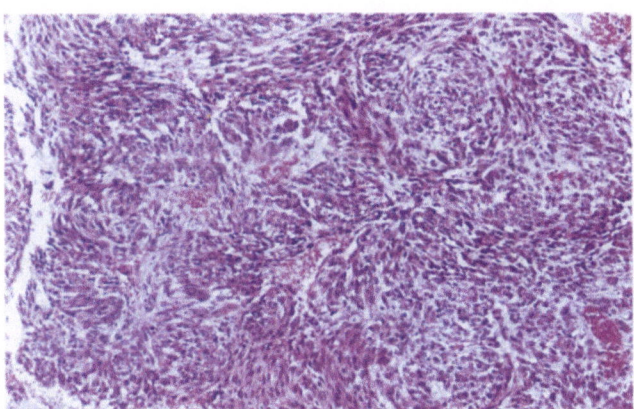

Figure 4.15 Oesophagus: smooth muscle tumour. The cellular whorled pattern present here is not difficult to diagnose though its malignancy is hard to assess. H & E × 125

7. Sweeney, E. C. and Cooney, T. (1980). Adenoid cystic carcinoma of the esophagus: a light and electron microscopic study. *Cancer*, **45**, 1516

8. Du Boulay, C. E. H. and Isaacson, P. (1981). Carcinoma of the oesophagus with spindle cell features. *Histopathology*, **5**, 403

9. Osamura, R. Y., Shimamura, K., Hata, J., Tamacki, N., Watanabe, K., Kubota, M., Yamazaki, S. and Mitomi, T. (1978). Polypoid carcinoma of the esophagus. A unifying term for 'carcinosarcoma' and 'pseudosarcoma'. *Am. J. Surg. Pathol.*, **2**, 201

10. Seremetis, M. C., Lyons, W. S., de Cuzman, V. C. and Peabody, J. W. Jr. (1976). Leiomyomata of the esophagus. Analysis of 838 cases. *Cancer*, **38**, 943

Using modern flexible instruments there is now no part of the stomach which cannot be biopsied under direct vision; gastroscopists are tending more and more to take biopsies from the first part of the duodenum with the same instrument (see pages 63 and 67) in the investigation of duodenitis and selected small bowel disorders.

On the basis of mucosal histology, the stomach is divisible into cardiac, body and antral (prepyloric and pyloric) regions. These lie roughly as shown in Figure 5.1, but there are no set anatomical landmarks and there is marked individual variation; in general the pyloric pattern of mucosa extends higher up the lesser curve in women than in men, and increases in extent relative to body mucosa in both sexes with advancing age. The regions cannot be reliably distinguished one from another endoscopically, though the body has a more rugose pattern, but the clinician should always record on the request form which region he believes to be the site of biopsy. Multiple small biopsies from the same region need not be numbered or identified separately and should be wrapped in porous paper and placed in fixative. When a generalized condition such as gastritis is suspected, both antral and body mucosa should be sampled. Localized ulcers should have at least four biopsies taken from the ulcer edge at 12, 3, 6 and 9 o'clock, as well as two biopsies from the base. Specimens are orientated in the laboratory. The usual precautions of using dissecting microscopy or a hand lens for correct orientation of small biopsies, of cutting a single section to check orientation before serializing, and of limiting the number of fragments embedded in a single block to avoid cutting right through one before reaching another, must be carefully observed.

Specialized Techniques of Value

Mucosubstances

Normal gastric mucin-secreting cells contain neutral mucin only and therefore stain red with PAS and diastase (Figure 5.2) but do not stain with Alcian blue: occasional mucus neck cells may stain faintly with Alcian blue at pH 2.5. Goblet cells are not normally present. Stains for sialomucins, usually Alcian blue at pH 2.5, are of great value in detecting minimal changes of intestinal metaplasia (Figure 5.3) and many pathologists, myself included, ask for a routine PAS following diastase and an Alcian blue at pH 2.5 on all gastric biopsies[1]. I prefer to do these separately rather than to combine them in a PAS–AB routine.

Immunocytochemistry

Immunocytochemical techniques are available for a large number of specialized functions. Commercial anti-gastrin serum is readily obtainable and I use a peroxidase–antiperoxidase (PAP) technique on paraffin-embedded material in selected patients with hyperacidity[2,3]. I also use antigastrin, antiglucagon and anti-insulin sera (Figure 5.4) on conventionally processed material for investigating the functional aspects of gastric endocrine cell tumours. Studies have been made on the ratio of Ig-secreting plasma cells and to define IgE cells[4] but I have rarely found these of value in the stomach. Other demonstrable cell components of which I have little personal experience are intrinsic factor[5], histamine[6], lysozyme[7] and pepsinogen[8].

Other Techniques

There are good descriptions available of the electron microscopic appearances of individual cells including endocrine cells[9] (Figure 5.5). I have not found scanning or transmission electron microscopy of great diagnostic help in gastric biopsy. There are also specialized techniques for the differential staining of body mucosal cells[10], but these are usually well delineated by H & E stains, especially in thin resin-embedded sections, or by PAS.

Gastric Mucosa

Cardiac Type Mucosa

Normal cardiac mucosa begins abruptly at the junction with the squamous cell lined oesophagus (Figure 5.6) and ends in a more gradual transition to body mucosa, forming a narrow ring between the oesophagus and body of the stomach. The majority of glands are simple-branching and often coiled, but occasional compound glands are seen. They open into shallow pits dipping down from the surface mucosa. Both glands and pits are lined by simple columnar cells which secrete neutral mucins (Figure 5.7). Goblet and other specialized cells are not present. At the transition to body-type mucosa specialized cells appear between the mucus cells, the glands lengthen and become straight and the epithelium changes to body type. In older people a scattering of lymphocytes and plasma cells sufficient to suggest a diagnosis of mild superficial gastritis is so common as to be regarded as normal: I have not seen enough cardiac material from adolescents and young adults to know how common a finding it is in them.

Body Mucosa

Normal body mucosa varies from 400 to 1500 μm in thickness. The inner three-quarters of this consists of straight non-branching tubules, often curled over as they abut onto the muscularis mucosae so that they are

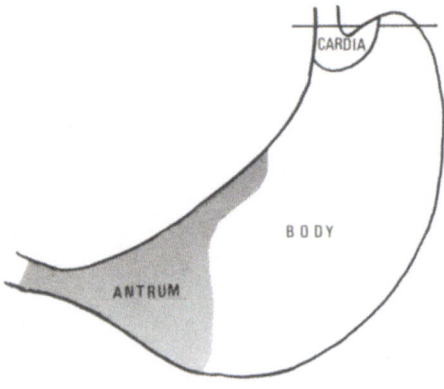

Figure 5.1 Diagram of histologically recognizable gastric zones. Considerable individual variations occur (see text)

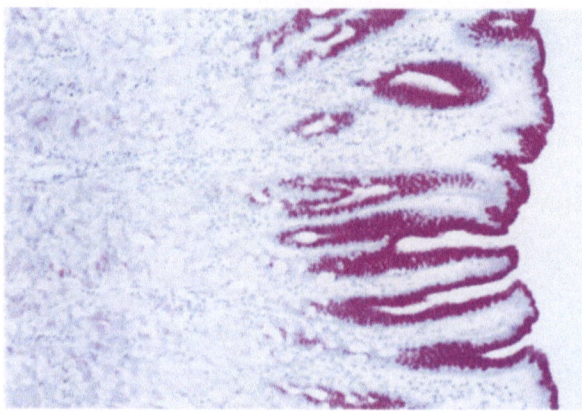

Figure 5.2 Body mucosa showing neutral mucins in surface mucosal and crypt cells.   Diastase–PAS × 125

Figure 5.3 Body mucosa in early atrophic gastritis, showing a small zone of intestinal metaplasia in which are goblet cells containing sialomucins.   Alcian blue at pH 2.5 × 125

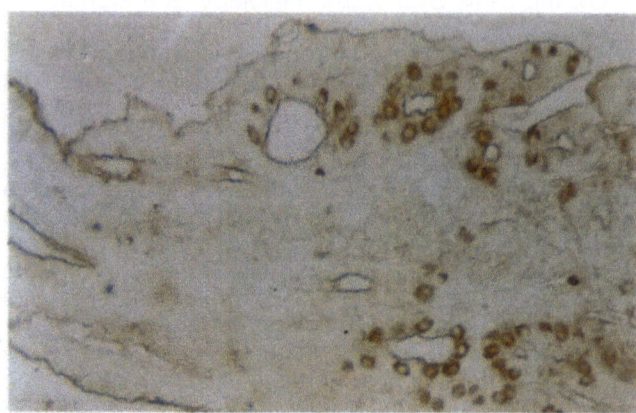

Figure 5.4 Normal antral mucosa showing gastrin-containing cells. Peroxidase–antiperoxidase (PAP) technique × 320

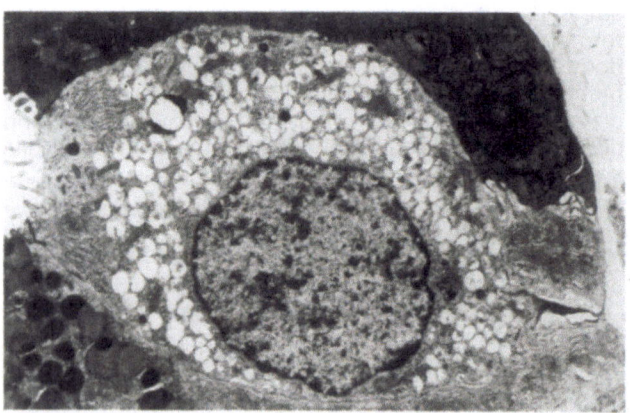

Figure 5.5 Transmission electron micrograph of gastrin-secreting cell. Some granules are opaque, others appear to contain finely granular material.   × 5000

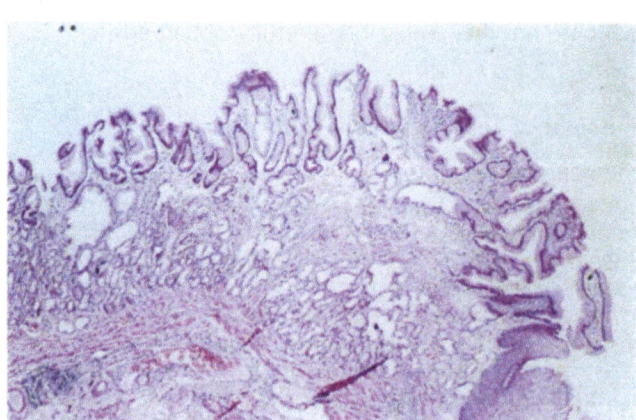

Figure 5.6 Normal cardio-oesophageal junction. The transition from squamous to glandular epithelium is normally abrupt as is shown here.   H & E × 80

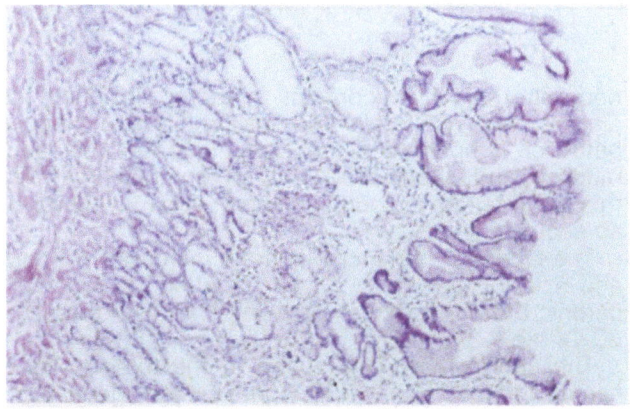

Figure 5.7 Higher magnification of the more distal cardiac mucosa in Figure 5.6, showing the simple mucus-secreting cells lining crypts and glands and the occasional dilated gland which is a normal finding.   H & E × 125

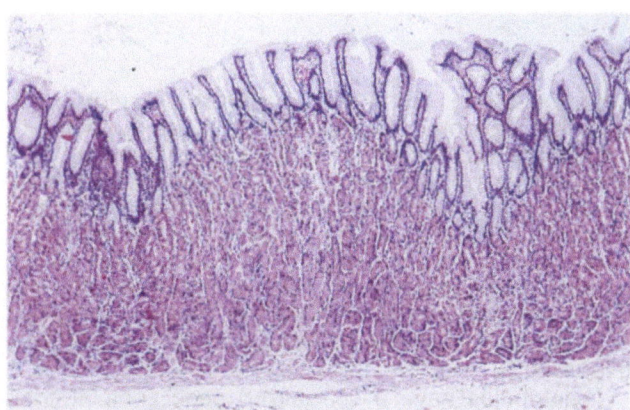

Figure 5.8 Normal body mucosa. The crypts are lined by columnar mucus-secreting cells without goblet formation and a variable number of tubules can be seen opening into them.   H & E × 65

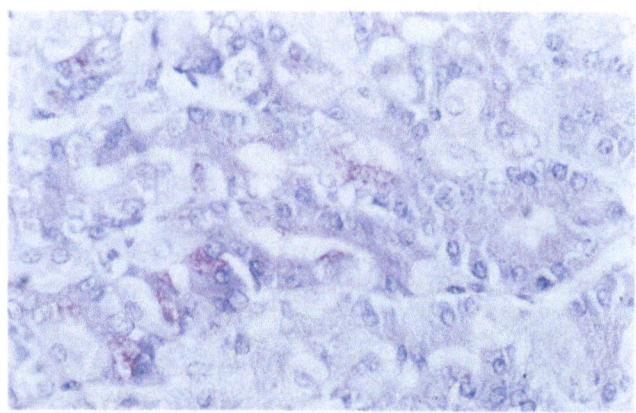

Figure 5.9 Normal body mucosa adjacent to muscularis. Using a PAS technique a few mucus-secreting cells containing neutral mucin are demonstrable. Pepsinogen-secreting cells, which predominate, have basal nuclei and granular cytoplasm, while the relatively few acid-secreting cells have a central nucleus and clear cytoplasm. These cells can also be separated on a well stained H & E or on thin resin sections.   Diastase–PAS × 320

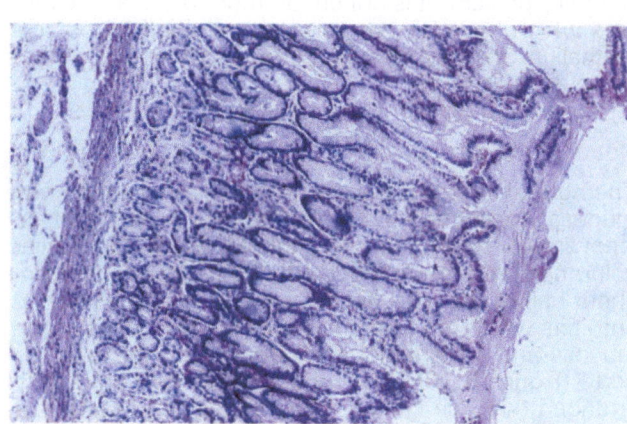

Figure 5.10 Normal antral mucosa. The broader deeper crypts are well shown and the tubules are less regularly arranged.   H & E × 100

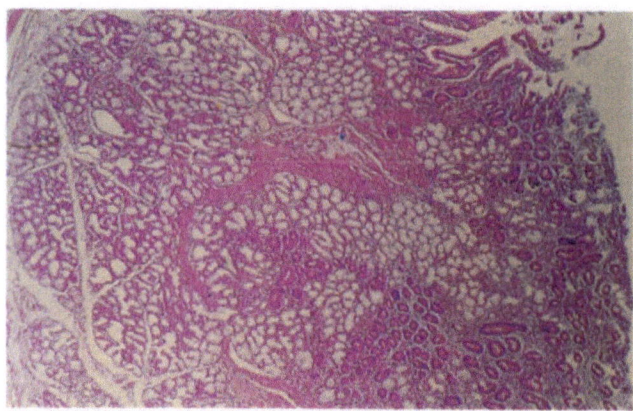

Figure 5.11 Normal pyloric mucosa. The splitting up of the deeper tubular zone by branching muscularis mucosae is obvious: many tubules appear in cross-section.   H & E × 65

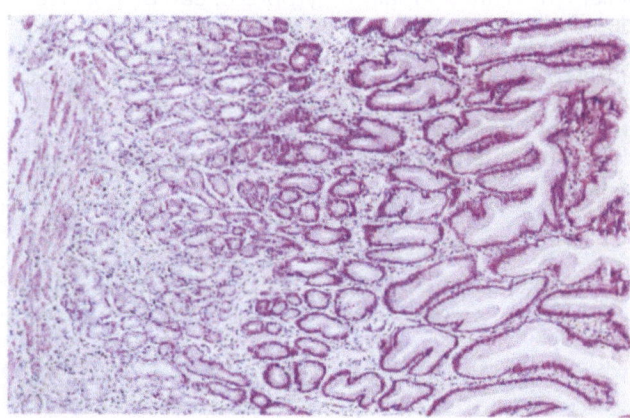

Figure 5.12 Normal body-antral junction. The superficial mucosa is antral in type with broad deep crypts but the tubules, although predominantly lined with mucus-secreting cells, still contain some acid and pepsinogen-secreting cells.   H & E × 80

cut transversely. Three or four tubules open into each crypt (pit, foveola) which is formed by an indipping of the surface mucosa (Figure 5.8) and are separated from one another by a delicate lamina propria which at its lower margin may be ingrown by strands of muscularis mucosae. The surface mucosa and the pits which dip down from it form the outer, luminal quarter of the mucosal thickness and are lined by tall columnar cells which secrete neutral PAS-positive mucin: no goblet cells or other specialized cells are present in this zone (Figure 5.2).

The tubules have a specialized neck zone at their upper end where cell replication occurs; deep to this each tubule is lined at the luminal end predominantly by parietal (oxyntic) cells which have eosinophilic cytoplasm and secrete both acid and intrinsic factor and at the lower end predominantly by pepsinogen-secreting chief cells which have a granular neutrophilic cytoplasm; neutral mucus-secreting columnar cells and occasional endocrine cells of varying types (Figure 5.9) are interspersed. Goblet cells and Paneth cells are not normally present. It is not uncommon to see a few tubules which have become dilated and lined by cubical epithelium in their deeper parts. I personally regard these as normal.

Antral Mucosa

The normal antral mucosa is slightly thinner than body mucosa, measuring 200–1100 μm. It consists of an inner zone of coiled branching tubules all lined by similar columnar cells secreting neutral mucin, which form about half of the total epithelial thickness. These open onto pits which are formed by indippings of the surface mucosa and are broader and deeper than those in the body (Figure 5.10). The tubules are more irregularly arranged than the straight body tubules and there is a marked tendency for muscularis mucosae to grow up between them; at the pylorus they become split up by the muscularis and eventually grow down deep to it to form the Brunner's glands of the duodenum (Figure 5.11). Proximally body and antral type mucosa merge in a transitional zone about 1 cm broad (Figure 5.12).

Although parietal cells have been said to be normally present in small numbers throughout antral mucosa[11] this has not been my experience. Gastrin-containing (G) cells, which are normally argyrophilic, can be positively identified using commercial antigastrin serum after standard fixation and lie in a band in the midzone of the antral region (Figure 5.4). Other endocrine cells, including cells secreting 5-hydroxytryptamine and somatostatin are diffusely present throughout.

The antral lamina propria has a fibrous and collagenous stroma which contains scattered lymphocytes, plasma cells, mast cells and eosinophils. Small aggregates of lymphocytes are commonly seen in adult mucosa and submucosa but, in contrast with ileal mucosa, are rare in young children[12] and may represent an acquired lesion.

The lamina proprial cell infiltrate increases with age and a lesion which might be regarded as superficial chronic antral gastritis in an adolescent is normal in a 60-year-old.

The approximate distribution of the three types of gastric mucosa is given in Figure 5.1. In general the transition from one to another occurs over a relatively short distance, usually not more than 1 cm.

References

1. Dawson, I. M. P. (1981). The value of histochemistry in the diagnosis and prognosis of gastrointestinal diseases. In Stoward, P. J. and Polak, J. M. (eds.) *Histochemistry: The Widening Horizons*, pp. 127–162. (Chichester: John Wiley & Sons)

2. Voillemot, N., Potet, F., Mary, J. Y. and Lewin, M. J. M. (1978). Gastrin cell distribution in normal human stomachs and in patients with Zollinger Ellison syndrome. *Gastroenterology*, **75**, 65

3. McIntyre, R. L. E. and Piris, J. (1980). Quantification of human gastric G cell density in endoscopic biopsy specimens: effect of shape of specimen. *J. Clin Pathol.*, **33**, 513

4. Kreuning, J., Bosman, F. T., Kuiper, G., van de Wal, A. M. and Lindeman, J. (1978). Gastric and duodenal mucosa in 'healthy' individuals. *J. Clin. Pathol.*, **31**, 69

5. Levine, J. S., Nakane, P. K. and Allen, R. H. (1980). Immunocytochemical localization of human intrinsic factor: the non-stimulated stomach. *Gastroenterology*, **79**, 493

6. Cross, S. A. M. (1977). Localization of histamine and histamine H$_2$-receptor antagonists in the gastric mucosa. *Histochem. J.*, **9**, 619

7. Isaacson, P. (1982). Immunoperoxidase study of the secretory immunoglobulin system and lysozyme in normal and diseased antral mucosa. *Gut*, **23**, 578

8. Samloff, I. M. (1971). Cellular localization of group pepsinogens in human gastric mucosa by immunofluorescence. *Gastroenterology*, **61**, 185

9. Rubin, W., Ross, L. L. Sleisenger, M. H. and Jeffries, G. H. (1968). The normal human gastric epithelia. A fine structural study. *Lab. Invest.*, **19**, 598

10. Maxwell, A. (1963). Technique for staining acid and pepsinogen cells in stomach. *Stain Technol.*, **38**, 286

11. Tominaga, K. (1975). Distribution of parietal cells in the antral mucosa of human stomachs. *Gastroenterology*, **69**, 1201

12. Watt, J. (1966). The pathology of multiple gastric ulceration in the newborn infant. *J. Pathol. Bacteriol.*, **91**, 105

Inflammatory change in gastric mucosa – as evidenced by the presence of polymorphs or by an increase in number of lymphocytes, plasma cells, mast cells or eosinophils – is a histological finding which by no means always corresponds with a history of dyspepsia, and in people over the age of 60 is so common that many pathologists and clinicians regard it as 'normal'. This cellular infiltration results from mucosal contact with irritants which include refluxed bile acid, alcohol, drugs and poisons and also from auto-immune type reactions, and, if the irritant is continuous or the mucosal defences alter, can be followed by epithelial erosion, ulceration and atrophy with loss of gland elements. These changes are initially reversible but become less so as they become more severe and long-continued. It is not uncommon for gastric mucosa so affected to undergo metaplasia to an intestinal pattern, which can eventually become dysplastic with an increased risk of carcinomatous change. It is therefore important to classify accurately the different patterns of gastritis, always relating the findings to the age of the patient.

Acute and chronic gastritis can develop in cardiac, body and antral mucosa though they are most common in the antrum; biopsies taken to confirm or exclude gastritis should always be taken from both body and antral regions. Since gastritis can be patchy, more than one area from each region should be sampled.

Acute Gastritis

Acute gastritis results from exposure of the mucosa to an acute insult of short duration – a large volume of alcohol in a short time, a dose of aspirin in those sensitive to it, the ingestion of other irritants, the taking of steroids which probably prevent the normally occurring small injuries from healing and as a concomitant of acute infections or uraemia; the list is not exhaustive. The mucosa as seen endoscopically is markedly congested and small surface erosions may be present (Figure 6.1). Involvement is often patchy and can affect body or antrum. Microscopically there is oedema, congestion and haemorrhage in the lamina propria, some of which may be the result of biopsy itself. Polymorphonuclear infiltration is variable (Figure 6.2). Erosion of surface mucosa is common and there is often necrosis of underlying glands (Figures 6.3 and 6.4) but this rarely extends to the full thickness of the biopsy; if biopsy is delayed there may be less severe inflammatory change and evidence of mucosal regeneration. Erosion may progress to acute ulcer but the mucosa usually returns to normal and a single episode is not thought to predispose to chronicity, though repeated ones may do so.

Chronic Gastritis

Chronic gastritis is a histological, not a clinical diagnosis, characterized by one or more of three important features: cellular infiltration of the lamina propria; damage to, followed by loss of gland elements; and epithelial metaplasia to an intestinal type. It is not always symptomatic, and, conversely, a number of patients with the symptoms of non-ulcer dyspepsia do not show the histological changes of gastritis. It may be related to reflux of bile, chronic alcohol abuse, or to the presence of parietal cell antibodies; in many patients there is no obvious causative factor and the condition certainly becomes more common with advancing age. Chronic gastritis can be generalized or patchy in distribution, and is a common finding around peptic ulcers and carcinomas; it can occur in body or antral mucosa. Histologically it can be active or quiescent, can regress in the early stages but is usually slowly though intermittently progressive. One end-result of progression is an atrophic mucosa with little evidence of active inflammation or cell destruction, usually known as gastric atrophy. This is a form of 'end stage' which can result either from inflammation or autoimmune reaction and is seen in pernicious anaemia, but in many patients the condition seems to stabilize as a quiescent chronic atrophic gastritis. Gastritis is usually graded histologically as superficial gastritis, atrophic gastritis or gastric atrophy but further classification into mild, moderate or severe, based on the degree of cellular infiltration and on presence or absence of gland atrophy and metaplasia[1], the type of epithelium in which it is present and the degree of activity or quiescence[2], can be helpful. The most important thing is for the clinician to understand what the pathologist means by the terms he uses and for a nomenclature to be agreed between them.

Assessment of Activity

This depends on the presence or absence of polymorphs and of active epithelial destruction and regeneration. Polymorphs in gastritis always mean an active lesion; they are found within the lamina propria, within the epithelium itself and contained within epithelial gland elements, particularly in gastric pits where they resemble the crypt abscesses seen in the large intestine. They are probably related to the degree of tissue damage.

Active epithelial destruction is seen particularly in surface mucosa and pits, though it can also involve deeper glands; it is usually associated with superficial erosion and the presence of polymorphs adjacent to the eroded epithelium (Figure 6.2). Concurrently there is regenerative activity in the crypt cells at the necks of glands, with nuclear hyperchromatism, increase in mitotic

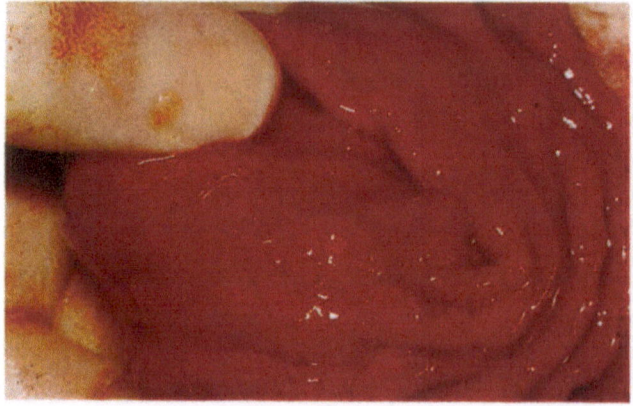

Figure 6.1 A resected stomach showing the marked mucosal congestion seen in acute gastritis. Small early surface erosions are also present

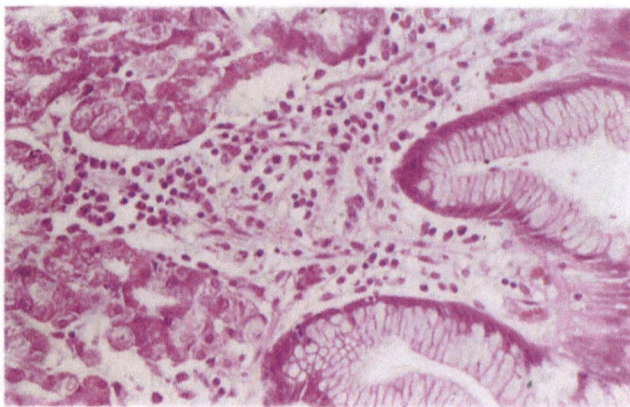

Figure 6.2 Body of stomach; a small collection of polymorphs and plasma cells in the lamina propria adjacent to an erosion.   H & E × 250

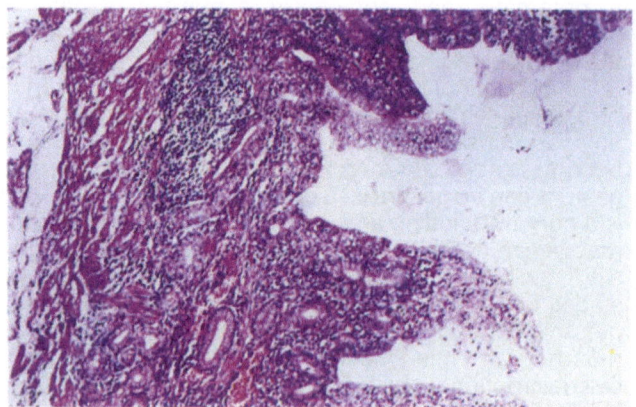

Figure 6.3 Gastric erosion. There is patchy ulceration of surface mucosa with some loss of gland elements which does not extend down to the muscularis. There is an increased incidence of mononuclear cells in the lamina propria.   H & E × 100

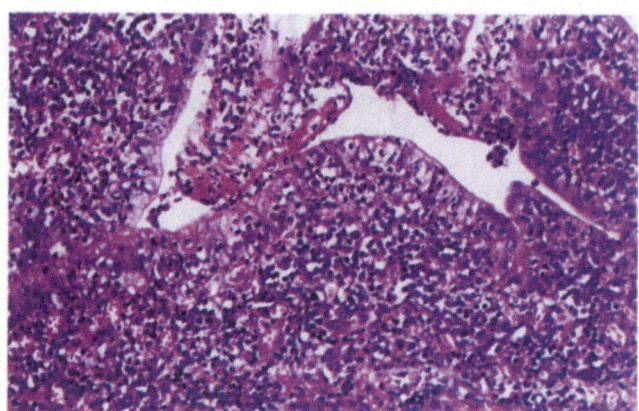

Figure 6.4 Higher-power view of an erosion showing some polymorph and mononuclear cell infiltration of the remaining surface epithelium.   H & E × 250

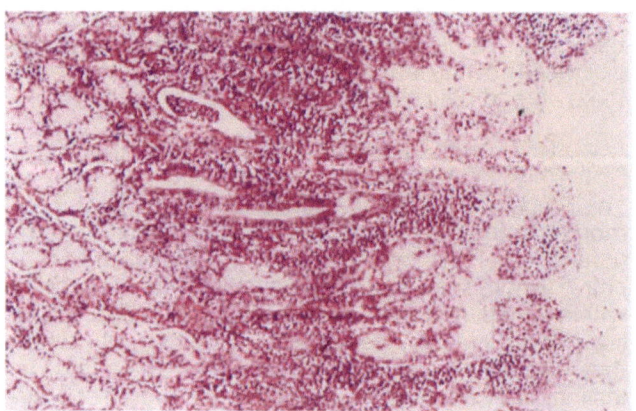

Figure 6.5 Antral region: active superficial chronic gastritis. The apparent patchy erosion of mucosa is probably traumatic and artifactual. The marked increase in round cells, some of which are present in a dilated gland, along with their superficial mucosal localization, is characteristic.   H & E × 125

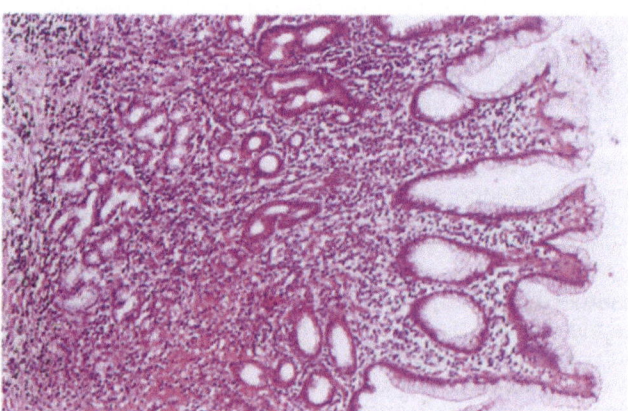

Figure 6.6 Body mucosa in active chronic gastritis: the mucosa is thinner than normal and only a few specialized cells remain.   H & E × 100

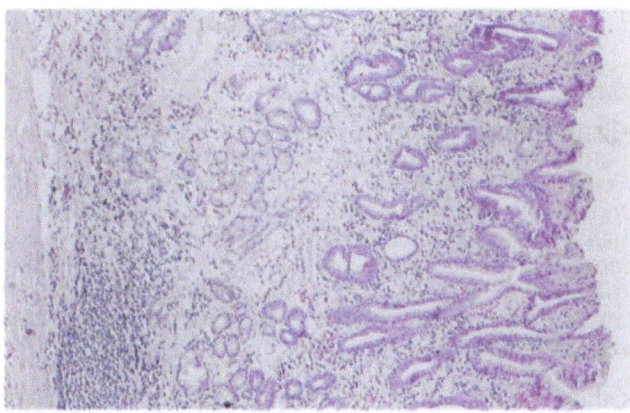

Figure 6.7 Body mucosa in quiescent chronic gastritis showing pyloric gland metaplasia.   H & E × 100

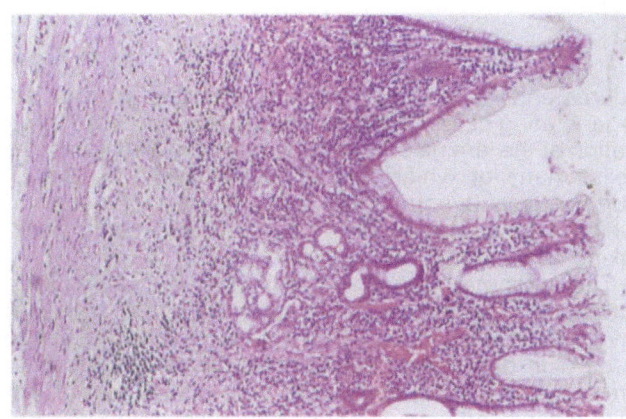

Figure 6.8 Antral mucosa: atrophic gastritis. The surface mucosa is intact, but glands are reduced in number and distorted. There is a heavy mononuclear infiltrate in the more superficial lamina propria and some fibrosis in the deeper mucosa.   H & E × 125

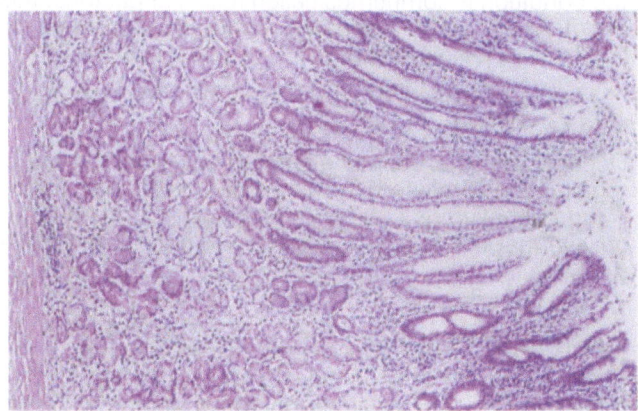

Figure 6.9 Body mucosa: chronic superficial gastritis. There is an increased mononuclear infiltrate in the superficial lamina propria but no loss of gland elements or of specialized cells.   H & E × 100

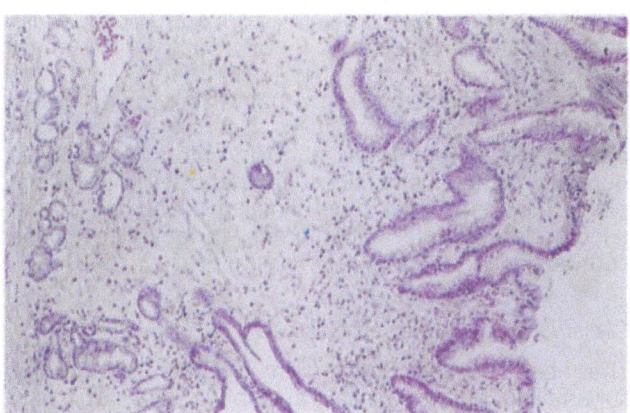

Figure 6.10 Antral mucosa: chronic active atrophic gastritis. Some gland elements remain and fibrosis is not a feature.   H & E × 125

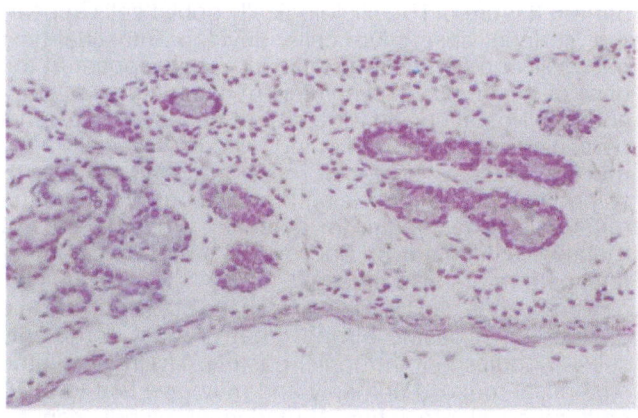

Figure 6.11 Antral mucosa: gastric atrophy. The mucosa is markedly thinned and few gland elements remain, but there is little or no inflammatory cellular infiltrate in the lamina propria.   H & E × 125

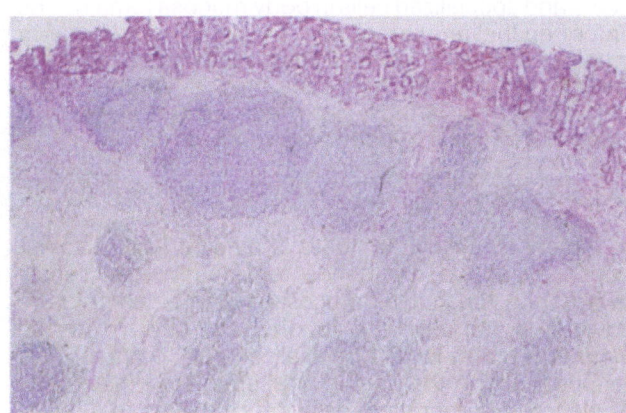

Figure 6.12 Body mucosa: lymphoid aggregates are present in lamina propria and submucosa.   H & E × 32

figures and sometimes irregularly arranged clumps of regenerating cells. Other features are an increased infiltration of the lamina propria by lymphocytes and plasma cells, many of which remain as the lesion becomes quiescent, and sometimes the presence of oedema which may be inflammatory but can also result from taking of the biopsy alone (Figure 6.5).

The outcome of continued epithelial destruction and attempted regeneration depends on the type of mucosa involved. In body mucosa regeneration does not keep pace with destruction and specialized gland elements are fairly rapidly lost, giving rise to a thinner epithelium with diminished acid and pepsinogen secretion (Figure 6.6). Much of the straight tubular appearance is lost and glands which remain appear more convoluted. There is commonly a metaplasia towards a simple pyloric pattern of mucus-secreting gland in which specialized cells are not seen (Figure 6.7).

In antral mucosa there is variable destruction of the simple mucus-secreting glands leading to a thinning of the mucosa, often with an increase in fibrous tissue within the lamina propria (Figure 6.8).

It is not normally a problem to separate body, antral and transitional mucosa. Difficulty occasionally arises when, in body mucosa, pyloric type metaplasia is extensive and no specialized cells remain. The simplest way is to look for gastrin-containing cells which are only present in genuine antral mucosa; antral mucosa also normally contains occasional parietal cells which metaplastic glands do not. The clinician taking the biopsy should also be able, within limits, to indicate its likely source.

Classification of Chronic Gastritis

The headings still conventionally used are chronic superficial gastritis, chronic atrophic gastritis and gastric atrophy. They can be incorporated into a more informative classification and report as follows.

Chronic Superficial Gastritis

An increased cellular infiltrate is present in the lamina propria, particularly beneath the surface and around the pits, but also often in the deeper parts (Figures 6.5 and 6.9). There is no diminution in numbers of gland elements and specialized cells in body mucosa remain. The type of epithelium can always be identified as body or antral but activity can only be assessed by the degree of cellular infiltration of the lamina propria. All these features should be carefully reported, e.g. active chronic superficial gastritis in body type mucosa.

Chronic Atrophic Gastritis

An increased cellular infiltrate is present in the lamina propria as above, but tends to extend more deeply towards the muscularis mucosae. Gland elements are reduced in number and tubules are often distorted (Figures 6.8 and 6.10). Specialized cells progressively disappear and in the body region are often replaced by simple mucus-secreting cells of pyloric type (Figure 6.7). There may be evidence of active gland destruction with occasional polymorphs present, though regenerative changes are usually not conspicuous. The type of epithelium can usually be identified (see above). These factors should be reported, e.g. quiescent atrophic gastritis in pyloric type mucosa.

Gastric Atrophy

Gland elements are atrophic and markedly reduced in number and the mucosa appears thin (Figure 6.11). There is no evidence of active tissue destruction or regeneration. Polymorphs are not seen and there is usually little or no excess of mononuclear cells in the lamina propria. In the presence of extensive pyloric metaplasia it can be difficult to tell atrophic body from atrophic antral mucosa. The condition is widespread rather than patchy.

Other features variably present in chronic gastritis are as follows.

Lymphoid Aggregates

Lymphoid follicles and aggregates, with or without germinal centres, are commonly present in the lamina propria, muscularis mucosae and submucosa in atrophic gastritis, especially when this surrounds a peptic ulcer (Figure 6.12). When these are extensive the condition is sometimes called follicular gastritis: this is not, in my view, a separate entity, but represents a local immunologic response.

Cyst Formation

Occasionally the deeper glands in the body or antral region become dilated, forming small cysts in which the lining epithelium is cubical or flattened (Figure 6.13). I believe that this is a normal feature especially in elderly people.

Regenerative Polyps

In some patients with active superficial or atrophic gastritis showing epithelial regenerative changes, small upgrowing polypoid lesions develop which are often cystic, can be multiple (Figure 6.14) and are often associated with intestinal metaplasia. The deeper glands may show atrophic change.

Intestinal Metaplasia

Intestinal metaplasia is a change of gastric epithelium, cardiac, body, transitional or antral to a true intestinal pattern (Figure 6.15). Histologically goblet cells appear, the surface absorptive cells develop intestinal-type microvilli and Paneth and endocrine cells appear at the base of the crypts. The epithelium has features of large and small intestine and villi are not a necessary or even a particularly common finding. Histochemically the mucins present in goblet cells are sialomucins or sulphomucins and an Alcian blue stain at pH 2.5 is the most reliable technique for detecting small patches of metaplasia (Figure 5.3). Enzymes of brush-border intestinal pattern are also present.

This change can occur in any of the stages of chronic gastritis or in gastric atrophy, but is most commonly seen in quiescent atrophic gastritis. It involves the superficial mucosa primarily and may give rise to polypoid mucosal projections but deeper glands can be affected; it is at first patchy and limited in extent but can evolve to cover large areas of mucosa. It is important as a potentially precancerous lesion and can sometimes become dysplastic (see page 51).

Other Forms of Gastritis

Acute Phlegmonous Gastritis

This condition, rarely seen nowadays, complicates severe streptococcal infections and is usually fatal. Endoscopically the mucosa is congested and sloughs may be present. Microscopically there is mucosal necrosis but the principal changes are in the submucosa where there is extensive oedema, polymorph infiltration and thromboses in small vessels (Figure 6.16).

Candidiasis

Gastric, like oesophageal, candidiasis is associated with altered immune status and is found in immunosuppressed patients particularly when treated coincidentally with steroids[3]. Lesions are usually raised discrete nodules which on biopsy consist of ulcerated mucosa with little surrounding inflammatory reaction; the fungus is readily visible on PAS staining (Figure 6.17).

Viral Gastritis

I have not seen herpetic infection in the stomach corresponding to those in the oesophagus though occasional cases are described[4]. Cytomegalovirus is sometimes found in debilitated patients in autopsy histology of the stomach; I have not seen it in biopsy material.

Granulomatous Gastritis

Crohn's disease occurs in the antral region of the stomach alone or as part of a more generalized gastrointestinal involvement. On endoscopy the mucosa can appear cobblestoned and fissured. Biopsy shows the fissuring ulceration and granulation tissue seen in intestinal biopsies and giant cell granuloma can be present (Figure 6.18).

Tuberculosis in the stomach is extremely rare and probably always secondary to open pulmonary disease. It usually produces ulceration rather than gastritis but occasionally tuberculous granulation tissue with caseation is present, and small discrete tubercles are seen in mucosa and submucosa.

'Food granulomas' are usually associated with peptic ulceration, particularly duodenal. They are due either to the presence of indigestible food material such as cereal husks which infiltrate through the edge of an ulcer to embed in surrounding submucosa or mucosa, or to the action of acid- and pepsin-containing gastric juice on muscularis mucosae denuded of covering epithelium. They are most common at the pylorus, are seldom recognized endoscopically but can cause great confusion in a biopsy. They consist essentially of amorphous material, sometimes resembling ova, surrounded by a granulomatous reaction in which are histiocytes and foreign body giant cells (Figure 6.19). Sometimes the central material is elongated and calcified and may resemble a worm (Figure 6.20); it can be double refractile. There is often considerable surrounding fibrosis.

Eosinophil Gastritis

Eosinophil gastroenteritis is probably an allergic manifestation and is seen principally in the pyloric region of the stomach and throughout the small intestine where it can cause obstruction[5]. The pyloric antrum appears thickened and oedematous. Microscopically the mucosa is normal; the submucosa is oedematous and heavily infiltrated by eosinophils; there is sometimes an accompanying arteritis which must be distinguished from polyarteritis nodosa but fibrosis is not a feature (Figure 6.21). Blood eosinophilia is usual.

Diffuse Varioliform Gastritis

This is a recently recognized condition which I am not entirely convinced is a genuine entity[6]. Endoscopically there is mucosal congestion and mucus deposition with enlargement of the mucosal folds of the body and sometimes also of the antrum with erosion on the summits of the folds. Microscopically the gastric pits are lengthened and erosion of less than full thickness is present surrounded by hyperplastic and dysplastic epithelium. There is no appreciable gland atrophy. Plasma cells and polymorphs are present in the lamina propria and immunological techniques show an increase in IgE-containing cells, suggesting a possible allergic origin. Without the use of immunocytochemical techniques I doubt whether this lesion is distinguishable from active superficial gastritis.

Ulcerative and Erosive Lesions

An erosion is a less than full thickness loss of mucosa which heals by regeneration from below. An ulcer is a full thickness loss of mucosa and heals, if at all, by ingrowth of epithelium from the sides. Erosive lesions usually result from an acute insult (see Figures 6.3 and 6.4); regeneration is usual. They are also seen in superficial and early carcinomas, where they are incorrectly called ulcers; this usage is so common that it is retained here. There is nearly always associated mucosal congestion and body or antral mucosa can be involved.

Peptic Ulcer

When an endoscopist sees an ulcerated lesion there are two common possibilities: peptic ulcer and ulcerated carcinoma. Biopsy should be taken from the ulcer edge at each of the four quadrants (3, 6, 9 and 12 o'clock) with two biopsies from the base. Chronic peptic ulcers occur in the antral or junctional mucosa; very rarely in body mucosa. The edge will show an abrupt transition from gastric mucosa of antral or junctional pattern usually with changes of an associated gastritis with or without intestinal metaplasia, to an ulcer base of necrotic slough and granulation tissue (Figure 6.22). Not infrequently when the biopsy is received the base has become detached from the epithelium as a separate fragment. There is sometimes hyperplasia of the epithelium at the ulcer edge with downgrowth through muscularis mucosae (Figure 6.23); the differential diagnosis of this from genuine neoplastic change which, though rare, does occasionally occur (Figure 6.24) must always be borne in mind. Look for alterations in nuclear–cytoplasmic ratio, increase in mitoses and irregularities in gland formation.

Zollinger–Ellison Syndrome

The classic syndrome of severe peptic ulceration involving duodenum and sometimes jejunum is associated with gastrin-secreting endocrine cell tumours of stomach and pancreas. A second syndrome has been described in which there is simple hyperplasia of normal gastrin-secreting cells in the antral region[7]. This can be confirmed, if suspected clinically, using peroxidase–antiperoxidase techniques (Figure 5.4). In ZE syndrome from either cause, body-type mucosa may extend more widely into the antral region.

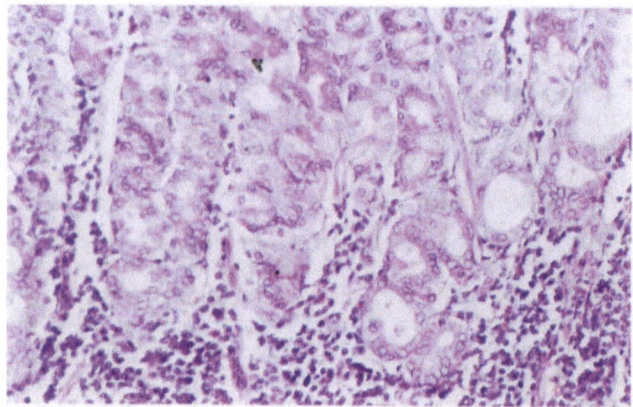

Figure 6.13 Cystic glandular dilatation (mild) in chronic active gastritis. Small cysts lie in the deeper gland elements abutting onto the muscularis mucosae.   H & E × 250

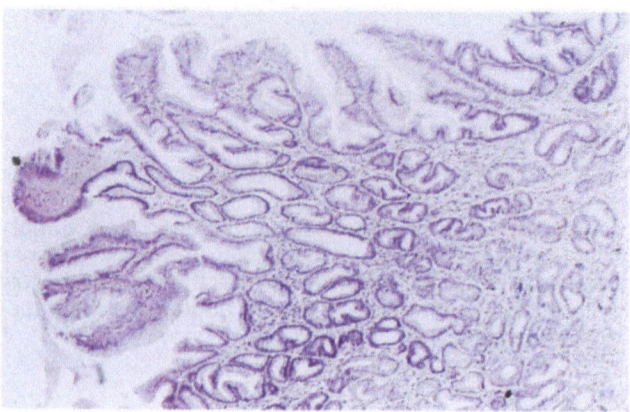

Figure 6.14 Antral mucosa: a regenerative polyp in a patient with an active atrophic gastritis. There is some distortion and cystic dilatation of gland elements and a 'crypt abscess' is present.   H & E × 125

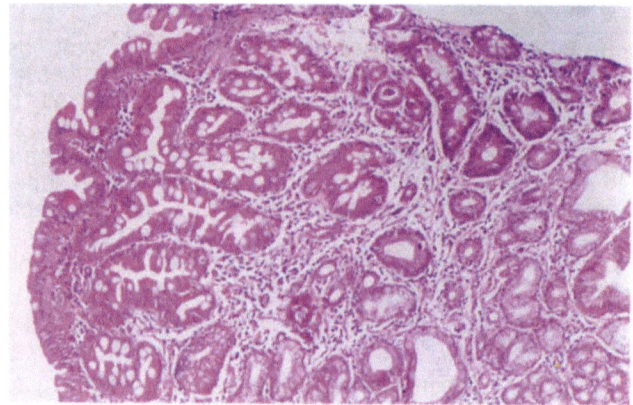

Figure 6.15 Antral region: intestinal metaplasia. Goblet cells are conspicuous but there is no attempt at villus formation.   H & E × 250

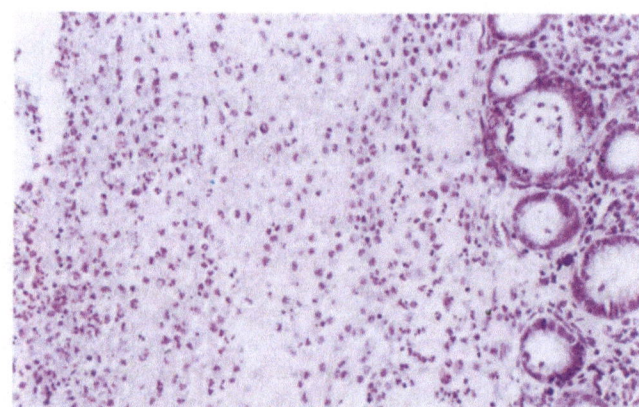

Figure 6.16 Acute phlegmonous gastritis. Note the submucosal oedema and presence of polymorphs with associated mucosal necrosis.   H & E × 320

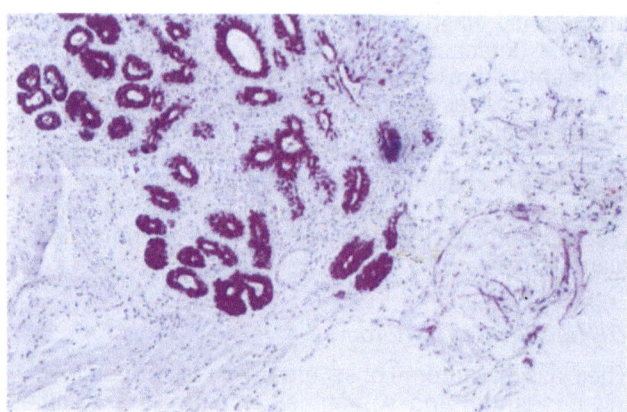

Figure 6.17 Gastric candidiasis showing fungi and relative absence of reactive inflammation. From a man aged 26 with Hodgkin's disease, stage 4, treated with antimitotic drugs.   H & E × 250

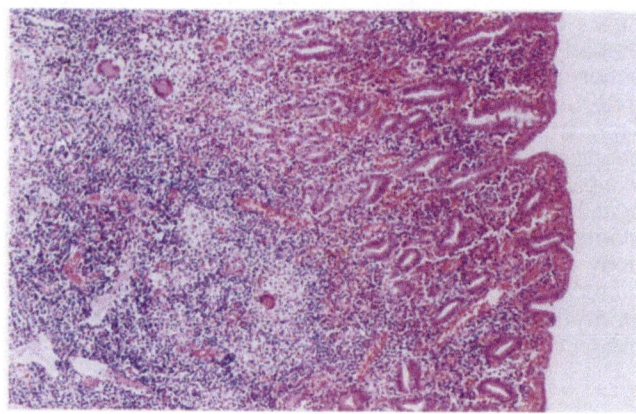

Figure 6.18 Antral region: Crohn's disease. Characteristic granulomas are present within thickened muscularis mucosae.   H & E × 125

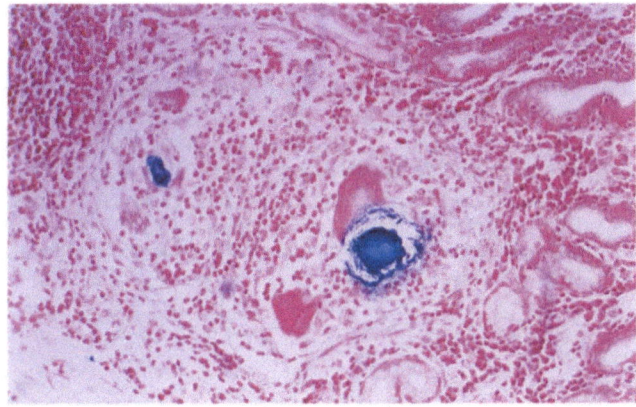

Figure 6.19 Antral (pyloric) region; foreign body granuloma. From a 55-year-old man who had a duodenal ulcer and a prepyloric mucosal swelling thought to be carcinoma. The nature of the material is uncertain: it contained calcium and iron. Perl's stain × 250

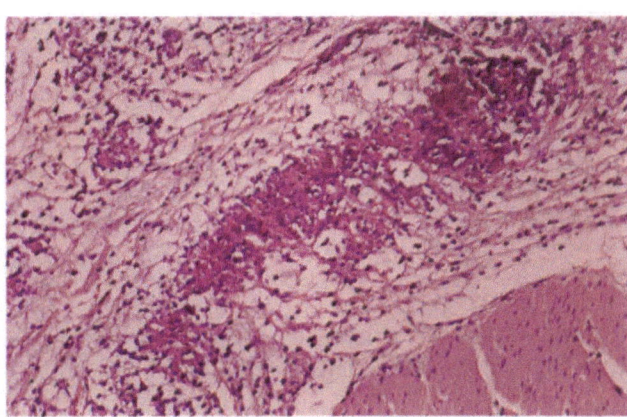

Figure 6.20 Antral region: foreign body granuloma in submucosa. This may be mistaken for a calcified worm; its nature remained undetermined. H & E × 250

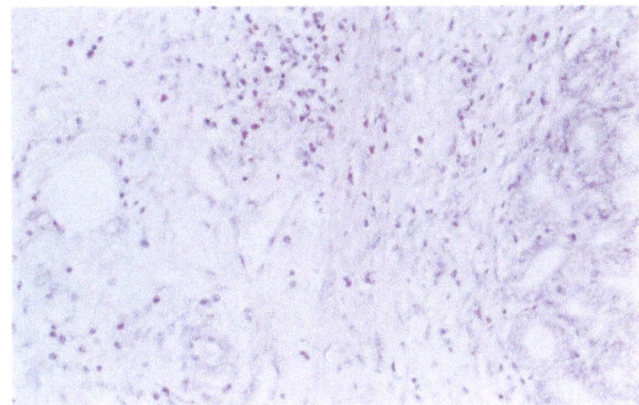

Figure 6.21 Eosinophil gastritis. There is marked oedema and eosinophil infiltration of the submucosa with relatively normal overlying mucosa, but no arteritis was present in this biopsy. H & E × 250

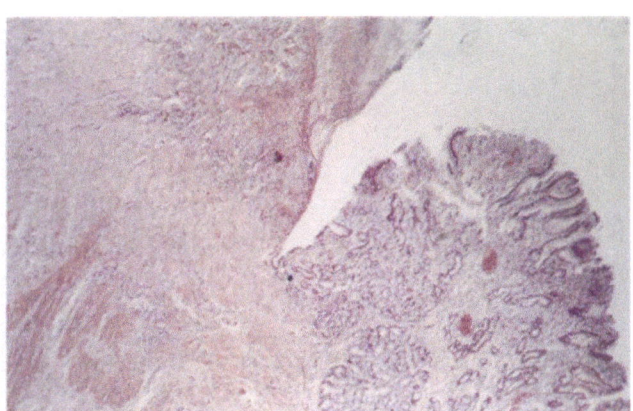

Figure 6.22 Early acute ulcer, pyloric region. On the right is pyloric mucosa showing intestinal metaplasia; on the left is ulcerated mucosa with partial destruction of muscularis mucosae and early chronic inflammatory change in the submucosa. H & E × 80

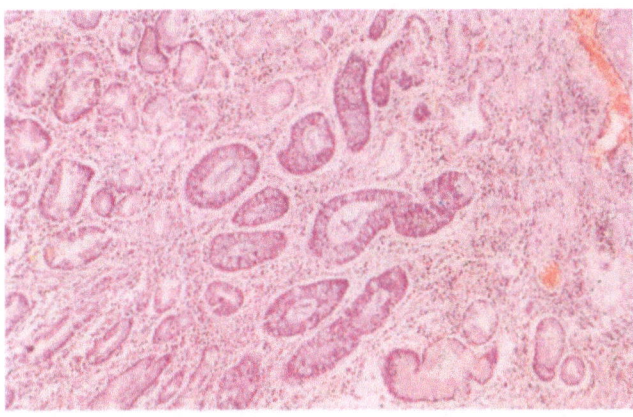

Figure 6.23 Mucosal proliferation of antral type glands at the edge of a chronic peptic ulcer. Compare with Figure 6.24. H & E × 250

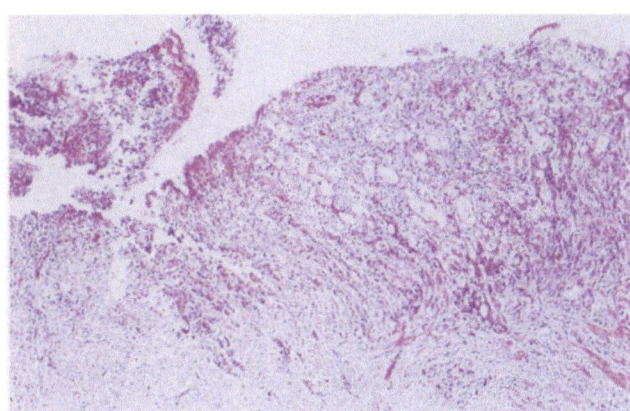

Figure 6.24 Carcinomatous change at the edge of a peptic ulcer. On the left the glands resemble those seen in non-neoplastic proliferation (see Figure 6.23) but towards the right they lose their relatively normal glandular appearance and are invading the deeper tissues. H & E × 80

References

1. Rao, S. S., Krausner, N. and Thomson, T. J. (1975). Chronic gastritis – a simple classification. *J. Pathol.*, **117**, 93

2. Morson, B. C. and Dawson, I. M. P. (1979). *Gastrointestinal Pathology*, 2nd edn, pp. 95–108. (Oxford: Blackwell)

3. Scott, B. B. and Jenkins, D. (1982). Gastroesophageal candidiasis. *Gut*, **23**, 137

4. Howiler, W. and Goldberg, H. I. (1976). Gastro-esophageal involvement in herpes simplex. *Gastroenterology*, **70**, 775

5. Johnstone, J. M. and Morson, B. C. (1978). Eosinophilic gastroenteritis. *Histopathology*, **2**, 335

6. Lambert, R., André, C., Moulinier, B. and Bugnon, B. (1978). Diffuse varioliform gastritis, *Digestion*, **17**, 159

7. Cowley, D. J., Dymock, I. W., Boyes, B. E., Wilson, R. Y., Stagg, B. H., Lewin, M. R., Polak, J. M. and Pearse, A. G. E. (1973). Zollinger–Ellison syndrome, type 1. Clinical and pathological correlations in a case. *Gut*, **14**, 25

Regenerative polyps are associated with chronic gastritis and have already been described (page 42) and illustrated (see Figure 6.14). Other non-neoplastic lesions can be hamartomatous, familial or both; they are uncommon but can cause confusion in biopsies and merit description.

Peutz–Jeghers' Polyps

These polyps appear in crops, often sequentially, principally in the stomach and upper small intestine, usually in young children. They are inherited as an autosomal dominant and melanin pigmentation around mouth and lips is also usual. Histologically there is widespread proliferation and branching of the muscularis mucosae; the branches are covered with the normal epithelium of the part which in the stomach can be antral or body mucosa (Figure 7.1). Secondary inflammatory changes occur, but malignant change, though it is well documented[1] is extremely rare. The essential diagnostic points are the tree-like branching of the muscularis and the normality of the polypoid epithelium (Figure 7.2). Further examples are illustrated in Chapters 14 and 19.

Juvenile and Familial Polyps

Interesting studies have been recently described on juvenile polyps in the stomach and intestinal tract[1-3]. Single or scattered polyps have long been recognized in the large intestine but are now increasingly described in small intestine and stomach in familial and non-familial forms, usually in the first 10 years of life. In the stomach the lesions begin as sessile polyps but rapidly become pedunculated with a narrow stalk (Figure 7.3). Histologically I have seen two forms. One consists of gland elements often lined by cubical epithelium and dilated to form cysts, set in an oedematous stroma of lamina propria in which inflammatory cells are numerous (Figure 7.4). They resemble those of large bowel and are easily recognized. A second pattern (Figure 7.5) consists apparently of hypertrophic mucosa without increase in the lamina propria and with little cyst formation. Recent studies[4] suggest that dysplastic and adenomatous change can occur at least in large intestinal

juvenile polyposis (see page 123). I have never seen it in the stomach.

Polyps Associated with Adenomatosis Coli

In this disorder, as in juvenile polyposis, recent studies have suggested that the upper gastrointestinal tract may also be affected. In the stomach small adenomatous polyps have been described in the antral mucosa and 'hyperplastic' polyps in body mucosa[5]. The 'hyperplastic' polyps of the body are described as containing acid-secreting cells with cystic dilated ducts and have also been described in women who do not have familial adenomatosis coli[6] (Figure 7.6). It seems clear that any patient who has multiple adenomas of the antrum or multiple hyperplastic polyps of the body of the stomach should be carefully screened for large bowel adenomatosis.

Adenomyomatous Hamartomas and Pancreatic Rests

These two related malformations are not uncommon along the greater curve of the stomach in body and antral regions as well as in the first part of the duodenum. Situated usually in the submucosa they can project into the lumen as a sessile polypoid lesion which sometimes ulcerates. I have seen several resected examples but only one biopsy, in which were gland elements, some with a myoepithelial pattern surrounded by irregular bands of muscle tissue and recognizable pancreatic tissue (Figure 7.7).

Polyps in Cronkhite–Canada Syndrome

In this syndrome gastrointestinal polyps are associated with alopecia, atrophy of nails and hyperpigmentation of skin. There is mucosal thickening with tubular dilatation and flattening of lining epithelial cells resembling colitis cystica superficialis (Figure 7.8).

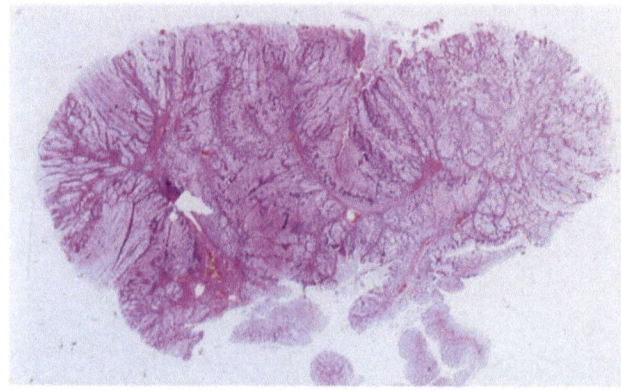

Figure 7.1 Peutz–Jeghers' polyp arising in antral mucosa. Note the tree-like appearances of the branching muscularis mucosae. Whole-mount section. H & E × 8

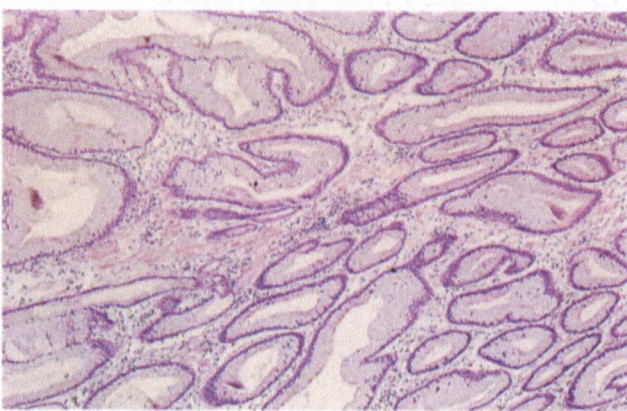

Figure 7.2 Higher-power view of Peutz–Jeghers' polyps showing normal antral type glands separated by strands of muscularis mucosae. H & E × 125

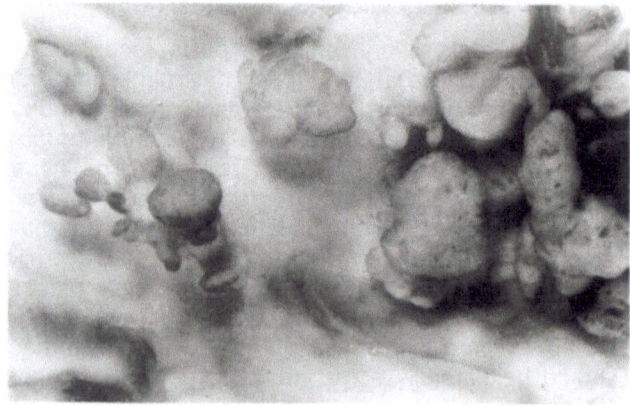

Figure 7.3 Postmortem specimen of stomach from a 1-year-old boy with non-familial juvenile polyposis involving stomach, small and large intestines. Sessile and pedunculated polyps are present.

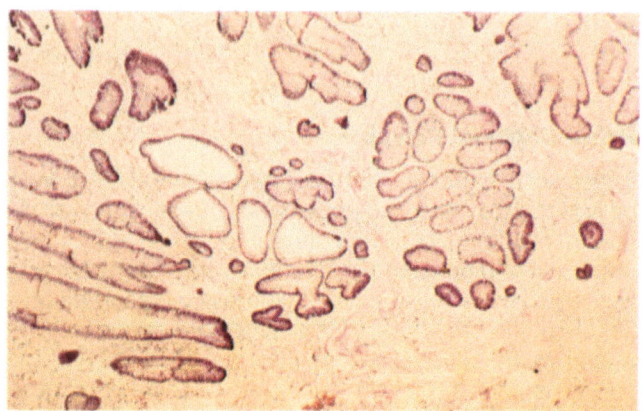

Figure 7.4 Histology of polyps illustrated in Figure 7.3. Simple pyloric-type glands are embedded in an oedematous stroma, and the whole resembles a large intestinal juvenile polyp. H & E × 80

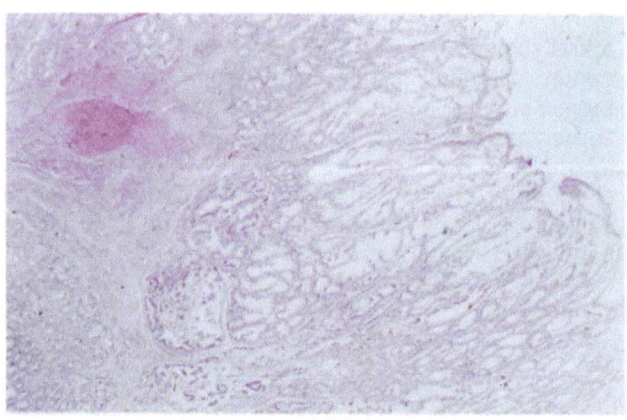

Figure 7.5 Antral juvenile polyp from a 4-year-old-girl. In this pattern there is generalized mucosal hypertrophy of normal-looking antral mucosa without oedema of lamina propria or inflammmatory changes. H & E × 65

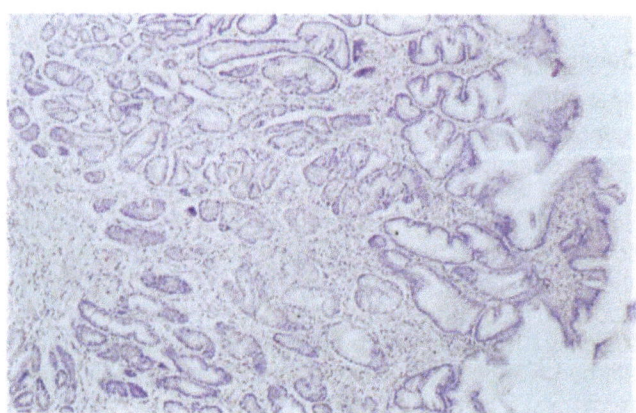

Figure 7.6 Body mucosa showing small hyperplastic polyp. Acid-secreting cells and dilated ducts are clearly visible. This patient did not, in fact, have adenomatosis coli. H & E × 100

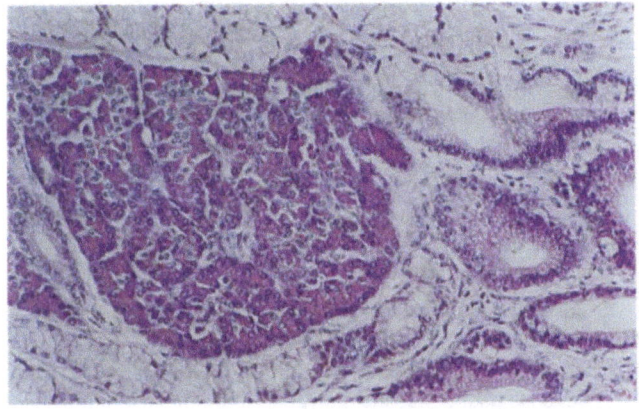

Figure 7.7 Biopsy of antral swelling showing a small island of pancreatic tissue. Subsequent resection showed a myoepithelial hamartoma with gland elements and further small islands of ectopic exocrine pancreas.   H & E × 250

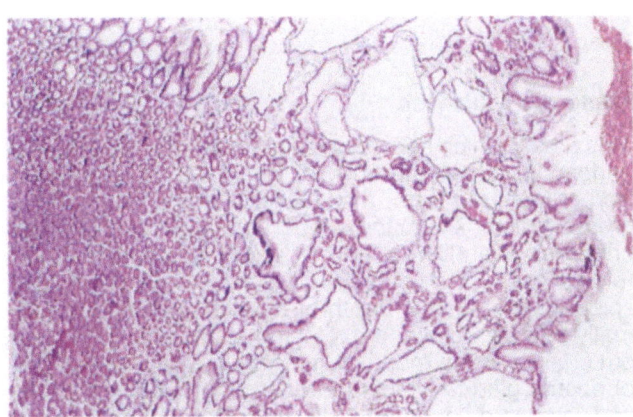

Figure 7.8 Cronkhite–Canada syndrome. There is cystic dilatation of superficial glands with epithelial flattening.   H & E × 80

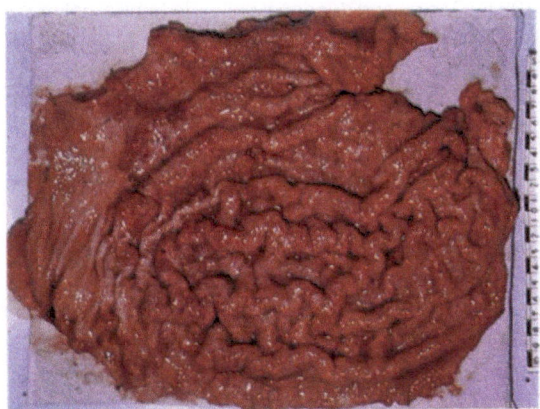

Figure 7.9 Stomach in Ménétrier's disease. The large thickened mucosal folds on the greater curve are clearly visible.

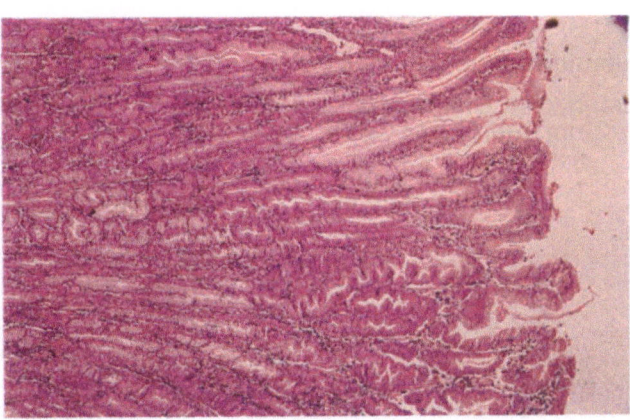

Figure 7.10 Stomach in Ménétrier's disease. Note the increased depth of mucosal pits and elongation of gastric glands.   H & E × 100

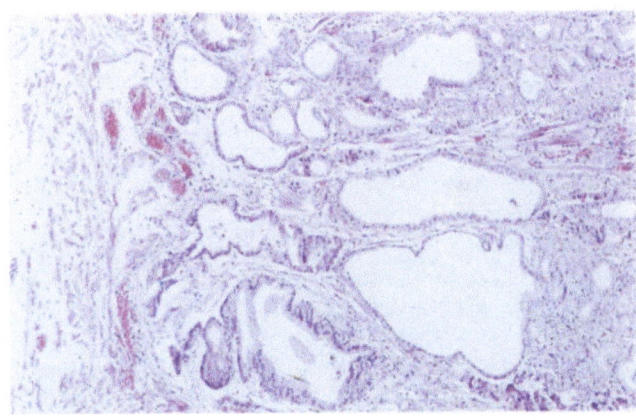

Figure 7.11 Stomach in Ménétrier's disease. Note the cystic dilatation of deep glands.   H & E × 125

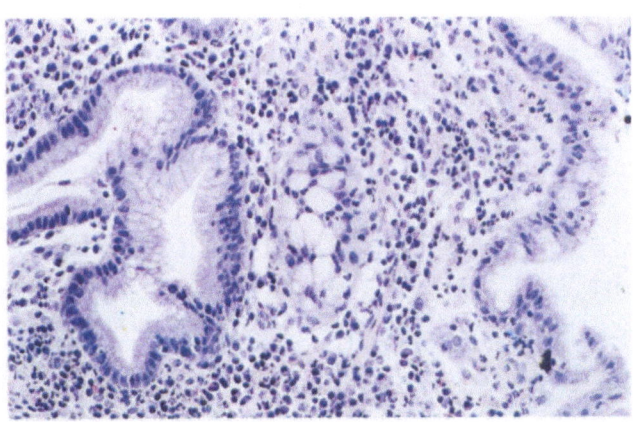

Figure 7.12 Xanthelasma: there are small collections of macrophages containing fat in the superficial lamina propria.   H & E × 250

Ménétrier's Disease

This order, which some consider a hamartoma, appears endoscopically in the body of the stomach in generalized or localized form; the latter is nearly always on the greater curve. The macroscopic appearance, often described as brain-like, is one of large thickened mucosal folds (Figure 7.9). On biopsy the chief features are conspicuous increase in depth of mucosal pits which normally occupy 25% of the total mucosal thickness, without change in the mucosal lining cells, some elongation of gastric glands which contain more mucus-secreting and less acid-secreting cells than normal, and cystic dilatation of the deep glands with some proliferation of the muscularis mucosae onto which they abut (Figures 7.10 and 7.11). The lamina propria shows the inflammatory changes of a mild superficial gastritis. There is risk of malignant change but I have not seen Ménétrier's disease and carcinoma in the same biopsy.

Xanthelasma

Grossly this condition is seen as tiny yellow plaques 1–2 mm in diameter which can be single or multiple.

Microscopically they consist of tiny collections of fat-containing macrophages in the lamina propria (Figure 7.12).

References

1. Bussey, H. J. R. (1970). Gastrointestinal polyposis. *Gut*, **11**, 970

2. Sachatello, C. R., Hahn, I. S. and Carrington, C. B. (1974). Juvenile gastrointestinal polyposis in a female infant. Report of a case and review of the literature of a recently recognised syndrome. *Surgery*, **75**, 107

3. Watanabe, A., Nagashima, H., Motoi, M. and Ogawa, K. (1979). Familial juvenile polyposis of the stomach. *Gastroenterology*, **77**, 148

4. Grigioni, W. F., Alampi, G., Martinelli, G. and Piccaluga, A. (1981). Atypical juvenile polyposis. *Histopathology*, **5**, 361

5. Ranzi, T., Castagnone, D., Velio, P., Bianchi, P. and Polli, E. E. (1981). Gastric and duodenal polyps in familial polyposis coli. *Gut*, **22**, 363

6. Tatsuta, M., Okuda, S., Tamura, H. and Taniguchi, H. (1980). Gastric hamartomatous polyps in the absence of familial polyposis coli. *Cancer*, **45**, 818

Stomach: Epithelial Dysplasia and Neoplasia

The increasing use of endoscopic biopsy has led to a more accurate distinction of dysplasia, intraepithelial and intramucosal carcinoma and invasive carcinoma. It is as well to define at once the terms used and their significance.

(1) *Dysplasia* is used to indicate an epithelial lesion confined by the muscularis mucosae in which proliferating glandular elements are irregular in shape and size and there is associated inflammatory change (further histological details are given below). The lesion is initially inflammatory and when mild or moderate in degree can revert to normal; severe dysplasia can be a precancerous lesion but by definition is not as yet neoplastic.

(2) *Intraepithelial carcinoma (carcinoma* in situ*)* is a lesion which commonly arises on a basis of pre-existing dysplasia but is itself neoplastic, with the potential of breaching the muscularis mucosae though still by definition confined by it. There is no sharp dividing line between the two lesions; the precise diagnosis is a matter of judgment for individual histopathologists.

(3) *Intramucosal carcinoma* is a lesion in which individual cancer cells, singly or in small groups, have invaded through the epithelial basement membrane into the lamina propria; in resected specimens this pattern of growth may be found to have infiltrated also into the submucosa and metastasized to lymph nodes, and may give rise to the well-recognized signet-ring patterns of carcinoma.

It is important to distinguish between precancerous *conditions*, such as pernicious anaemia, in which the *risk* of cancer developing is increased, and precancerous *lesions*, such as severe dysplasia, where the *histological pattern* indicates that malignant change is likely to supervene[1]. All assessments made on biopsy material which does not include muscularis mucosae must be cautious, since it is not possible to determine whether or not invasion has occurred.

Epithelial Dysplasias

These occur in antral or body type mucosa, usually on the basis of a preceding chronic atrophic gastritis with intestinal metaplasia. Gland elements become increasingly irregular in size and shape (Figures 8.1 and 8.2). Individual crypts show irregular branching and the glands themselves expand into the lamina propria producing a 'back-to-back' appearance similar to that seen in endometrial dysplasia and carcinoma (Figure 8.2). Individual cells show an increase in nuclear–cytoplasmic ratio, nuclear pleomorphism, hyperchromatism, stratification and an accompanying decrease in specialized cells. Mild degrees of dysplasia are not readily distinguishable from chronic inflammation and severe dysplasia can merge imperceptibly into true intraepithelial (*in situ*) carcinoma.

Intra-epithelial *(in situ)* Carcinoma

The biopsy diagnosis of this lesion, which commonly develops on a basis of severe dysplasia, is a matter of judgment. There is no absolute separating line from severe dysplasia (Figure 8.3) on one hand, and (unless muscularis mucosae is included and invasion can be assessed) from invasive carcinoma on the other. Since many lesions diagnosed on biopsy as severe dysplasia or intraepithelial carcinoma will come to resection, which allows an accurate assessment of invasion, most pathologists who are prepared to make careful comparisons of biopsy findings with resected material will form their own criteria by experience.

Benign Epithelial Neoplasms

Tubular and tubulovillous adenomas are uncommon but well recognized[2]; pure villous adenomas are, in my experience, extremely rare. They project into the lumen as sessile polypoid growths which rarely become pedunculated. They are commonly surrounded by a zone of atrophic gastritis which often shows intestinal metaplasia, and at the base of the adenoma there are often gland elements showing moderate or severe dysplasia. Histologically the tubular and tubulovillous patterns are reminiscent of large intestinal adenomas (Figures 8.4 and 8.5). When biopsy does not include muscularis mucosae it can be difficult or impossible to distinguish

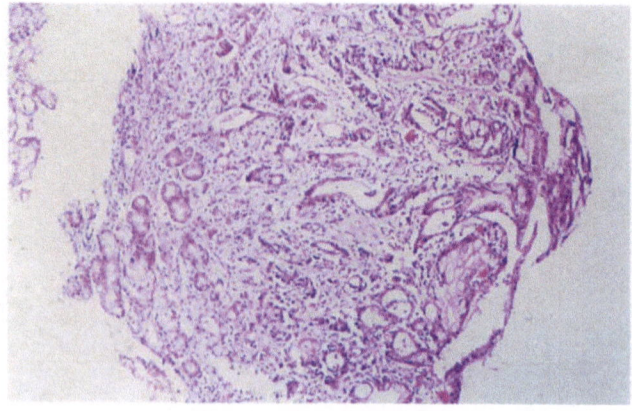

Figure 8.1 Epithelial dysplasia. Gland elements are irregular in size and shape and there is nuclear pleomorphism. The changes are more marked in the superficial mucosa (right) but only fragments of muscularis are included (left) which highlights the difficulty of being certain whether or not invasion has taken place. H & E × 80

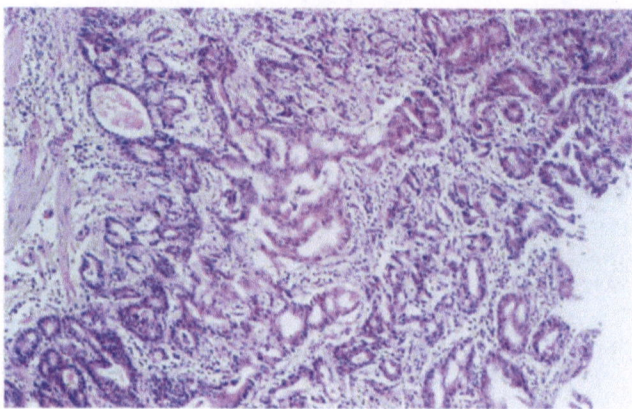

Figure 8.2 More severe epithelial dysplasia with back-to-back appearance in some glands. This is very much a borderline lesion histologically but the muscularis (far left) was not in fact breached. H & E × 125

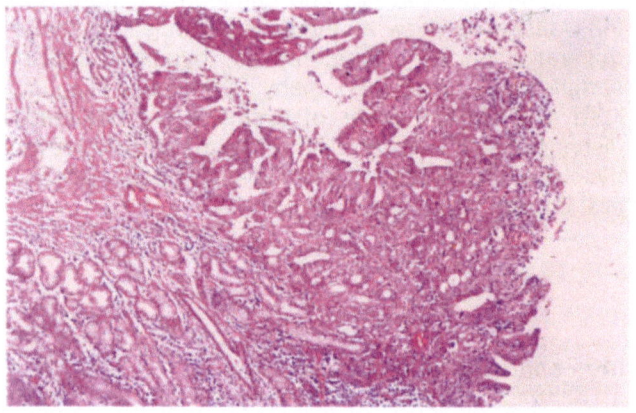

Figure 8.3 Intra-epithelial carcinoma. There was no indication here that the muscularis had been breached, and the diagnosis has to be made on the degree of glandular irregularity, cellular pleomorphism, mitoses, etc. H & E × 100

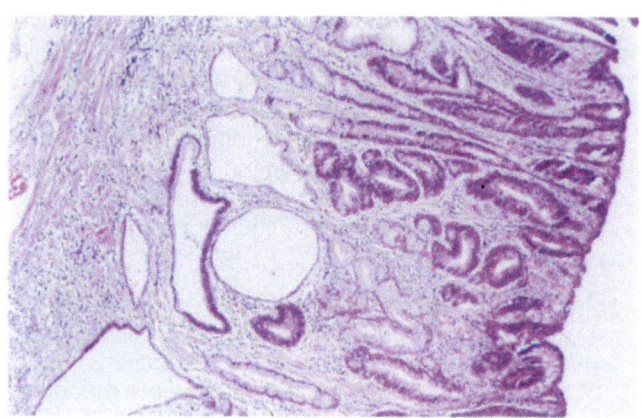

Figure 8.4 Early tubular adenoma. This presented as a slightly raised plaque at endoscopy. The adenoma is arising from the superficial epithelium. H & E × 125

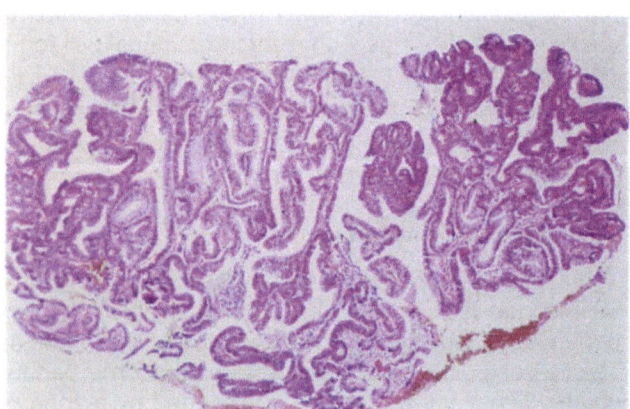

Figure 8.5 Tubulovillous adenoma. The general pattern resembles the more familiar tumour in the large bowel. H & E × 65

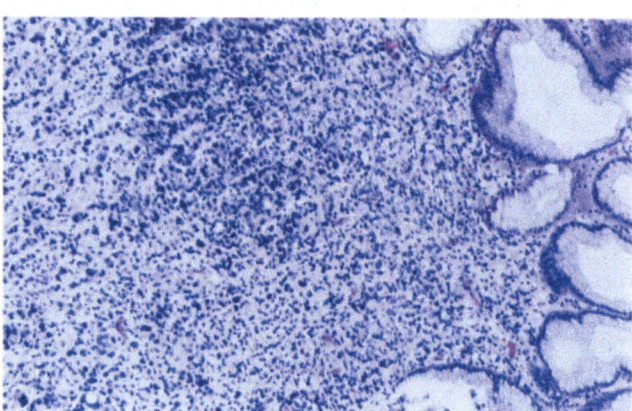

Figure 8.6 Intra-epithelial carcinoma. Individual carcinoma cells have invaded the lamina propria. H & E × 125

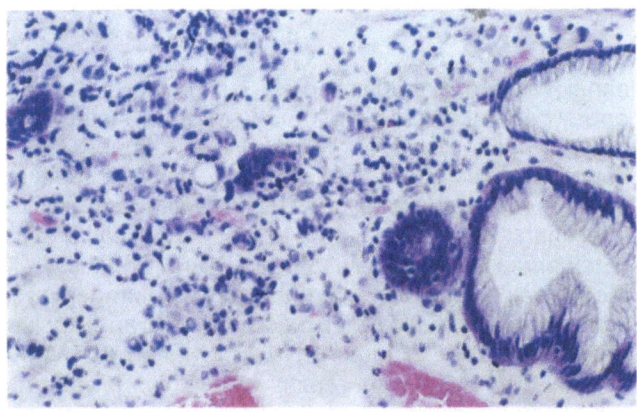

Figure 8.7 Intra-epithelial carcinoma. At first sight the biopsy appears normal, but single mucus-secreting cells of signet-ring type are present scattered throughout the lamina propria. A PAS stain would help here. H & E × 250

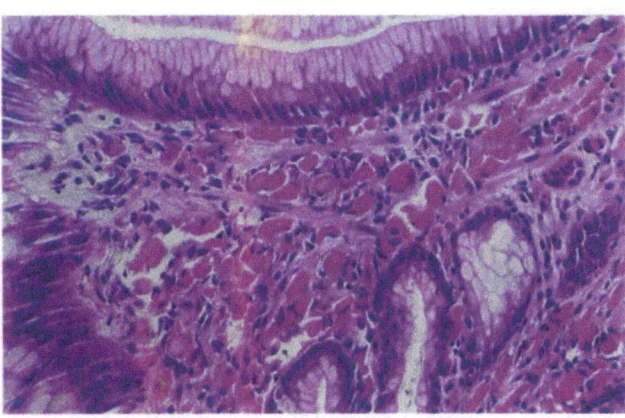

Figure 8.8 Muciphages in antral mucosa. They are larger than carcinoma cells and nuclei are less compressed. H & E × 250

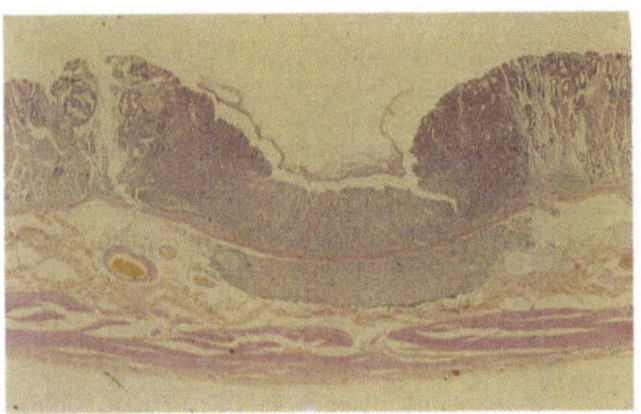

Figure 8.9 Early invasive adenocarcinoma. Glandular irregularity is present in the deeper epithelium on the right and there is early infiltration of the submucosa. H & E × 25

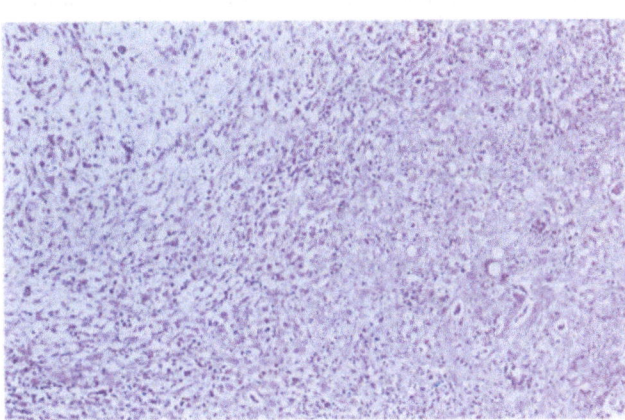

Figure 8.10 Stomach: carcinoma, diffuse type. An anaplastic small-celled pattern with a suggestion of gland formation in places and a number of signet ring cells. H & E × 100

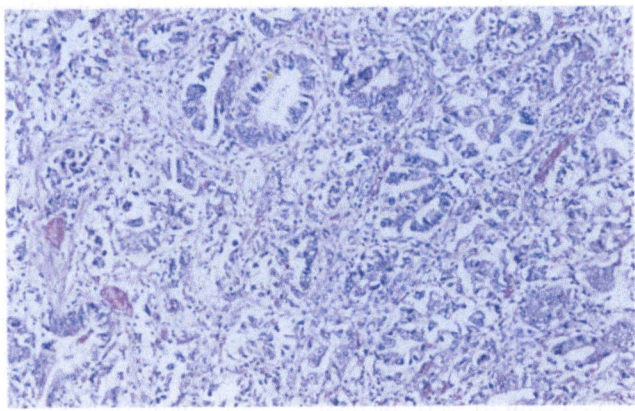

Figure 8.11 Stomach: carcinoma, intestinal type. Gland elements are better formed, though there is no conspicuous pseudovillous formation and the pattern cannot be designated for certain on biopsy alone. H & E × 100

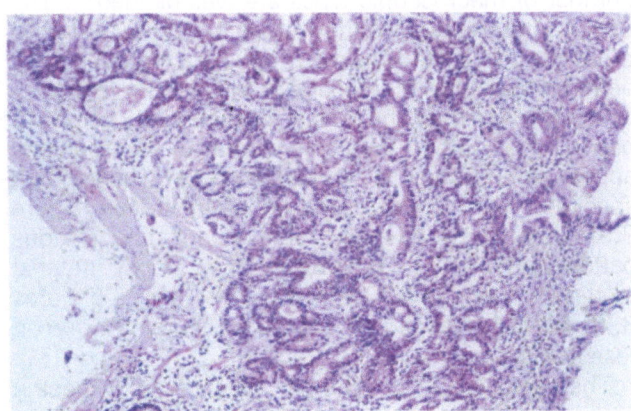

Figure 8.12 Intestinal pattern of adenocarcinoma. There is marked glandular irregularity with some stromal reaction, and though invasion is not visible in this biopsy it was present in the subsequent resected specimen. H & E × 125

invasive malignant change from dysplasia at the base of the lesion.

Intramucosal Carcinoma

Intramucosal carcinomas are defined as carcinomas in which the lamina propria is invaded by carcinoma cells, which either singly or in small groups have breached the glandular basement membrane (Figures 8.6 and 8.7). The submucosa and muscle coats can also be infiltrated and there can be lymph nodal metastases; intramucosal refers to the fact that carcinoma cells are present on biopsy in the lamina propria, not that they are confined to it. There is not necessarily a corresponding degree of glandular irregularity, and glands can appear histologically normal since the site of the carcinoma is not necessarily included in the biopsy. Careful search should be made on all gastric biopsies for intramucosal carcinoma cells. A PAS stain is often helpful in detecting them, but they must not be confused with muciphages which, though rare, can be seen in gastric epithelium (Figure 8.8). Muciphages usually lie immediately beneath surface epithelium while carcinoma cells tend to lie deeper, adjacent to the muscularis mucosae. If preservation techniques permit, muciphages can be shown to contain acid phosphatase histochemically which gastric carcinoma cells do not.

Invasive Adenocarcinomas

As a result of improved gastroscopes and the stimulus of Japanese and other workers[3-5] there is widespread recognition of the possibility of detecting gastric carcinoma in an operable stage with some hope of improving the prognosis. Early carcinoma is usually defined as being confined to mucosa and submucosa and a number of macroscopic types are well defined[3,4]. The biopsy interpretation of these does not present special problems beyond those already outlined, though it must be remembered that, because of their innate tendency to ulcerate and heal, the clinical diagnosis may be one of peptic ulcer rather than carcinoma. A number will appear as intramucosal, though study of the resected specimen will also show submucosal infiltration (Figure 8.9). Others have a recognizable adenocarcinomatous pattern and it may be possible even on biopsy material to classify them as diffuse or intestinal in type (Figures 8.10 and 8.11), though this is more accurately done on resected specimens.

The association of chronic gastritis with gastric carcinoma is well known. Careful studies[6] have shown that in most carcinomas there is associated generalized antral atrophic gastritis with intestinal metaplasia which, immediately adjacent to the carcinoma, often becomes hyperplastic or dysplastic. This finding accords with the classical studies of Lauren[7] who separated carcinomas into diffuse or intestinal on a histological basis. Diffuse carcinomas are made up of groups and clusters of cells either with no glandular lumens or lumens which are poorly defined and showed mucin secretion stainable as neutral mucin with PAS. They have an equal sex incidence, spread widely in tissues, excite a fibrous reaction and are not particularly associated with pre-existing intestinal metaplasia (Figure 8.10). Intestinal pattern carcinomas have a male preponderance and a well-recognizable glandular pattern with columnar cells which show some cellular pleomorphism and nuclear hyperchromasia (Figures 8.11–8.13). They secrete little mucin, which often stains with Alcian blue at pH 2.5. They are more definitely associated with previous atrophic gastritis and intestinal metaplasia and are considered to have a better prognosis than the diffuse type.

Other Patterns of Epithelial Carcinoma

Adenosquamous Carcinomas

These contain adenomatous and squamous cell neoplastic elements and are found rarely in the stomach, usually towards the cardiac end. They may be of mixed gastric and oesophageal origin or may represent a variable degree of squamous metaplasia in a primary adenocarcinoma, when they are sometimes called adenoacanthomas (Figure 8.14). It is rare indeed to find both elements in a single biopsy.

Carcinomatous Change in Peptic Ulcer – Ulcer Cancer

This has already been discussed on page 43. Biopsies of the edge of benign peptic ulcers can show epithelial hyperplasia with glandular irregularity produced by surrounding fibrous tissue. The hyperplastic epithelium does not show true dysplastic change, and a biopsy of the ulcer floor will not show any epithelial elements. True carcinomatous change occasionally occurs and must be judged mainly on changes in individual cells characteristic of carcinoma and by involvement of the ulcer floor (Figures 8.15 and 8.16).

Neuroendocrine Tumours

Neuroendocrine tumours are well recognized in gastric mucosa, and have recently been described in association with pernicious anaemia. They show a variety of patterns ranging from an anaplastic oat cell type, through ribbon patterns to a more characteristic carcinoid pattern with cell nests[8-10], sometimes intermixed with glandular elements (Figures 8.17 and 8.18). Many are non-functional; others secrete a wide variety of hormones and biological amine products. Argentaffin cells showing aldehyde-induced fluorescence are rare, but a number of tumours contain granules which are argyrophil and/or stain with lead haematoxylin (Figure 8.19). Some will react with antigastrin, antiglucagon or anti-insulin sera in a peroxidase technique (Figure 8.20). They can present difficulties in differentiation from carcinoma, and in any biopsy in which there are groups, clumps or trabeculae of suggestive cells it is worth using both argyrophil and lead haematoxylin techniques. Electron microscopy can also help in identifying the presence and more precise nature of granules.

Secondary Carcinoma

Secondary deposits of carcinoma are rare in gastric mucosa but can be most confusing when they do occur. I have seen them from lung and breast (Figure 8.21). They should be suspected when small groups of dysplastic cells, sometimes with mitotic figures, which are not suggestive of primary carcinoma, are found within the lamina propria.

References

1. Morson, B. C., Sobin, L. H., Grundmann, E., Johansen, A., Nagayo, T. and Serck-Hanssen, A. (1980). Precancerous conditions and epithelial dysplasia in the stomach. *J. Clin Pathol.*, **33**, 711

2. Ming, S.-C. (1977). The classification and significance of gastric polyps. In Yardley, J. H., Morson, B. C. and Abell, M. R. (eds.) *The Gastrointestinal Tract; International Academy of Pathology Monograph*, pp. 149–177. (Baltimore: Williams and Wilkins)

3. Murakami, T. (1971). Pathomorphological diagnosis: definition and gross classification of early gastric cancer. In Murakami, T. (ed.) *Early Gastric Cancer* (Gann monograph on cancer research, II). (Tokyo: University of Tokyo Press). (This monograph contains much useful information on early gastric carcinomas)

4. Morson, B. C. and Dawson, I. M. P. (1979). *Gastrointestinal Pathology*. 2nd edn, pp. 155–173. (Oxford: Blackwell)

5. Green, P. H. R., O'Toole, K. M., Weinberg, L. M. and Goldfarb, J. P. (1981). Early gastric cancer. *Gastroenterology*, **81**, 247

6. du Plessis, D. J. (1974). The distribution of gastritis in carcinoma of the stomach. *Br. J. Surg.*, **61**, 521

7. Lauren, P. (1965). The two histological main types of gastric carcinoma: diffuse and so-called intestinal-type carcinoma. *Acta Pathol. Microbiol Scand.*, **64**, 31

8. Jones, R. A. and Dawson, I. M. P. (1977). Morphology and staining patterns of endocrine cell tumours in the gut, pancreas and bronchus and their possible significance. *Histopathology*, **1**, 137

9. Chejfec, G. and Gould, V. E. (1977). Malignant gastric neuroendocrinomas. Ultrastructural and biochemical characterisation of their secretory activity. *Hum. Pathol.*, **8**, 433

10. Sweeney, E. C. and McDonnell, L. (1980). Atypical gastric carcinoids. *Histopathology*, **4**, 215

Figures 8.13–8.21 will be found overleaf.

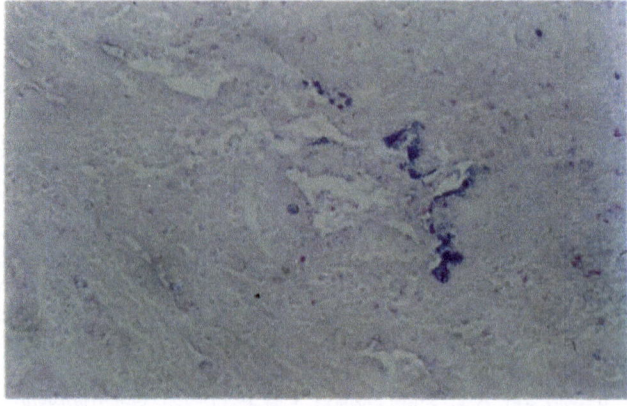

Figure 8.13 Intestinal pattern of adenocarcinoma. Some sialomucin (blue) is present, indicating an intestinal pattern.   Alcian blue (pH 2.5)-PAS technique × 150

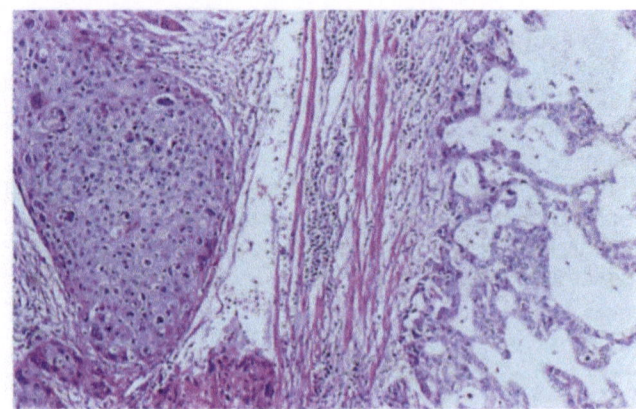

Figure 8.14 Adenosquamous carcinoma. This very uncommon example comes from a tumour at the cardia. There is obvious squamous carcinoma on the left and equally obvious adenocarcinoma on the right.   H & E × 125

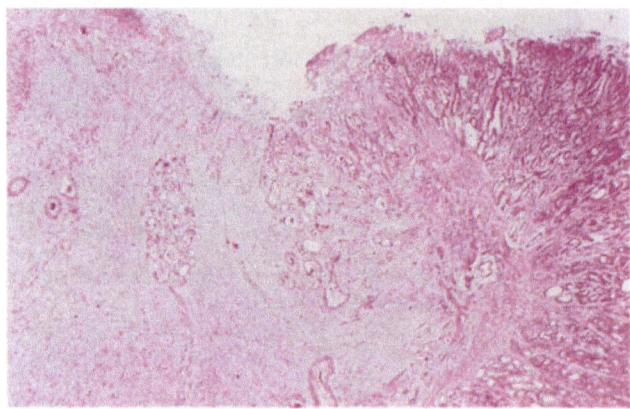

Figure 8.15 Ulcer cancer. There is clearly invasion of the base of a chronic peptic ulcer by cancer originating in the epithelium at the ulcer edge.   H & E × 30

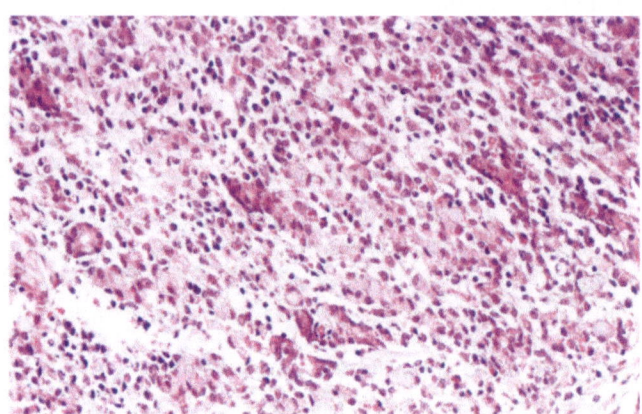

Figure 8.16 Ulcer cancer. A high power view of the edge of a peptic ulcer showing an invasive adenocarcinoma of diffuse pattern. A small normal gland element remains on the left.   H & E × 150

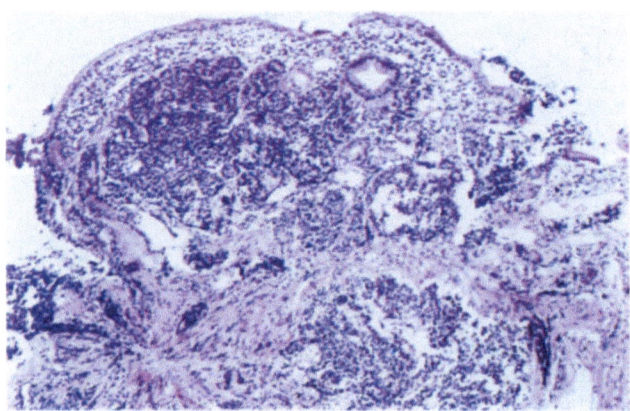

Figure 8.17 Anaplastic oat cell pattern of gastric endocrine cell tumour. H & E × 65

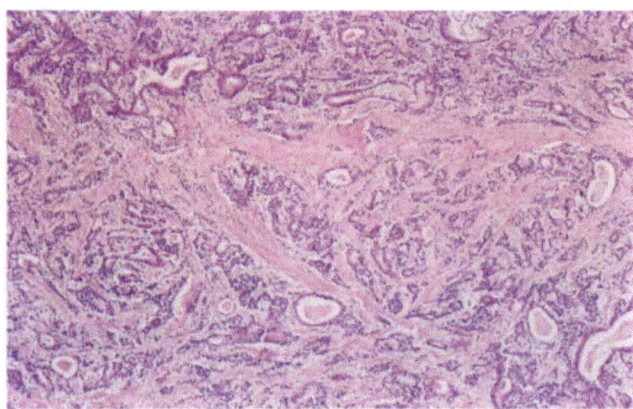

Figure 8.18 Mixed glandular and carcinoid pattern in a gastric endocrine cell tumour. H & E × 65

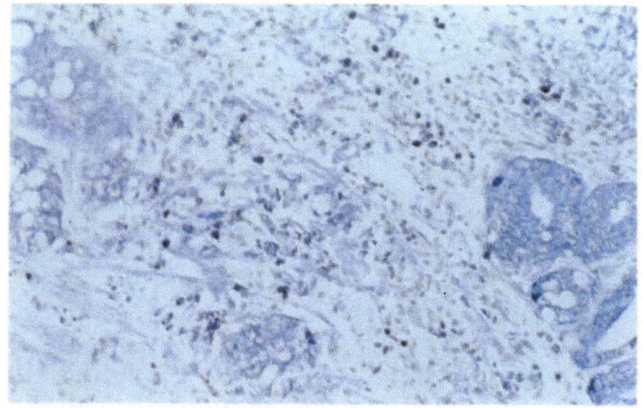

Figure 8.19 Endocrine cell tumour infiltrating the body mucosa. On the right are normal endocrine cells (granules stain dark blue) in a gland; many tumour cells in the centre contain similarly stained granules. Lead haematoxylin × 150

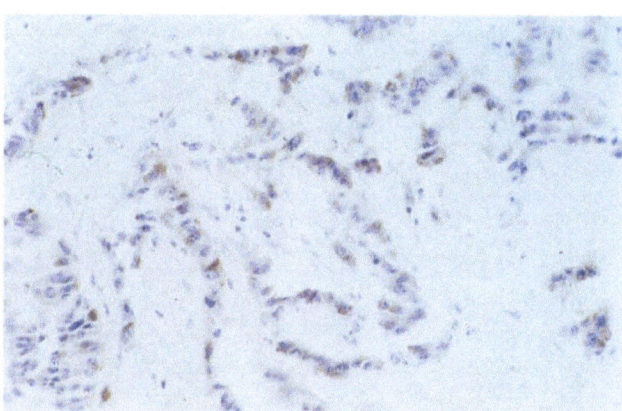

Figure 8.20 Glucagonoma, to show glucagon-containing cells. PAP technique × 150

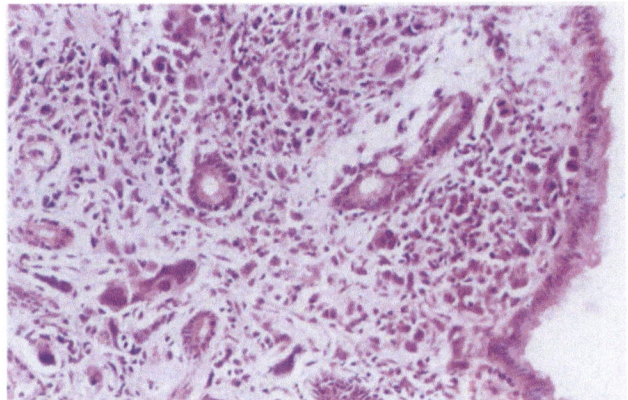

Figure 8.21 Secondary carcinoma of breast; small groups of pleomorphic carcinoma cells lie within the lamina propria. H & E × 125

Hyperplasia and Neoplasia of Lymphoid Tissue

Reactive lymphoid follicles are found in the mucosa and submucosa of the stomach in association with chronic gastritis and with peptic ulcer. Many have a long history, and show a characteristic follicular pattern with germinal centres. They are benign[1,2] (Figure 9.1) and are sometimes referred to as pseudolymphomas. A similar lesion in which the follicles do not show germinal centre formation and more resemble the pattern of follicular lymphoma is also found (Figure 9.2), sometimes but not always in association with hypogammaglobulinaemia[3]. This condition is sometimes referred to as nodular lymphoid hyperplasia (see page 83), and can infiltrate submucosa and muscle coats, though this is probably not a common occurrence (Figure 9.3). It is not possible to say how many lymphomas begin as follicular hyperplasias and rarely in a superficial biopsy which does not include submucosa can an unequivocal diagnosis of lymphoma be made, but some general points may be of value.

Secondary deposits of lymphomas whose primary site of origin is elsewhere are more common than primary gastric lymphomas. Primary lymphomas are variously classified, and one man's histiocytoma[4] can be another man's immunoblastic tumour[5,6]. There is general agreement that Hodgkin's disease rarely if ever occurs as a primary gastric lesion. Some gastric lymphomas present as sheets of uniform small lymphocytic cells infiltrating the lamina propria (Figure 9.4) while others show an infiltration of more pleomorphic cells with some giant cells which are not true Reed-Sternberg cells but have been mistaken for them (Figure 9.5). They are variously categorized as immunoblastic, immunocytic and histiocytic; the arguments for and against such categorization are more fully presented on page 86.

Plasma cell tumours, both solitary plasmacytomas and secondary deposits of myeloma, also occur in gastric mucosa (Figure 9.6) but do not usually present a problem in diagnosis.

Leiomyomatous Tumours

Tumours of muscularis propria or more rarely muscularis mucosae are not uncommon in the stomach[7]. They commonly protrude into the lumen, ulcerate secondarily and bleed (Figure 9.7) and the edge of the ulcer crater is then biopsied. There is little problem in diagnosing typical examples as leiomyomatous (Figure 9.8) but it is impossible on biopsy material to assess their malignancy; the actual size of the lesion is a better guide.

There is a variant of smooth muscle tumour which can give rise to diagnostic difficulty. This is the so-called epithelioid leiomyoma or leiomyoblastoma[8]. It is composed of sheets of polygonal cells without fibrils which sometimes have a vacuolated cytoplasm and resemble epithelial rather than smooth muscle cells (Figure 9.9).

Neurogenic Tumours

Tumours of nerve sheaths and neuroblastic tumours derived from autonomic nerve plexuses occur rarely in the stomach[9]. I have seen a single example in a biopsy from the edge of a peptic ulcer in a woman known to have neurofibromatosis (Figure 9.10).

Inflammatory Fibroid Polyps

These are well described in the stomach[10] and are thought by some[11] to represent degenerate neurogenic tumours, a view which I cannot share. They usually lie in antral submucosa and are made up of loose, often oedematous, fibrous tissue with numerous arterioles, and a diffuse infiltrate of eosinophils (Figure 9.11). There is no blood eosinophilia and the condition is not to be confused with eosinophil gastroenteritis.

Glomus Tumours

Glomus tumours are well recognized in the stomach[12] and can project into the lumen. I have seen biopsies taken from two examples, in both of which the subsequent bleeding necessitated partial gastrectomy (Figure 9.12). The appearances are characteristic and do not usually give rise to diagnostic difficulty provided that the possibility of seeing one is kept in mind.

References

1. Wright, C. J. E. (1973). Pseudolymphoma of the stomach. *Hum. Pathol.*, **4**, 305

2. Stroehlein, J. R., Weiland, L. H., Hoffman, W. N. and Judd, E. S. (1977). Untreated gastric pseudolymphoma. *Am J. Dig. Dis.*, **22**, 465

3. Munro, A. and Simpson, J. G. (1974). Nodular lymphoid hyperplasia of the stomach and small intestine in hypogammaglobulinaemia. *Br J. Surg.*, **61**, 953

4. Isaacson, P., Wright, D. H., Judd, M. A. and Mepham, B. L. (1979). Primary gastrointestinal lymphomas. A classification of 66 cases. *Cancer*, **43**, 1805

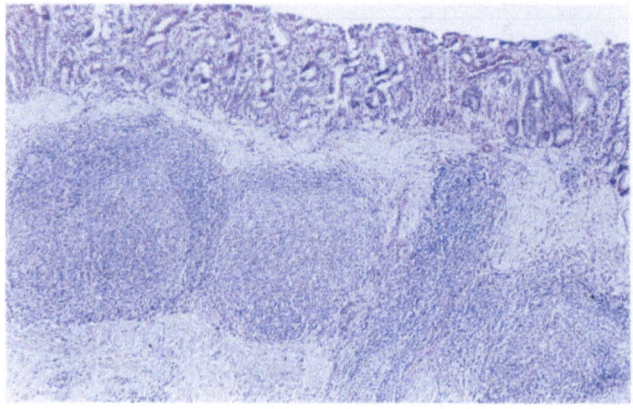

Figure 9.1   Reactive lymphoid follicles. This biopsy came from near the edge of an ulcer. There is chronic gastritis in the overlying mucosa, and large lymphoid follicles with active germinal centres are present in the sub-mucosa.   H & E × 65

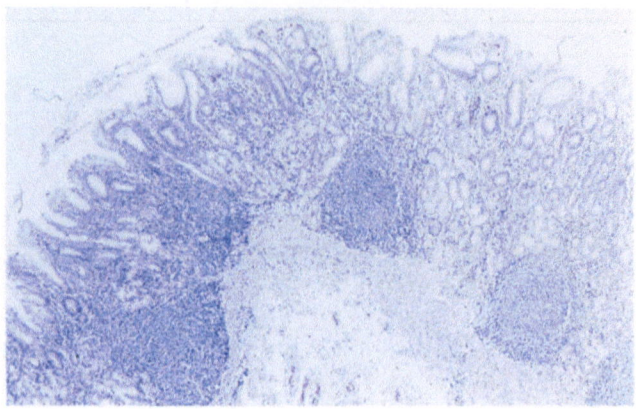

Figure 9.2   Reactive lymphoid follicles. Here most of the follicles are intra-mucosal and some do not have germinal centres.   H & E × 65

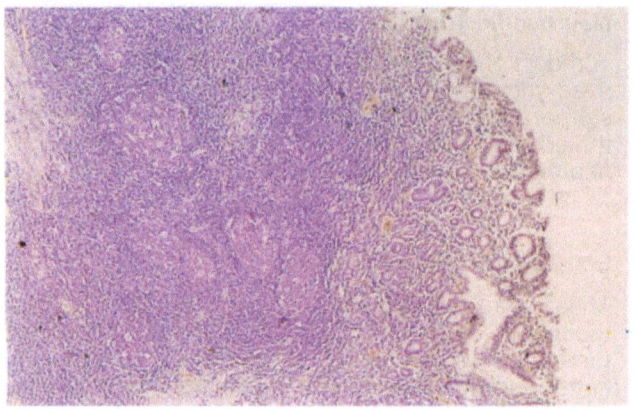

Figure 9.3   Reactive lymphoid follicles of nodular lymphoid hyperplastic pattern. Some of the follicles do, some do not, have germinal centres and there is obvious infiltration into the submucosa.   H & E × 100

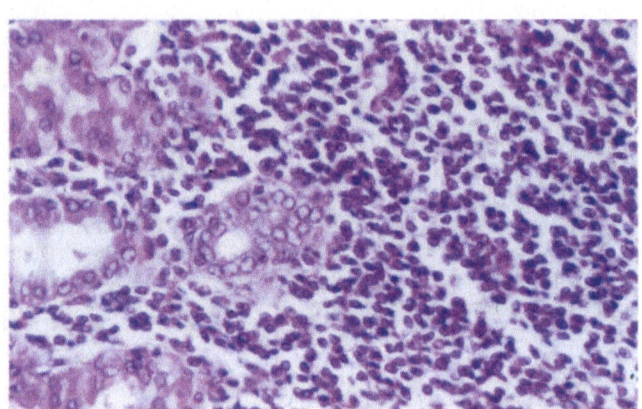

Figure 9.4   Lymphoma of uniform small cell type.   H & E × 125

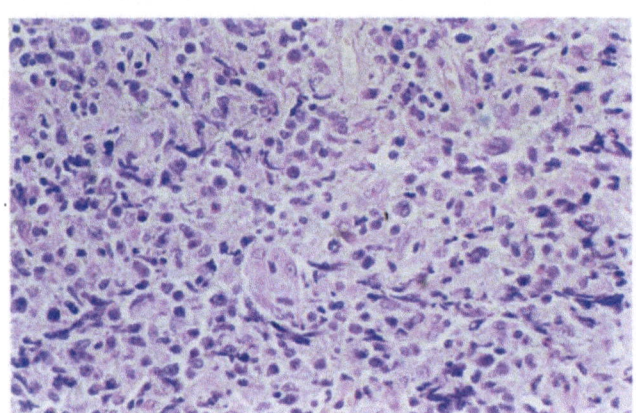

Figure 9.5   Lymphoma with a pleomorphic pattern which includes tumour giant cells, some of which resemble Reed–Sternberg cells.   H & E × 125

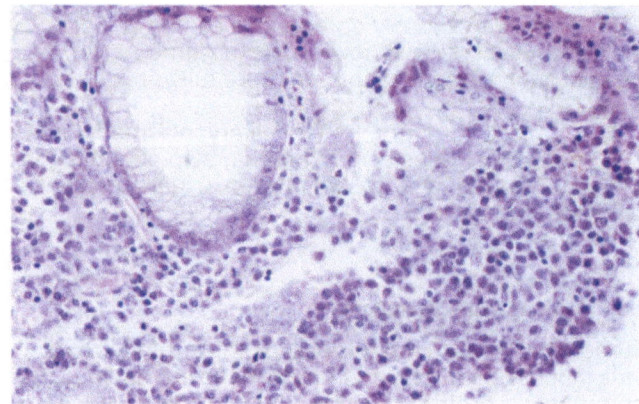

Figure 9.6   Plasmacytoma. The cells here resemble normal plasma cells. H & E × 200

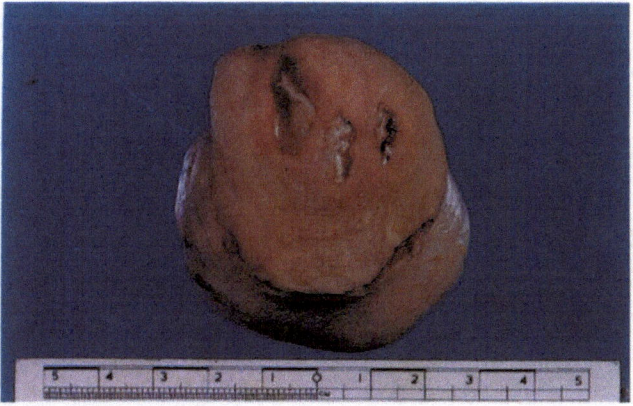

Figure 9.7 Leiomyomatous tumour, resected, mucosal surface towards the viewer. There are three deep ulcers on the mucosal surface, and this patient was admitted with severe haemorrhage

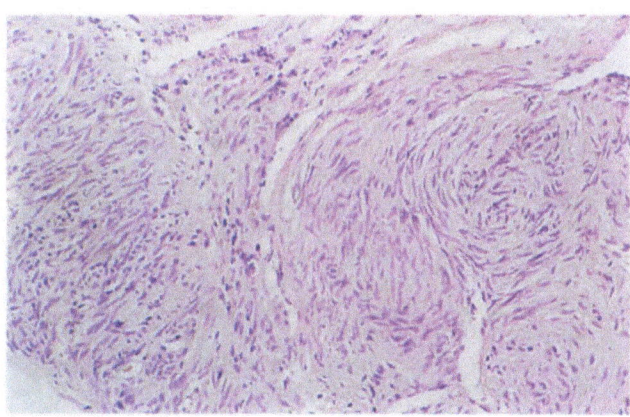

Figure 9.8 Leiomyomatous tumour. The appearance of whorled bundles of smooth muscle fibres is fairly characteristic. H & E × 125

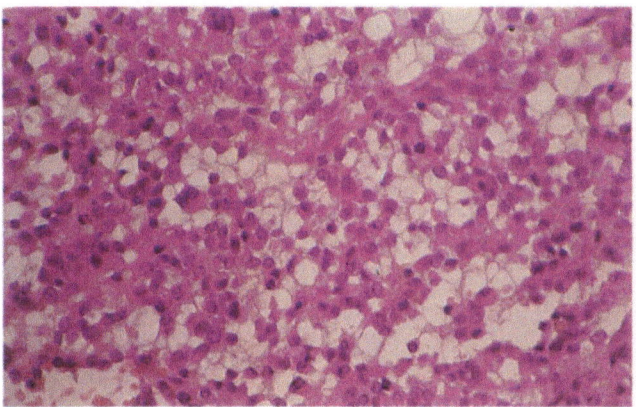

Figure 9.9 Atypical leiomyomatous tumour. This variant has an epithelioid pattern and many cells have a vacuolated cytoplasm suggesting a signet ring type of neoplasm. H & E × 250

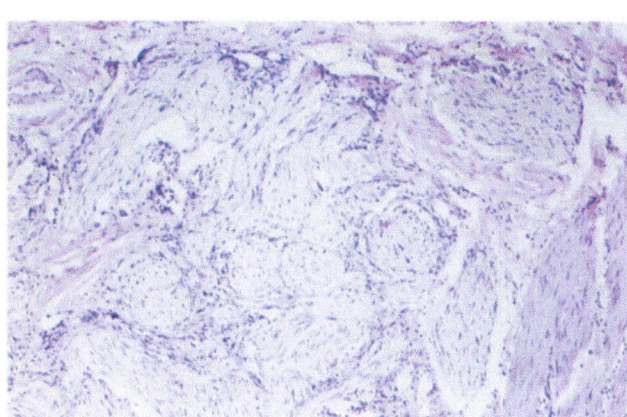

Figure 9.10 Gastric neurofibromatosis. This biopsy shows the characteristic bundles of whorled fibres lying in the submucosa just beneath the muscularis mucosae. H & E × 100

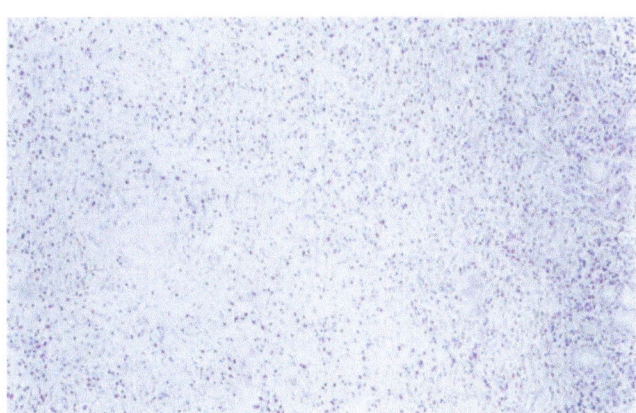

Figure 9.11 Inflammatory fibroid polyp. There is a stroma of oedematous fibrous tissue infiltrated with eosinophils and covered with antral mucosa (far right). H & E × 80

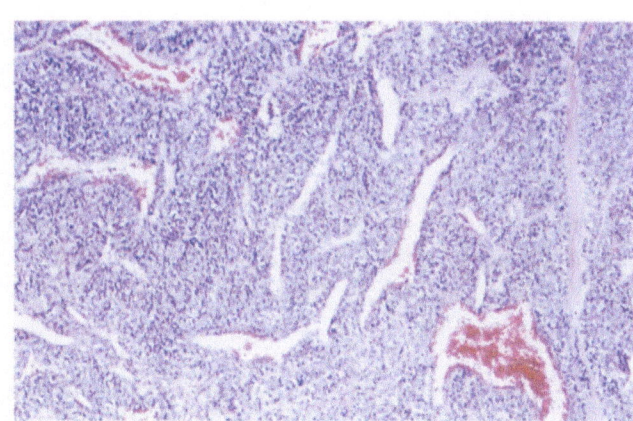

Figure 9.12 Glomus tumour. It shows the characteristic vascular spaces and glomus type cells. H & E × 80

5. Henry, K. and Farrer-Brown, G. (1977). Primary lymphomas of the gastrointestinal tract. 1. Plasma cell tumours. *Histopathology*, **1**, 53

6. Van den Heule, B., van Kerkem, C. and Heimann, R. (1979). Benign and malignant lymphoid lesions of the stomach. A histological reappraisal in the light of the Kiel classification of non-Hodgkin's lymphomas. *Histopathology*, **3**, 309

7. Skandalakis, J. E., Gray, S. W., Shepard, D. and Bourne, G. H. (1962). *Smooth Muscle Tumours of the Alimentary Tract*. (Springfield, USA: Thomas)

8. Appelman, H. D. and Helwig, E. B. (1976). Gastric epithelioid leiomyoma and leiomyosarcoma (leiomyoblastoma). *Cancer*, **38**, 708

9. Rutter, A. P. M. (1965). Neurogenic tumours of the stomach. *Br. J. Surg.*, **52**, 920

10. Johnstone, J. M. and Morson, B. C. (1978). Inflammatory fibroid polyp of the gastrointestinal tract. *Histopathology*, **2**, 349

11. Goldman, R. L. and Friedman, N. B. (1967). Neurogenic nature of so-called inflammatory fibroid polyp of the stomach. *Cancer*, **20**, 134

12. Harig, B. M., Rosen, Y., Dallemand, S. and Farman, J. (1975). Glomus tumour of the stomach. *Am. J. Gastroenterol.*, **63,** 423

10

Small Intestine: Normal Biopsy Appearances

There are two practical ways of sampling small intestinal mucosa. Commonly a Crosby or similar capsule is swallowed, allowed to pass the ligament of Trietz and its level checked radiographically. A single 'blind' biopsy is taken, though some instruments allow multiple biopsies. Because visualization is impossible, only generalized lesions present at this level can be sampled. Increasingly, with the development of fibreoptics and gastroscopy, instruments are being passed through the pylorus, and duodenal biopsies taken under direct vision. It is probable that direct duodenal biopsy will have at least partly replaced blind jejunal biopsy within a few years and a knowledge of normal duodenal morphology is becoming essential to the practising histopathologist.

Specialized investigations can be helpful in selected small intestinal biopsies, and for each clinical diagnosis, clinician and pathologist should have a predetermined agreement as to which, if any, are to be carried out, so that tissues can be processed appropriately. For example, in suspected lactase deficiency it is preferable to hand the biopsy unfixed to the clinical chemist for analysis. Tables 1.1 and 1.2 (pages 11 and 14) indicate those conditions in which special techniques may help and how material should be preserved. It is essential to have an adequate clinical history which must include ethnic origin, age, sex, recent habitat, precise site of biopsy and details of any previous biopsies: all of these can influence the assessment of biopsy appearances.

Single biopsies are usually removed from the capsule immediately by the clinician. Unless minute they should be placed, mucosal surface upwards, on a flat permeable surface such as a square of filter paper or plastic mesh; to orientate them, especially if the biopsy is flat, a hand lens or dissecting microscope is needed. I prefer to use filter paper, which allows penetration of fixative; the natural serous exudate from the under-surface of the biopsy is sufficient for adhesion. Unless the biopsy is to be quenched unfixed, immerse filter paper and biopsy in neutral or buffered 10% formalin precooled if possible to 4 °C and fix for 4–6 h. Fixation can be prolonged overnight if conventional embedding is to follow: if hydrolytic enzyme techniques are to be used, cool immediately to 4 °C and transfer after 4 h to cold gum sucrose for overnight storage. Make any dissecting microscope observations as soon as possible. Small fragments and small multiple duodenal biopsies should be wrapped in porous paper, placed in fixative and sent to the laboratory for orientation.

Special Techniques of Value

Enzymes

In my hands the demonstration of alkaline phosphatase and/or aminopeptidase in cold fixed cryostat-sectioned material has been of value in selected biopsies from children below the normal height and weight percentiles but without other evidence of malabsorption[1]. These enzymes can also be helpful in assessing apparently refractory gluten-induced enteropathy (see below). Attempts to demonstrate early phagolysosomal damage by using acid phosphatase techniques have not proved as helpful as I had first hoped. Techniques for selected disaccharidases are practicable[2] but less easy and probably less reliable than biochemical analysis and reagents can be expensive. I do not use them. Techniques for ganglion cells (see page 15) are rarely needed in small bowel biopsies.

Immunocytochemistry

In those few gluten-induced enteropathies (g.i.e.) associated with immune deficiency (hypogammaglobulinaemic sprue), in giardiasis and in primary immune deficiency disorders it may occasionally be necessary to delineate plasma cells producing IgA or IgM and to demonstrate complement and secretory piece. I have occasionally been asked to locate and count secretin-containing or other endocrine cells in g.i.e. and to look for heavy chains in suspected α-heavy chain disease or macroglobulinaemia. If fluorescent techniques with conjugated antisera are used the biopsy is best quenched unfixed; if peroxidase methods are chosen, preferably fix for a short time in neutral buffered formalin or Zenker's fluid: alternatively use conventionally fixed paraffin-embedded material with or without trypsinization[3]. In general these techniques are not difficult provided that good-quality antisera are available and proper controls are used.

Techniques for Endocrine Cells

For identifying 5-hydroxytryptamine, use diazo or argentaffin silver techniques or aldehyde-induced fluorescence on aldehyde-fixed material; when screening for endocrine cells use lead haematoxylin and an argyrophil technique: I prefer that of Grimelius[4]. More specific identification depends on the use of specific antisera (see above) or transmission electron microscopy.

Scanning and Transmission Electron Microscopy

Scanning electron microscopy is fascinating for research workers but except in specialized units does not as yet play a significant part in diagnostic histopathology: transmission electron microscopy is useful in confirming the presence of viruses and the small bacteria of Whipple's disease, in studying abnormalities in microvilli and in the identification of granules within endocrine cells[5] but is not essential for routine diagnosis.

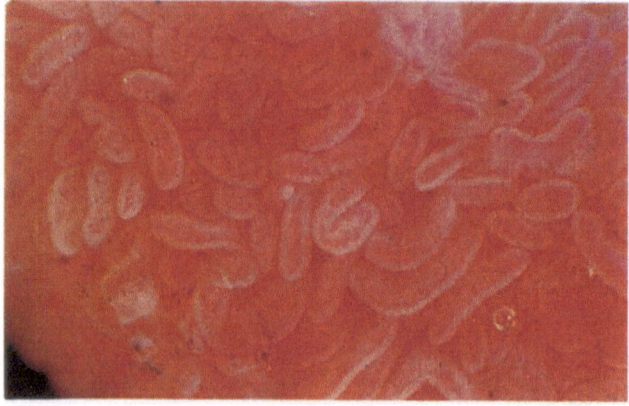

Figure 10.1 Dissecting microscopy, normal Caucasian male. Finger-shaped villi predominate but leaf and spade forms are also present

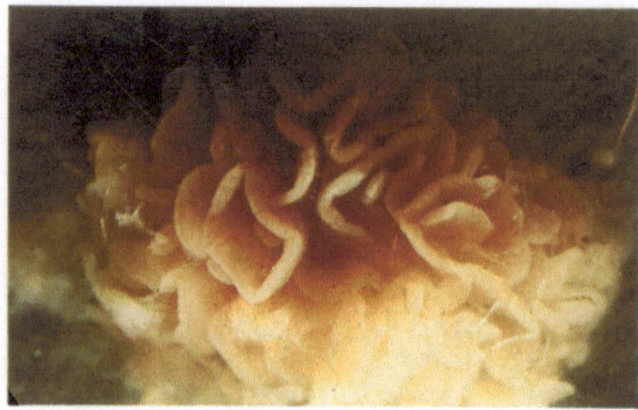

Figure 10.2 Dissecting microscopy; normal Nigerian male. No finger-shaped forms are visible and the biopsy shows only ridges and convolutions but these are not thickened or reduced in height. Compare with Figures 10.3 and 10.4

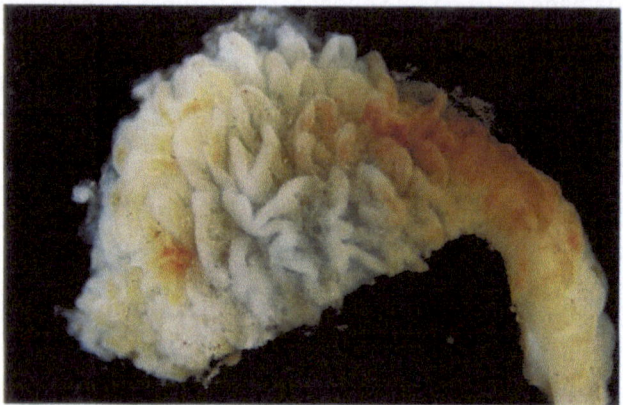

Figure 10.3 Dissecting microscopy in tropical sprue. The biopsy consists of ridges and convolutions which show some thickening and reduction in height. Compare with Figure 10.2

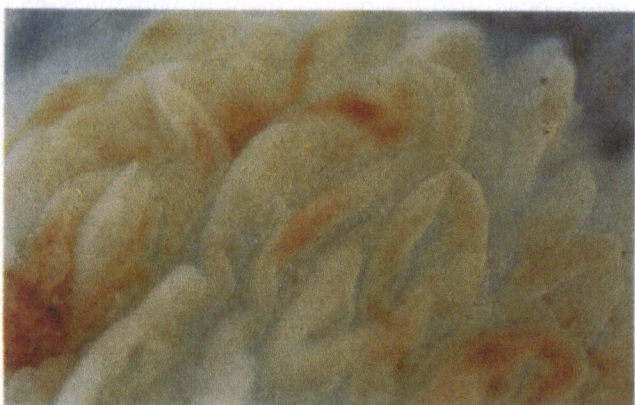

Figure 10.4 Dissecting microscopy in tropical sprue. The convolutions are not greatly thickened but shortening is obvious

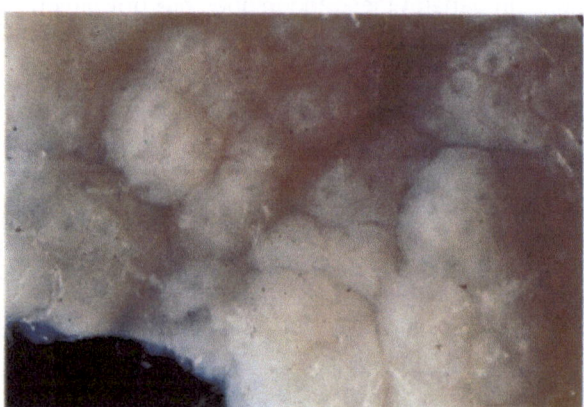

Figure 10.5 Dissecting microscopy in gluten-induced enteropathy (g.i.e.). The mucosa is virtually flat and shows a mosaic appearance

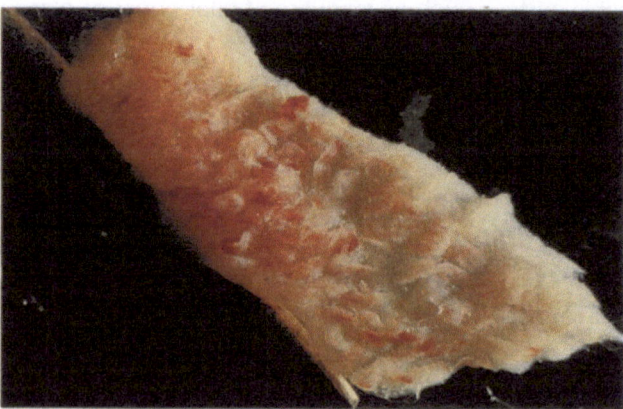

Figure 10.6 Dissecting microscopy in g.i.e. The mucosa is flat and submucosal capillaries are visible through it

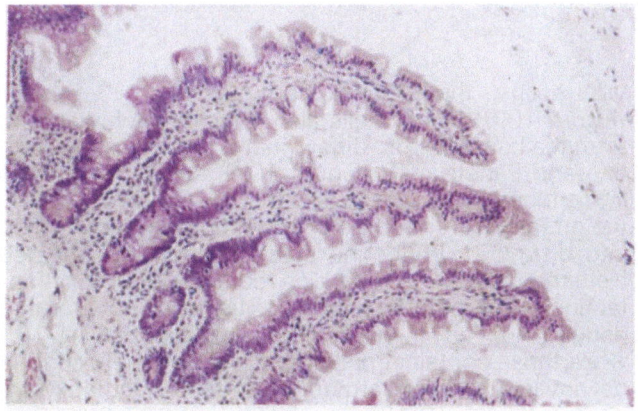

Figure 10.7 Jejunal biopsy, normal Caucasian. It is usually considered that four consecutive normal villi indicate a normal biopsy. H & E × 100

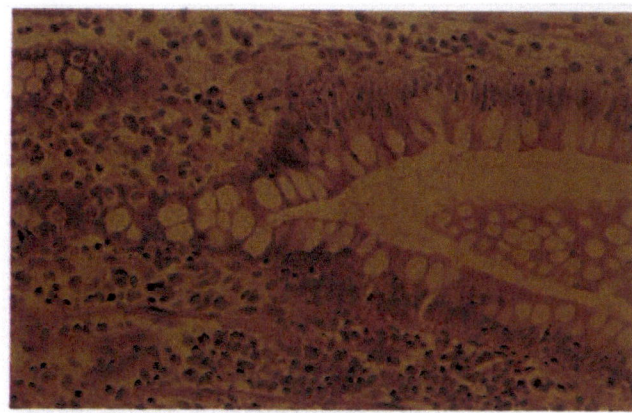

Figure 10.8 Normal crypt zone opening out into the bottom of a crypt. H & E × 250

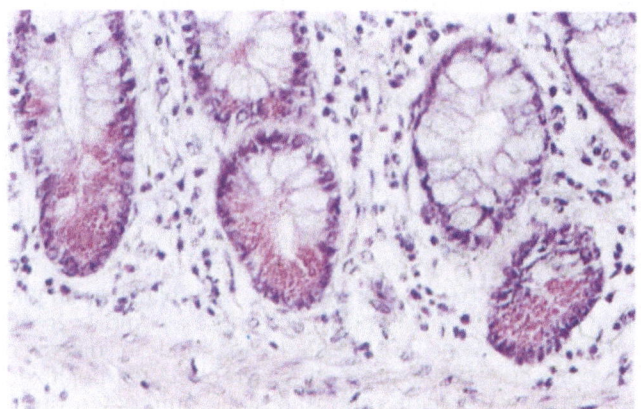

Figure 10.9 Paneth and mucus-secreting cells in basal glands. H & E × 250

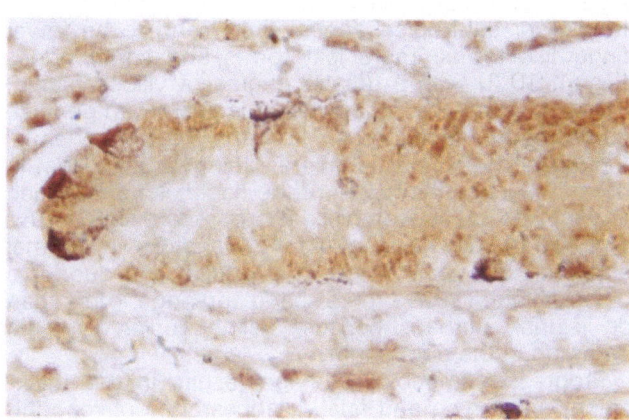

Figure 10.10 Endocrine cell at base of jejunal gland. Grimelius' argyrophil technique × 320

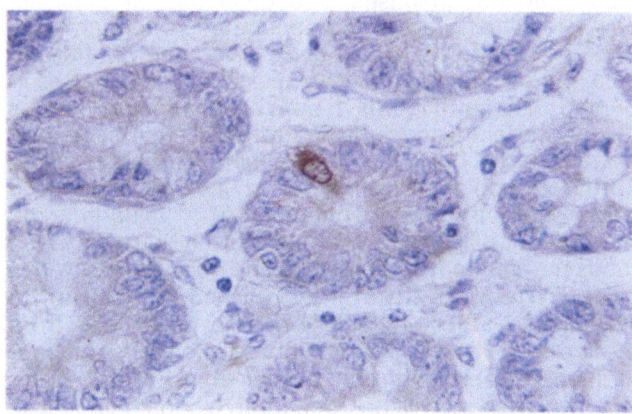

Figure 10.11 Endocrine cell containing glucagon. PAP technique × 250

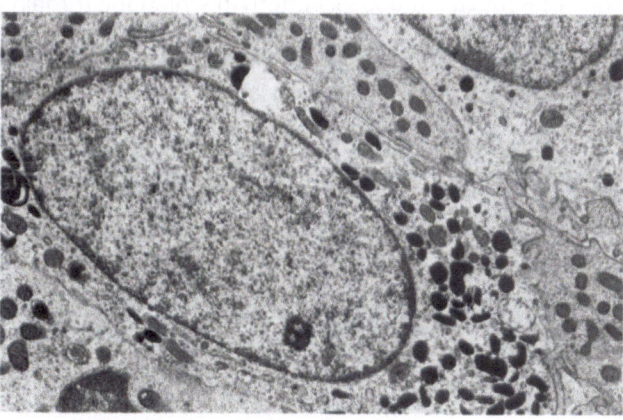

Figure 10.12 Endocrine cell containing 5HT. Note the variability in size of individual granules and the angularity of many. Electron micrograph × 10 000

Morphologic Techniques

Simple counts of numbers of cells, such as intra-epithelial lymphocytes are often of value in g.i.e.: beyond a micrometer eyepiece they do not call for specialized equipment or skills. More complex morphometry, sometimes linked with immunocytochemistry, is only likely to be needed in specialized children's units[6–8].

Dissecting Microscopic Appearances

I am at variance with many workers in believing that the chief value of the dissecting microscope is in orientation rather than in diagnosis: I do not think that morphological description of biopsies is of great value and it must certainly never replace careful histological assessment. Three categories of appearance are recognizable.

In Caucasians domiciled in England, the USA and northern Europe, finger-shaped villi predominate, with a small number of spade or leaf forms (Figure 10.1). In Asiatics and many Blacks, and in others domiciled in tropical or subtropical zones, there tend to be fewer finger-like forms, more leaf forms and some ridges (Figure 10.2) with a greater degree of villous fusion. This picture can be difficult to distinguish from genuine partial flattening (Figures 10.3 and 10.4): a helpful though not fully reliable differentiating factor is that in normal mucosa the height of the ridges is not reduced and they do not appear thickened (compare Figure 10.2 with 10.4). There is a greater variation in normal appearances in children than in adults, and duodenal biopsies tend to have more spade and ridge forms than do jejunal, perhaps because villous fusion is more common in the duodenum.

Progressive mucosal damage results in the thickening, shortening and final disappearance of recognizable villi. Under the dissecting microscope this is seen first as a disappearance of finger-like villi, and an increase in number of spade forms, followed by the appearance of ridges and convolutions, apparently due to non-separation of villi; these are decreased in height (Figures 10.3 and 10.4) in comparison with ridges seen in normal biopsies.

Partial flattening progresses with the gradual disappearance of ridges and convolutions and the appearance of a mosaic mucosal pattern in which the remains of crypt openings can be seen (Figure 10.5) and through which submucosal capillaries are often visible if the biopsy is examined fresh or after short fixation (Figure 10.6).

Normal Histological Appearances in the Jejunum

Partial and complete mucosal flattening present no problem in recognition though their differential aetiology can be difficult to determine; minor variations from normal can be important and difficult to diagnose and a knowledge of the range of normal appearances is essential.

The normal jejunal mucosa consists essentially of a crypt regeneration zone which gives rise to an underlying basal layer, in which are the basal glands, and to surface villi which project into the lumen and increase the absorptive area (Figure 10.7). The regenerative zone is an active mitotic zone producing new cells which migrate up the sides of the villi, mature into enterocytes and goblet cells, and are shed from the villous tips, the process normally taking 3–5 days (Figure 10.8). Crypt cells also migrate downwards to form the basal glands, differentiating into mucus-secreting and Paneth cells (Figure 10.9) and probably also into endocrine cells; the belief that the endocrine cells in the gut are all of neuroectodermal origin[9] is now falling into disfavour. Endocrine cells can be demonstrated histochemically; those which contain 5-hydroxytryptamine are argentaffin, diazo-positive and show formaldehyde-induced fluorescence (Figures 1.14–1.16), while those containing polypeptides are usually though not invariably either argyrophil or lead haematoxylin-positive (Figure 10.10) though their more precise definition in terms of what they secrete must be determined by immunocytochemistry (Figure 10.11) or electron microscopy (Figure 10.12). It is possible with practice to assess the overall mitotic activity of crypt zones, and to make actual counts of mitotic cells when necessary[10].

The connective tissue element of the small intestine, the lamina propria, forms a narrow continuous zone between the basal glands and extends upwards to form the cores of the villi; it contains blood vessels, lymphatics and a sprinkling of lymphocytes, plasma cells, macrophages and eosinophils (Figure 10.13). Plasma cells can be classified using immunocytochemical techniques into those which secrete IgA, IgG and IgM (Figure 10.14). The ratios of these cells in normal epithelium vary from author to author[11] but figures of IgA : IgM : IgG of 32 : 6 : 1, are generally acceptable. Lymphocytes are continually emigrating and immigrating between intact enterocytes along the sides of the villi (Figure 10.15), presumably sampling antigenic material in the gut lumen[12]; the normal ratio is 8–40 lymphocytes per 100 enterocytes and in diseased mucosa is better expressed as lymphocytes per fixed length of muscularis mucosae since enterocyte numbers themselves are reduced in a flattened mucosae (see page 17)[13].

The villi themselves consist of a lamina proprial zone covered by a single layer of enterocytes and goblet cells (Figure 10.8) in a ratio of 8–12 : 1. The enterocytes have vesicular basal nuclei and a slightly opaque cytoplasm; from the luminal aspect of each cell protrude microvilli (Figure 10.16) forming a brush border in which are localized a number of enzyme systems including aminopeptidases, disaccharidases and lipases, some of which can be demonstrated histochemically (Figures 10.17–10.19). Goblet cells contain neutral and acid non-sulphated epithelial mucins, but little if any sulphated material (Figures 1.5–1.7). In addition there is on the surface, and indistinguishable microscopically from the brush border, a mucus coat – probably derived both from goblet cell mucin and mucus glycocalyx.

Morphometry and quantitation are of value in some mucosal biopsies, and examples of cell numbers and ratios have already been given. The normal villus varies from 320 μm to 570 μm in height and from 85 μm to 140 μm in width; the basal zone thickness varies from 120 μm to 270 μm, giving height : width ratios of about 4 : 1 and villous height : basal layer thickness of about 2.5 : 1. In general villi become more elongated and less straight, and also lose their surface indentation as one descends the small bowel aborally; fusion of villi, on the contrary, is more common in the upper part, especially the duodenum.

Aggregations of lymphoid tissue are common in the submucosa but also occur in the lamina propria (Figure 10.20) and may occasionally appear to produce flattening; they can or need not show germinal centres.

Normal Histological Appearances in the Duodenum

Some differences are present in the mucosa of the first part of the duodenum. Villi are shorter than in the jejunum, and more often show branching and fusion, while biopsies from the first part usually have a deep layer of Brunner's glands (Figure 10.21). Individual villi however have a similar structure to those in the jejunum (Figure 10.22).

It is not uncommon to find in duodenal biopsies from symptom-free patients a sprinkling of inflammatory cells in the lamina propria, including some polymorphs. Endoscopic and biopsy studies have been made on patients with normal duodenal appearances, with reddening of the first part of the duodenum suggesting duodenitis and with visible duodenal ulceration and attempts made to correlate clinical with histopathological and morphometric findings[14] for various reasons discussed more fully on page 79, these have not been entirely successful, and the interpretation of histopathological evidence of mild inflammation and increased lamina proprial cellularity must be cautious.

Second, it is also not uncommon to find islets of gastric-type mucosa in the first part of the duodenum. Some of these are metaplastic and secondary to chronic inflammation but some appear to be heterotopic[15]. The latter are probably of no significance but can be misinterpreted as evidence of duodenitis.

Normal Histological Appearances in the Ileum

Ileal villi are rarely biopsied. Villi tend to be longer and less straight and do not show the saw-toothed appearance seen in jejunal villi (compare Figures 10.7 with 10.23).

References

1. Dawson, I. M. P. (1981). The value of histochemistry in the diagnosis and prognosis of gastrointestinal diseases. In Stoward, P. J. and Polak, J. M. (eds.) *Histochemistry: the Widening Horizons*, pp. 127–162. (Chichester: John Wiley & Sons)

Figures 10.13–10.23 will be found overleaf.

2. Lojda, Z. (1974). Cytochemistry of enterocytes and of other cells in the mucous membrane of the small intestine. In Smyth, D. H. (ed.) *Biomembranes 4A. Intestinal Absorption*. (London: Plenum Press)

3. Robinson, G. (1982). Immunohistochemistry. In Bancroft, J. D. and Stevens, A. (eds.). *Theory and Practice of Histological Techniques*, 2nd Edn. pp. 406–427. (Edinburgh: Churchill Livingstone)

4. Grimelius, L. (1968). A silver nitrate stain for $\alpha 2$ cells in human pancreatic islets. *Acta Soc. Med. Uppsala*, **73**, 243

5. Toner, P. G., Carr, K. E. and Wyburn, G. M. (1971). *The Digestive System – An Ultrastructural Atlas and Review*. pp. 55–204. (London: Butterworth)

6. Ferguson, A., Sutherland, A., MacDonald, T. T. and Allan, F. (1977). Techniques for microdissection and measurement in biopsies of human small intestine. *J. Clin Pathol.*, **30**, 1068

7. Slavin, G., Sowter, C., Robertson, K., McDermott, S. and Paton, K. (1980). Measurement in jejunal biopsies by computer-aided microscopy. *J. Clin. Pathol.*, **33**, 254

8. Rosenkrans, P. N. C., Meijer, C. J. L. M., Polanco, M., Mearin, M. L., van der Wal, A. M. and Lindeman, J. (1981). Long term morphological and immunohistochemical observations on biopsy specimens of small intestine from children with gluten sensitive enteropathy. *J. Clin. Pathol.*, **34**, 138

9. Pearse, A. G. E. and Polak, J. M. (1971). Neural crest origin of the endocrine polypeptide (APUD) cells of the gastrointestinal tract and pancreas. *Gut*, **12**, 783

10. Wright, N. A., Appleton, D. R., Marks, J. and Watson, A. J. (1979). Cytokinetic studies of crypts in convoluted human small intestinal mucosa. *J. Clin Pathol.*, **32**, 432

11. Brandtzaeg, P. and Baklein, K. (1976). Immunohistochemical studies of the formation and epithelial transport of immunoglobulins in normal and diseased human intestinal mucosa. *Scand. J. Gastroenterol.*, **11**, Suppl. 36

12. March, M. N. (1980). Studies of intestinal lymphoid tissue III. Quantitative analysis of epithelial lymphocytes in the small intestine of human control subjects and of patients with coeliac sprue. *Gastroenterology*, **79**, 481

13. Guix, M., Skinner, J. M. and Whitehead, R. (1979). Measuring intraepithelial lymphocytes, surface area and volume of lamina propria in the jejunal mucosa of coeliac patients. *Gut*, **20**, 275

14. Hasan, M., Sircus, W. and Ferguson, A. (1981). Duodenal mucosal architecture in non-specific and ulcer-associated duodenitis. *Gut*, **22**, 637

15. Lessels, A. M. and Martin, D. F. (1982). Heterotopic gastric mucosa in the duodenum. *J. Clin. Pathol.*, **35**, 591

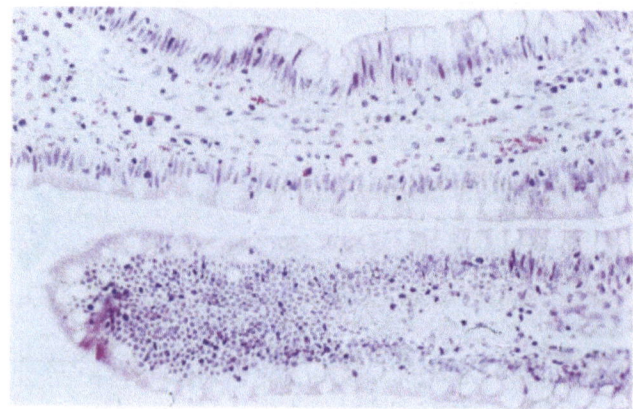

Figure 10.13 Normal ileal villus. There are lymphocytes, plasma cells and occasional eosinophils in the lamina propria.   H & E × 200

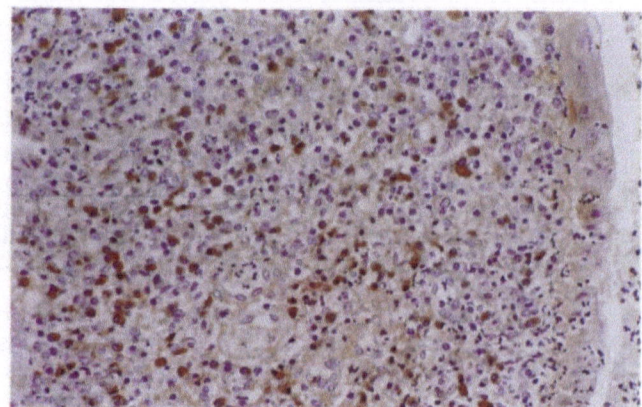

Figure 10.14 Normal lamina propria. Plasma cells containing IgA.   PAP technique × 125

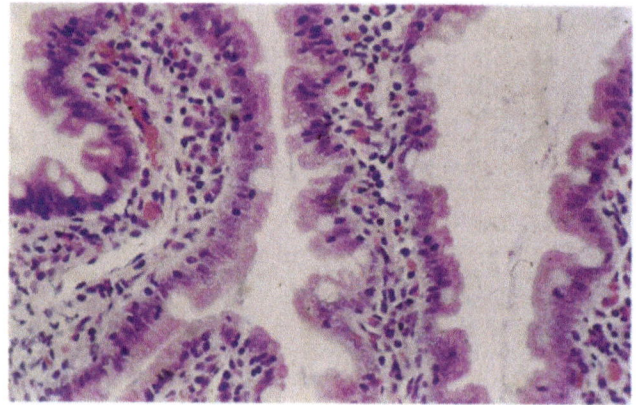

Figure 10.15 Normal villi. The small deeply stained nuclei of migrating lymphocytes are clearly visible.   H & E × 200

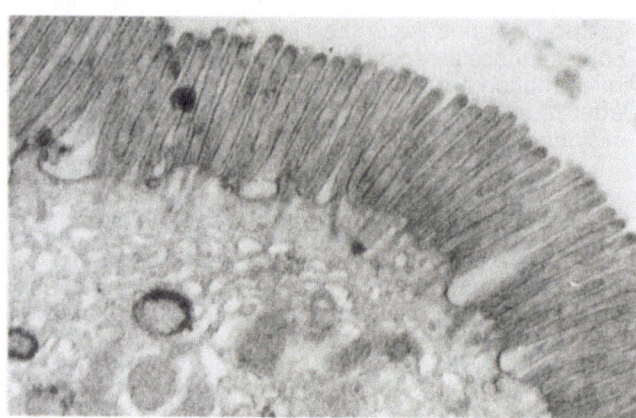

Figure 10.16 Normal surface enterocyte showing normal microvilli. Electron micrograph × 5000

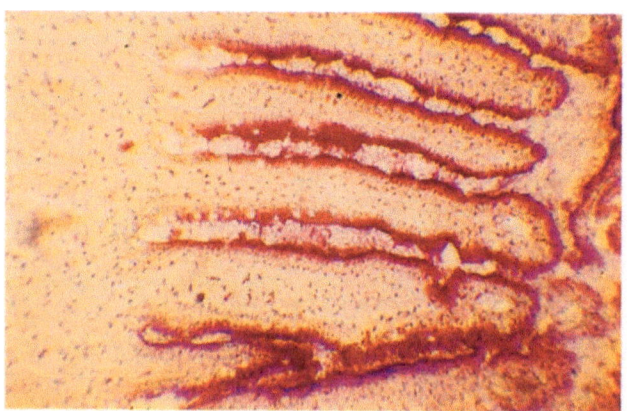

Figure 10.17 Brush border location of aminopeptidase. The technique for this enzyme produces a more 'smudgy' effect than that for alkaline phosphatase, so that I usually use the latter.   × 150

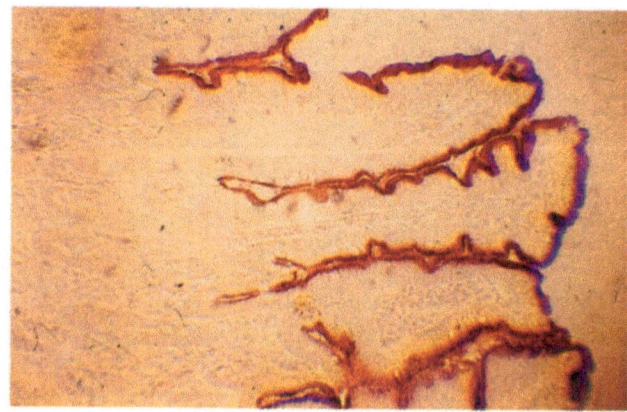

Figure 10.18 Brush border location of alkaline phosphatase. The localisation is much clearer than that in Figure 10.17. It extends upwards from the crypt zone but is not found in the basal layer. Localization can be made even clearer by the use of phase contrast microscopy (see Figure 10.19)   × 150

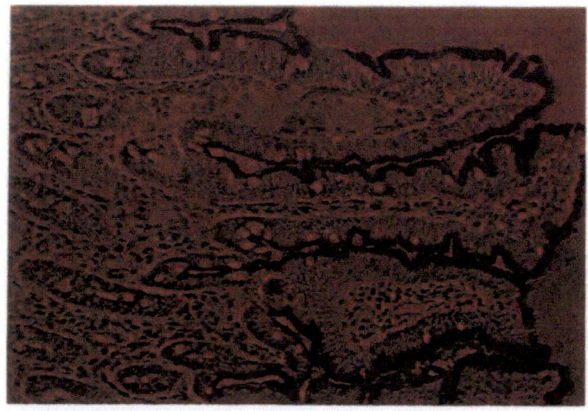

Figure 10.19 Section shown in Figure 10.18 viewed in phase contrast. The location of enzyme relative to gland elements is now clearly visible   × 150

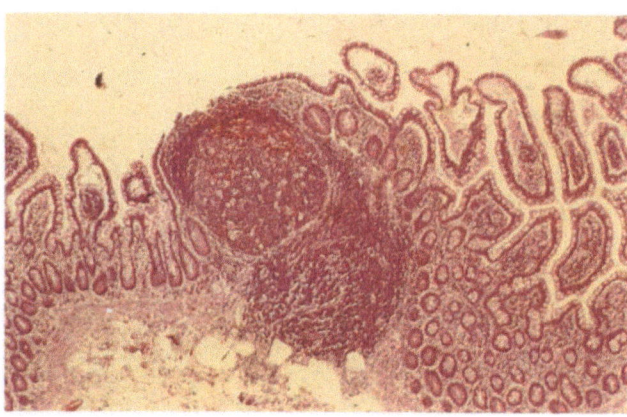

Figure 10.20 Normal jejunum. Lymphoid aggregates in lamina propria. H & E × 100

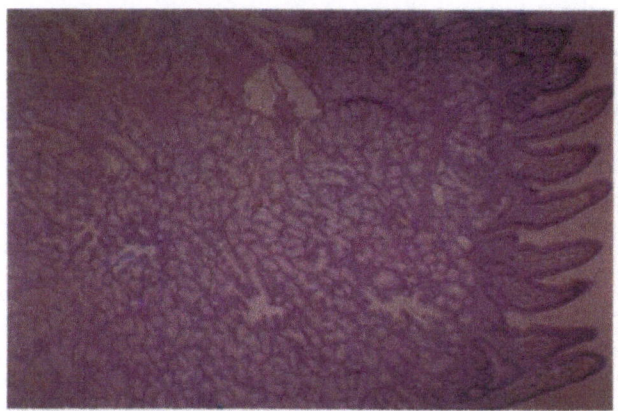

Figure 10.21 Normal duodenum. The villi are shorter than those in the jejunum and Brunner-type glands lie immediately beneath the mucosa interrupting the muscularis mucosae. Branched and fused villi, as seen here, are a normal finding.   H & E × 80

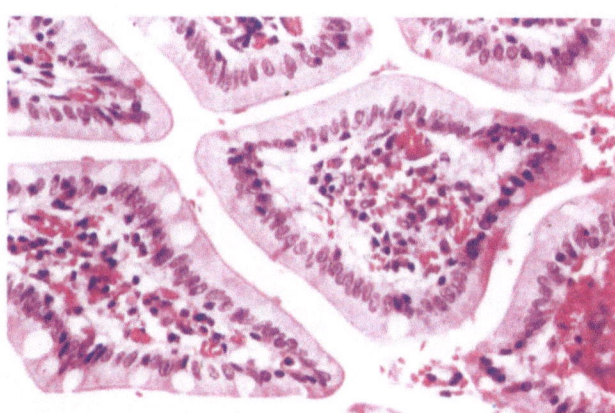

Figure 10.22 Cross-sectional view of a duodenal villus. The enterocytes and lamina propria are similar to those in the jejunum. Migrating lymphocytes are clearly visible.   H & E × 125

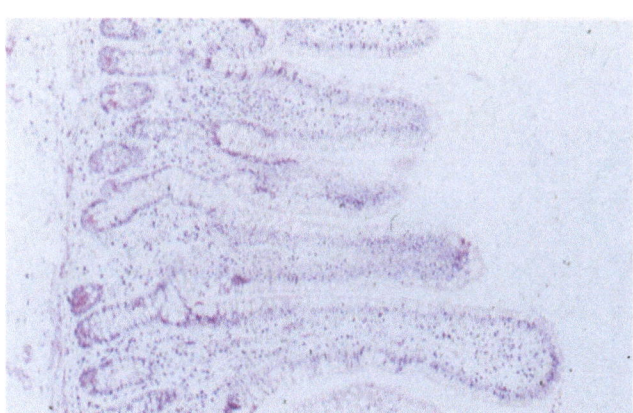

Figure 10.23 Normal ileum. The top villus is longer than a jejunal villus and there are no 'saw tooth' constrictions.   H & E × 125

11

Small Intestine: Patterns of Non-infective Mucosal Damage

All patterns of mucosal damage, whether infective or not, tend to produce flattening with decrease of absorptive surface. This leads to defective absorption which can present in a number of ways, particularly as weight loss, diarrhoea and foul-smelling stools which often have an increased content of unabsorbed fat. Just as 'all that waddles is not dystrophy' so 'all that flattens is not sprue'[1]. Capsule biopsies sample blindly and cannot be directed at focal lesions, and since in generalized conditions there is commonly variability in severity of damage, the degree of flattening present in a single biopsy may not be representative. Among the more common disorders which can cause generalized flattening, are gluten-induced enteropathy (g.i.e.), idiopathic steatorrhoea, tropical sprue, acute and chronic infective enteritis, bacterial overgrowth in stagnant loop syndromes, abnormal sensitivity to soy and cows' milk protein, immunodeficiency syndromes with or without giardiasis or neoplasia, malnutrition including kwashiorkor, irradiation and the use of certain drugs; the list is not exhaustive.

In all these conditions there are several possible ways of producing mucosal flattening. The most common is by increasing the rate of destruction and shedding of surface enterocytes, probably more often by a direct damaging effect on them, caused for example by toxic breakdown products of gluten or by bacterial or viral action, than by immunological mechanisms. This stimulates hyperactivity in the crypt zone in an attempt to replace damaged cells as they are shed. Should the hyperactivity fail to keep pace with the loss, villi become shorter and broader, the covering enterocytes are more irregularly arranged and crowded together and the mucosa becomes ridged, convoluted and eventually flat; I prefer the term 'flat' to 'atrophic' since the crypt activity is hyperplastic. At the same time, and because of the increased crypt activity, more cells migrate downward as well as upward. Since basal glands are not damaged to the same extent by external agents operating in the gut lumen there is less destruction of cells and the basal layer thickens. All degrees of flattening and basal thickening can be seen depending on the degree of involvement in the particular area sampled.

A less common causative factor is failure of the crypt zone to replicate sufficiently to compensate for normal enterocyte shedding. This can be seen in some forms of severe adult malnutrition, in which the villous flattening is not accompanied by crypt zone activity or basal thickening. In kwashiorkor there appears to be direct mucosal damage stimulating crypt zone response, combined with some crypt zone failure (see below).

In some disorders, such as α-heavy chain disease and Whipple's disease, the disorder is not primarily epithelial; plasma cells, lymphocytes or macrophages pack the lamina propria producing broadening and flattening of villi without primarily damaging surface enterocytes or crypt zones.

It will be clear that a number of conditions can produce similar end patterns of mucosal damage. Biopsy interpretation can be further complicated because greater or less degrees of severity in a single biopsy do not necessarily reflect the overall picture even in a localized zone of small intestine, while different diseases preferentially affect different regions of the bowel. There are, however, particular histological changes and patterns to look for and certain special investigations which may help in the differential diagnosis; these are described below.

Because in Britain gluten-induced enteropathy is the most common cause of non-infective mucosal flattening, I have described it first and compared or contrasted the changes in other disorders with what is seen in it.

Mucosal Flattening resulting from Increased Enterocyte Destruction with Compensatory Crypt Zone Hyperplasia

Gluten-induced Enteropathy (g.i.e.)

A certain fraction of any population appears to be sensitive to certain of the breakdown products of gluten. The actual damage to surface enterocytes, which results in more rapid destruction and shedding than normal and to varying degrees of mucosal flattening, is probably a direct toxic one[2] but there appears to be a genetic predisposition associated with two non-linked gene loci for HLA-B and HLA-DW3 antigens[3]. The condition can be found initially in children, adolescents or young adults, who commonly show evidence of malabsorption, anaemia which can be micro- or macrocytic or dimorphic with associated folate but not B_{12} deficiency, and steatorrhoea with failure to reach normal height and weight percentile. There may also be evidence of lack of fat-soluble vitamins A and D.

Mucosal biopsy shows a varying degree of flattening under the dissecting microscope; in my experience most biopsies are flat and in those which show convolutions these are reduced in height compared with normal leaf and spade forms though they are not always thickened. Apart from showing some degree of abnormality and assisting orientation, the dissecting microscope is of no value in differential diagnosis, and can be misleading: I have seen a diagnosis of a 'flat' biopsy made on normal jejunal mucosa which was orientated upside down and the submucosal surface regarded as a flat mucosa!

Microscopically I always first look for normal villi; if any are present, even if there is partial flattening of others, and the biopsy is jejunal, a diagnosis of g.i.e. –

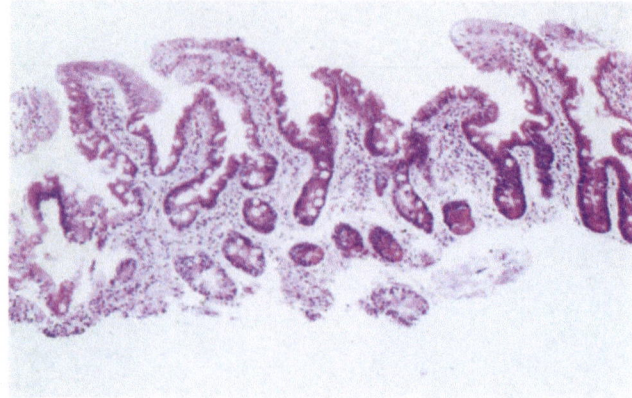

Figure 11.1 Slight flattening, probably not gluten-induced. Some villi are slightly short and thickened and one is branched, indicating some degree of abnormality, but at least two villi, though not consecutive, are normal. The child from whom this biopsy came was later shown to have an infective enteritis. H & E × 25

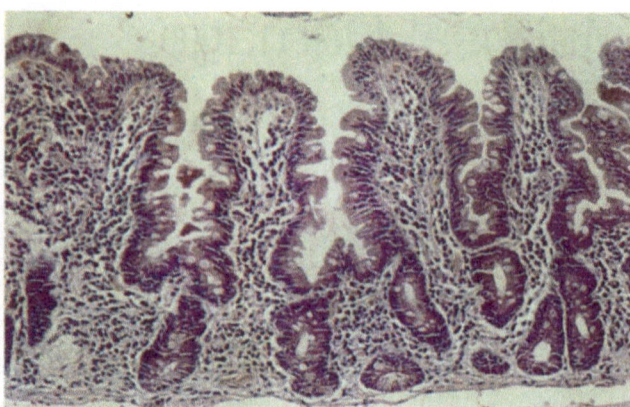

Figure 11.2 Partial flattening. All villi are shorter and broader than normal, there is crowding of surface enterocytes especially at the villous tips with an increased round cell infiltrate in the lamina propria. H & E × 100

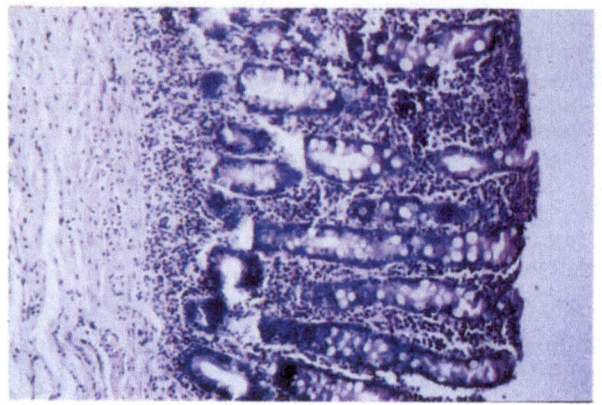

Figure 11.3 Severe flattening. No recognizable villi remain, surface enterocytes are distorted, there is a marked increase in cells in the lamina propria and the whole mucosa resembles large bowel. H & E × 100

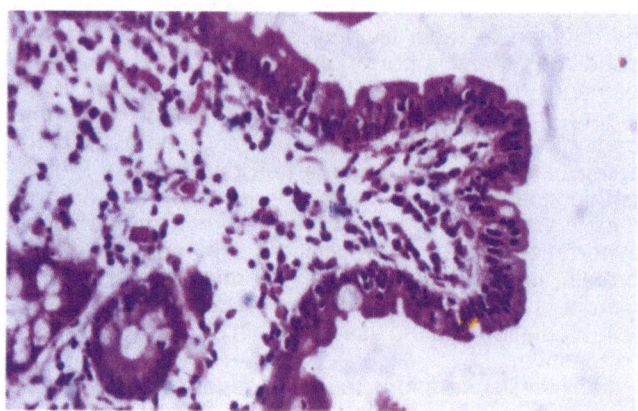

Figure 11.4 Partial flattening. Note the moderate distortion and crowding of surface enterocytes and an increase in number of plasma cells, mainly just beneath the surface epithelium. H & E × 250

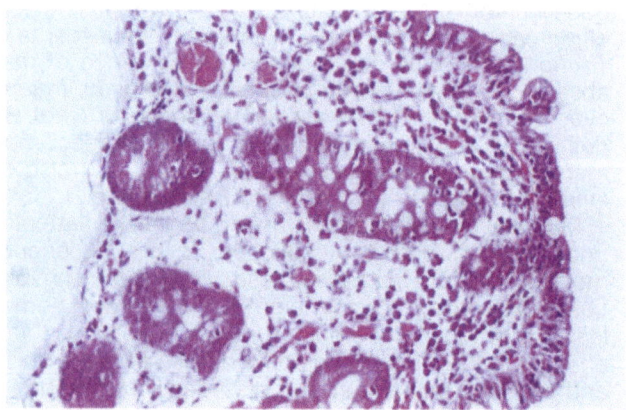

Figure 11.5 Severe flattening. Note the crowding of surface enterocytes and increased numbers of intra-epithelial lymphocytes in the surface epithelium. H & E × 250

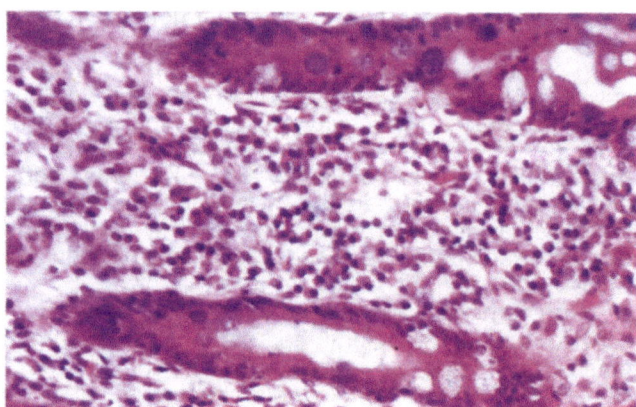

Figure 11.6 Partial flattening. An elongated crypt (top) shows hyperplastic activity. Plasma cell numbers are increased in the lamina propria. H & E × 250

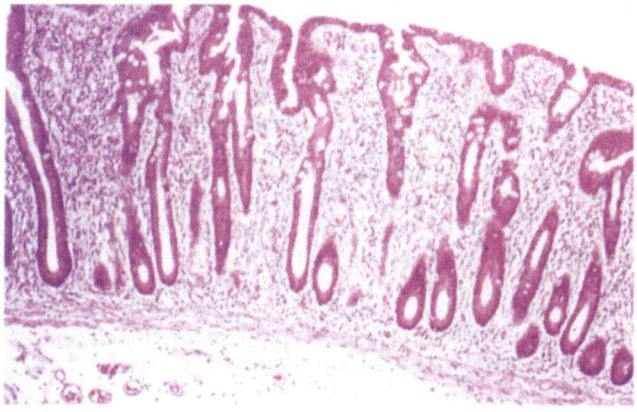

Figure 11.7 Severe flattening. The basal layer is increased in thickness and forms about two-thirds of the total mucosal width. H & E × 80

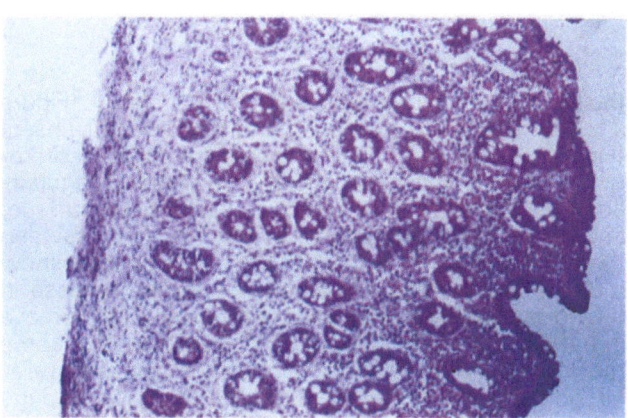

Figure 11.8 This tangentially cut section, not ideal for reporting, shows clearly that the cellular infiltrate is most marked immediately beneath the surface epithelium. H & E × 100

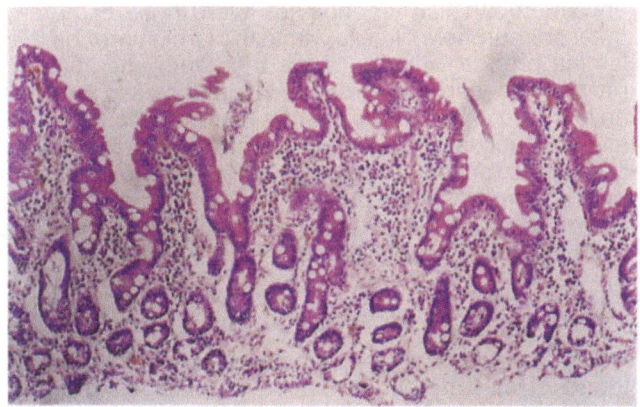

Figure 11.9 Gluten-induced enteropathy (g.i.e.) 3 months after gluten withdrawal. Villi are beginning to reappear, and one (right) is relatively normal. The basal layer is still thickened. Cellular infiltrate and migrating lymphocyte numbers are also returning to normal. H & E × 80

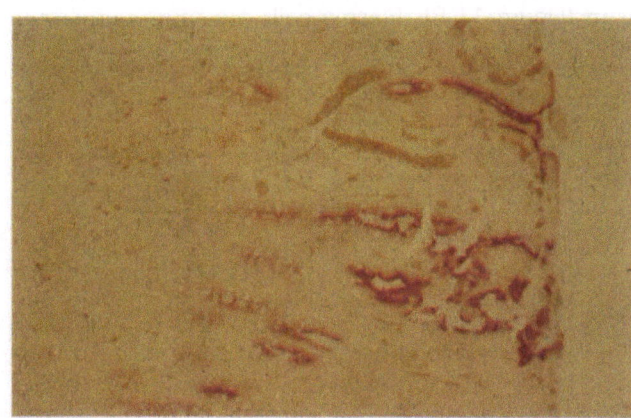

Figure 11.10 G.i.e. 4 months after gluten withdrawal. The mucosa in this patient has remained flat and alkaline phosphatase is present only in the more superficial glands, indicating the likelihood of a poor response. Azo dye technique without counterstain × 125

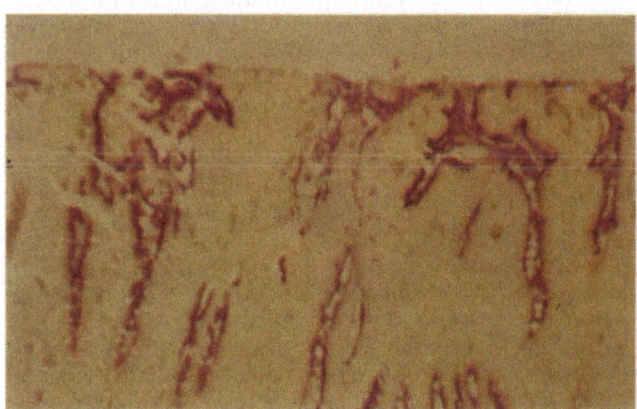

Figure 11.11 G.i.e. 2 months after gluten withdrawal. The mucosa remains flat but there is alkaline phosphatase activity almost throughout the mucosa, suggesting a better prognosis for mucosal recovery. A further biopsy 4 months later revealed a considerable degree of mucosal regeneration. Azo dye technique without counterstain × 125

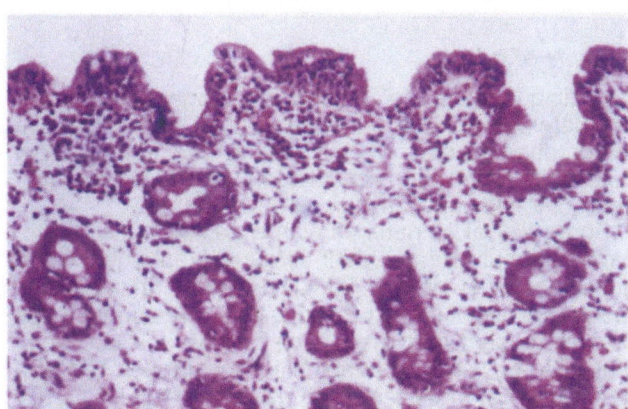

Figure 11.12 Idiopathic steatorrhoea. There is marked flattening though the remains of villi can be made out. Relatively few plasma cells are present in the lamina propria. The differential diagnosis from g.i.e. had to be made mainly on a lack of response to a gluten-free diet. H & E × 250

though not absolutely excluded – is unlikely (Figure 11.1). If all villi are shortened and thickened or absent (Figures 11.2 and 11.3) look first at the surface enterocytes. In g.i.e. these are distorted in shape, irregularly crowded together particularly at the luminal surface, and have many interepithelial lymphocytes between them (Figures 11.4 and 11.5). The crypt zones show moderate to marked hyperactivity with an increase in the normal crypt column length and usually an increase in mitotic index (Figure 11.6). These changes become more marked as the flattening increases, and are a reliable guide to the degree of surface enterocyte damage and loss. The basal cell layer shows an increase in thickness with a relatively normal histological appearance (Figure 11.7). The former assertion that a decrease in Paneth cells indicated the likelihood of a poor response to gluten-free diet has not been true in my experience, and I cannot confirm or deny that secretin-secreting and 5HT cells are increased in number, as has been reported[4,5].

Within the lamina propria the normal cellularity increases, particularly immediately beneath the epithelium (Figure 11.8). Plasma cells are more numerous, though the normal IgA : IgG : IgM ratios are retained unless the patient has an associated IgA deficiency. Lymphocytes are often visibly increased, though this can be masked by greatly increased immigration and emigration between enterocytes, and there are often more eosinophils than usual.

Some workers like to grade biopsies which are not normal into three groups:

(1) mild degree of flattening: villi are recognizable but there is some shortening and broadening and some distortion of surface enterocytes with crowding together and some increase in cellularity of lamina propria;

(2) moderate degree of flattening: as above with recognizable villi but more severe changes;

(3) completely flat: with no, or virtually no, trace of villous formation.

Such a grading is usually subjective and not confirmed by actual measurement: it can be of value for comparison when performed by the same observer on carefully processed material but does not necessarily allow of comparison between different groups of workers.

Variants of g.i.e.

In 'collagenous sprue' a band of collagenous material lies between surface enterocytes and lamina propria. Minor degrees are not uncommon and are probably reversible; broad bands of collagen are thought by some authors to indicate a less good outlook[6].

Some 2% of all patients with g.i.e. have also hypogammaglobulinaemia which is usually an isolated IgA deficiency with normal IgM production. In them the mucosa is usually flat and appearances resemble those of g.i.e. except that the lamina propria is less cellular than in g.i.e. and immunological techniques reveal a deficiency of IgA-secreting plasma cells. Giardial infestation may also be present.

Gluten Withdrawal and Challenge

Withdrawal of gluten from the diet, provided that it is absolute, usually brings about a rapid clinical improvement and a slower return to normal of biopsy appearances which do not always correlate with the clinical findings, perhaps because sampling is random and recovery patchy. There is usually a return to normal of lamina proprial cellularity and of numbers of migrating lymphocytes before the villi recover their normal width and length or crypt zones return to normal activity (Figure 11.9). In patients who have thus improved, the administration of gluten, either in the diet or by installation through a tube, can cause a rapid reversal to a flat mucosa, but may produce little observable clinical deterioration though some relapse is usually seen[7]. Special investigations may be of value (see below).

Morphological Measurements

In my opinion these are rarely needed in untreated g.i.e. when the flattening is severe, but can sometimes be helpful in partial flattening, in patients on a gluten-free diet who are undergoing assessment and in patients who have undergone gluten challenge. Flattening is associated with an alteration in numbers of enterocytes and a diminution in volume of lamina propria. It is therefore clearly impracticable to compare numbers of migrating interepithelial lymphocytes with those of enterocytes, or numbers of cells within the lamina propria with lamina proprial volume, since the same alterations in ratio can as readily be produced by a decrease in one as an increase in the other. The one feature which does not alter in mucosal flattening, and is included in most biopsies, is the muscularis mucosae. It is desirable to count the numbers of cells present in, and to measure the lamina proprial volume of the mucosa which overlies, a fixed measured length of muscularis mucosae.

Histochemical Investigations

Alkaline phosphatase and aminopeptidase are normally found in all enterocytes above crypt level: they are faintly present in some cells in the crypt zone and are not found in glands in the basal layer. My own (unpublished) observations on flat mucosa in g.i.e. have shown two patterns of enzyme distribution. In one (Figure 11.10) both enzymes are confined to the surface epithelium and superficial glands; in this group clinical response to a gluten-free diet has been slow; I have not seen enough repeat biopsies to know for certain what happens to the mucosa. In a second group both enzymes are present throughout the glands of the basal layer (Figure 11.11); in this group the clinical response to diet has been good. The distinction is not absolute and my numbers are not large, but the technique is easy and may have some prognostic value.

Dermatitis Herpetiformis

Approximately 60% of patients with dermatitis herpetiformis (d.h.) also have g.i.e. Approximately 90% of patients with g.i.e. but no overt skin lesions have impairment of glycine and l-alanine absorption and some degree of epidermal ridge atrophy of the skin which are features of d.h. Some patients with d.h. but no evidence of malabsorption who have normal jejunal biopsies develop mucosal flattening when fed diets high in gluten. The histological appearances in those patients with d.h. who have g.i.e. are identical in all respects with patients who have g.i.e. but no skin lesion, and the two conditions are clearly associated.

Idiopathic Steatorrhoea

A small number of adults appear not to respond to a gluten-free diet even when strictly controlled in hospital. Biopsy findings are usually a flat mucosa resembling that in g.i.e. but plasma cells in the lamina propria are fewer and migrating lymphocytes not greatly increased (Figure 11.12). There may be an increased tendency to diffuse lymphoma. If the ileum is sampled changes are as severe there as in the jejunum, contrary to g.i.e. in which mucosal changes become less severe as one descends the bowel aborally. Morphological studies may be helpful (see below).

Enzyme Defects Producing Malabsorption

Enzyme systems within enterocytes or on brush borders can be congenitally absent or reduced in demonstrable amount due to inherited defects, or may be temporarily or permanently lost or reduced in acquired disease, particularly infection.

Disaccharidase Deficiencies

In infants these usually manifest themselves as a specific inherited deficiency of lactase; in adults the condition is usually acquired and affects many or all disaccharidases[8,9]. The mucosa is either histologically normal or shows the changes of the infective condition which produced the hypolactasia; there are no histological changes specific for lactase deficiency. Histochemical techniques are described but the reagents for them are expensive and the results obtained not entirely reliable. It is probably still preferable to hand the biopsy over intact to the biochemists.

Aminopeptidase Deficiencies

Some workers think that there are defects in peptidase secretion paralleling those seen in disaccharidase deficiency[10]; there are no apparent histological abnormalities and I know of no histochemical studies on aminopeptidases, though these are easy to perform and reliable (but see below).

Children below Normal Height and Weight Percentiles

We have recently studied, using intestinal biopsy, a small group of children who are below the normal height and weight percentiles for their age, without obvious clinical reason and without overt malabsorption. Histologically all biopsies were superficially normal but histochemical techniques for aminopeptidase and alkaline phosphatase have shown a patchy loss of enzyme in surface enterocytes (Figure 11.13) in about 50% which is not present in control material and does not appear to be artefact as we at first thought. We are not sure of the meaning of this change, which resembles what we have seen in some infections (see page 78), but it may be that in these children enterocytes degenerate prematurely before they are shed.

Defects in Protein Synthesis

The disorder a-β-lipoproteinaemia and related hypo-β-lipoproteinaemic syndromes[11,12] are characterized by acanthocytosis, often with retinopathy and central nervous system manifestations. Jejunal biopsies show a curious foamy vacuolation of the enterocytes covering the upper part of the villi, which in cryostat sections will stain with conventional lipid stains (Figure 11.14). A similar vacuolation, less marked and less extensive, is rarely seen in gluten-induced enteropathy (Figure 11.15).

Damage due to Drugs and Chemicals

A number of antibiotics and other drugs can give rise clinically to steatorrhoea but there are few reliable biopsy studies. The only two of which I have personal experience are neomycin[13] and methotrexate[14]. Some patients and experimental animals given neomycin showed broadening and shortening of villi apparently due to oedema and round-cell infiltration, while patients on methotrexate show vacuolation and patchy necrosis of surface enterocytes with some reduction in crypt activity[15]. It is probable that these changes result from direct toxic effects on crypt epithelium.

Damage secondary to other Primary Diseases

Aside from infections, which are considered on page 78, and immunological disorders (page 83), few other diseases give rise to recognizable mucosal damage demanding biopsy. A possible exception is diabetes mellitus, and there are a number of biopsy reports available[16]. Most patients have had histologically normal biopsies but in occasional individuals there has been a flat biopsy indistinguishable from g.i.e. and a coexistence of the two conditions has been suggested.

Mucosal Flattening resulting from Decreased Crypt Activity

Adult Malnutrition

This occurs in people too poor to afford an adequate diet, and especially in women in the childbearing age who become pregnant frequently and breast-feed their children. It is also seen in those who adopt inadequate diets for religious or other reasons. I have seen it in parts of West Africa but not in Britain, although Vegans are said to show it on occasion. The total mucosal thickness is reduced and villi appear short and flattened, but enterocytes are not crowded together, there is no crypt zone proliferation, no increase in cellularity of the lamina propria and intra-epithelial lymphocytes are normal in number (Figure 11.16). The condition responds to a normal diet.

Kwashiorkor

The small intestinal changes in kwashiorkor lie somewhere between those of malnutrition and of epithelial destruction with crypt hyperactivity. My own material has more resembled the adult pattern but Professor Kaschula in Cape Town[17], whose experience is much greater than mine, has allowed me to study some of his material. The mucosal changes in it closely resemble g.i.e., though there is less conspicuous increase in inter-epithelial lymphocytes (Figure 11.17). Sometimes gas cysts develop in the submucosa (Figure 11.18).

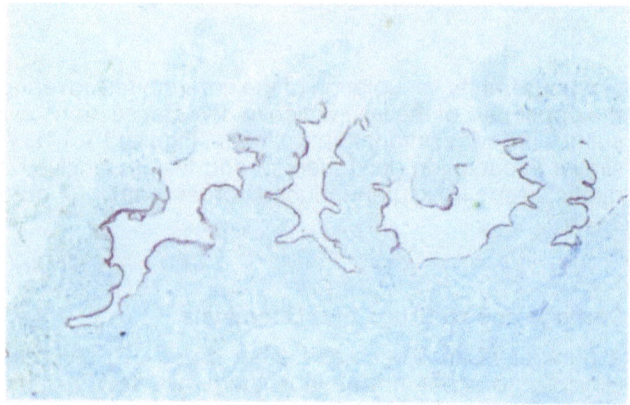

Figure 11.13 Some children below the normal height and weight percentiles have a histologically normal mucosa, but villi show an absence of alkaline phosphatase and aminopeptidase at the villous tips. This is not an artefact and may represent premature enterocyte degeneration. Azo dye technique for alkaline phosphatase × 80

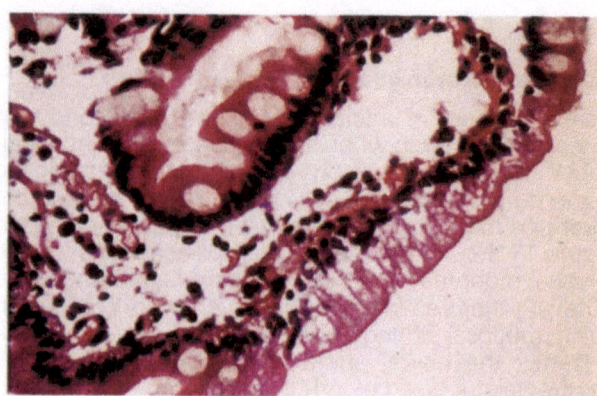

Figure 11.14 A-β-lipoproteinaemia. Enterocytes covering the upper parts of villi show foamy vacuolation. H & E × 250

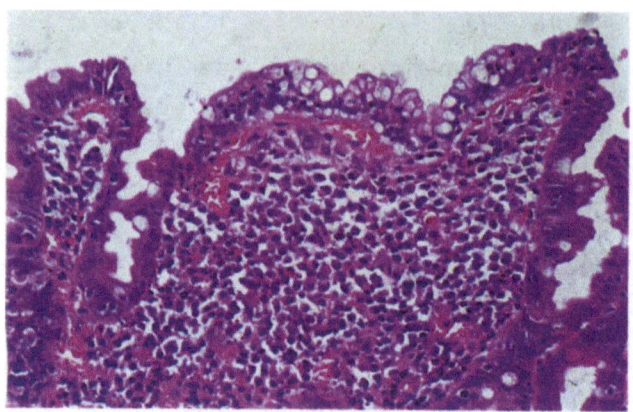

Figure 11.15 Lipid vacuolation of surface enterocytes in g.i.e. This is a rare finding; the vacuoles are rounder and more suggestive of lipid content than those in Figure 11.14. H & E × 250

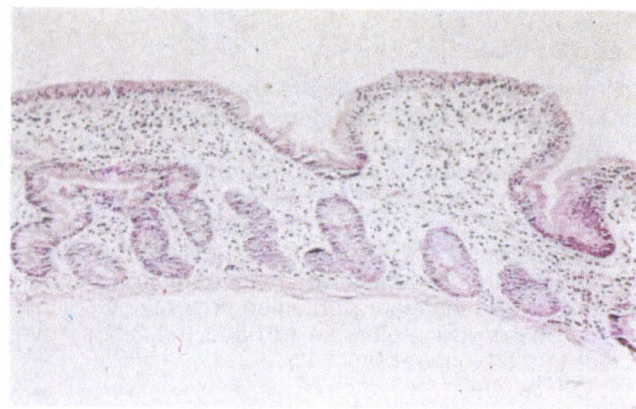

Figure 11.16 Adult malnutrition. The mucosa is flat but there is no enterocyte distortion or crowding, no crypt zone proliferation or lymphocyte emigration and no increased cellularity in the lamina propria. H & E × 65

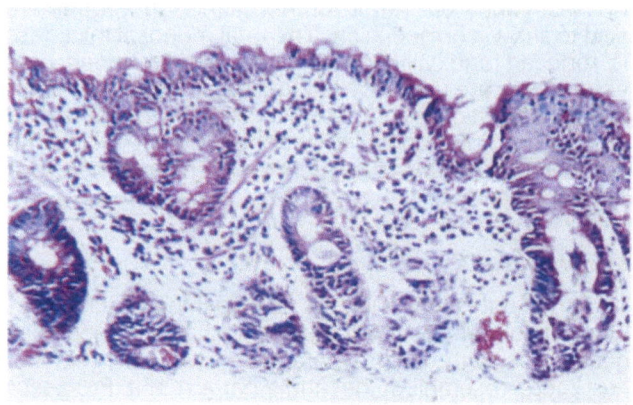

Figure 11.17 Infantile kwashiorkor. The mucosa is flat but histological changes lie midway between g.i.e. and adult malnutrition, and there is some crypt hyperactivity. H & E × 100

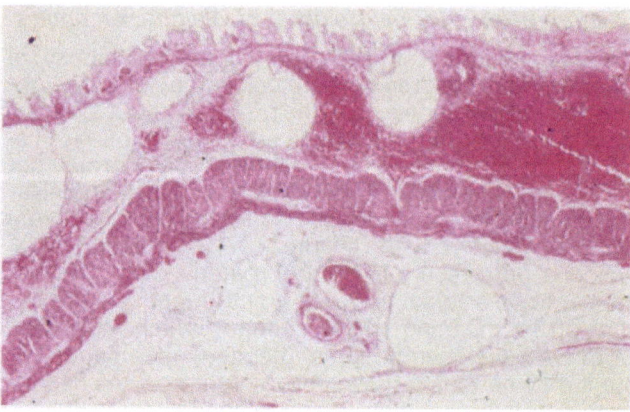

Figure 11.18 Infantile kwashiorkor. A full-thickness postmortem section which shows the submucosal gas cysts. H & E × 25

References

1. Katz, A. J. and Grand, R. J. (1979). All that flattens is not 'sprue'. *Gastroenterology*, **76**, 375

2. Dissanayake, A. S., Truelove, S. C. and Whitehead, R. (1974). Jejunal mucosal recovery in coeliac disease in relation to the degree of adherence to a gluten-free diet. *Q. J. Med.*, N.S. XLIII, **161**, 185

3. Pena, A. S., Mann, D. L., Hague, N. E., Heck, J. A., van Leeuwen, A., van Rood, J. J. and Strober, W. (1978). Genetic basis of gluten-sensitive enteropathy. *Gastroenterology*, **75**, 230

4. Polak, J. M., Pearse, A. G. E., van Noorden, S., Bloom, S. R. and Rossiter, M. A. (1973). Secretin cells in coeliac disease. *Gut*, **14**, 870

5. Challacombe, D. N. and Robertson, K. (1977). Enterochromaffin cells in the duodenal mucosa of children with coeliac disease. *Gut*, **18**, 373

6. Bossart, R., Henry, K., Booth, C. C. and Doe, W. F. (1975). Subepithelial collagen in intestinal malabsorption. *Gut*, **16**, 18

7. Kumar, P. J., O'Donaghue, D. P., Stenson, K. and Dawson, A. M. (1979). Reintroduction of gluten in adults and children with treated coeliac disease. *Gut*, **20**, 743

8. Bayless, T. M. (1972). Intestinal lactase deficiency. In Bergsma, D. (ed.). *Birth Defects. Part XIII*. pp. 4–11. (New York: National Foundation–March of Dimes)

9. Sahi, T. (1978). Dietary lactose and the aetiology of human small-intestinal hypolactasia. *Gut*, **19**, 1074

10. Sadikali, F. (1971). Dipeptidase deficiency and malabsorption of glycyl-glycine in disease states. *Gut*, **12**, 276

11. Greenwood, N. (1976). The jejunal mucosa in two cases of a-beta-lipoproteinaemia. *Am. J. Gastroenterol.*, **65**, 160

12. Scott, B. B., Miller, J. P. and Losowsky, M. S. (1979). Hypo beta lipoproteinaemia – a variant of the Bassen–Kornzweig syndrome. *Gut*, **20**, 163

13. Pryse Davies, J. and Dawson, I. M. P. (1964). Some observations on the enzyme histochemistry of the small intestine in human malabsorption states, with some experimental studies on the effect of neomycin on rats. *Acta Gastroenterol. Belg.*, **27**, 537

14. Gwavava, N., Pinkerton, C. R., Glasgow, J. F. T., Sloan, J. M. and Bridges, J. M. (1981). Small bowel enterocyte abnormalities caused by methotrexate treatment in acute lymphoblastic leukaemia of childhood. *J. Clin. Pathol.*, **34**, 790

15. Pinkerton, C. R., Camerson, C. H. S., Sloan, J. M., Glasgow, J. F. T. and Gwavava, N. J. T. (1982). Jejunal crypt cell abnormalities associated with methotrexate treatment in children with acute lymphoblastic leukaemia. *J. Clin. Pathol.*, **35**, 1272

16. Malins, J. M. and Mayne, N. (1969). Diabetic diarrhoea: a study of 13 patients with jejunal biopsy. *Diabetes*, **18**, 858

17. Barbezat, G. O., Bowie, M. D. and Kaschula, R. O. C. (1957). Studies on the small intestinal mucosa of children with protein–calorie malnutrition. *S. Afr. Med. J.*, **41**, 1031

Most adult patients with infective enteritis involving the small bowel are not biopsied unless diarrhoea becomes intractable, as in coccidiosis. Viral and bacterial infections, often combined, are more common in infants and children, can be epidemic, and biopsies are sometimes taken. Experimental studies on lambs infected with rotavirus[1] and in human volunteers given 'Norwalk' virus[2] suggest that there is damage to, followed by sloughing of, mature enterocytes from villus tips leading sometimes to partial flattening and followed by complete healing. I have seen this type of change (Figures 12.1 and 12.2) sometimes with mild degrees of mucosal flattening in the mucosa of young children investigated for persistent diarrhoea and failure to thrive in whom gluten-induced enteropathy (g.i.e.) has not been suspected clinically (see also Figure 11.13). Viral studies were not done but repeat biopsies in a few of the children showed a normal mucosa a few months later. Appearances are similar to those already described in some children who are below the normal height and weight percentile for no apparent reason (page 75). Both conditions may be the result of viral infection, but the apparent healing we have sometimes seen may equally be due to a patchy lesion with variable sampling.

In children with proven *E. coli* infections biopsies can be normal, but sometimes show blunting and slight broadening of intestinal villi with increased cellularity of the lamina propria, which may contain polymorphs (Figure 12.3). Some workers have described focal necrosis as is seen in viral infections, with or without intracapillary thrombi, but one must remember that *E. coli* and viral infections frequently coexist.

Tropical Sprue

The diagnosis of tropical sprue depends more upon the clinical history and the place of domicile of the patient than upon the biopsy appearances; clinical features differ in the Caribbean from those in India or Malaysia. The disorder is probably primarily infective since it responds to broad-spectrum antibiotics and is possibly produced by a coliform organism[3]. It occurs in countries and latitudes in which bowel infections and infestations are common and the spectrum of dissecting microscopic and histological changes regarded as within normal limits is a broad one, so that minor changes are difficult to interpret and although it produces a degree of broadening and flattening of villi this is seldom complete. It is therefore not surprising that some studies have suggested that in many patients there is no real qualitative difference between the mucosa of a patient with tropical sprue and that of the indigenous population[4], though the same does not necessarily hold for Europeans domiciled in or recently returned from a region where sprue is endemic.

Under the dissecting microscope ridges, convolutions and spade forms are common but flattening may not be severe enough to differ from what is normal for the area; a flat mucosa is rare, and one must always remember that g.i.e. can occur wherever gluten is available in the diet. Microscopically there are no specific diagnostic changes but appearances are those of the less severe examples of g.i.e. Sometimes the oedema and cellular infiltrate in the villi are out of proportion to the degree of flattening and suggest an inflammatory process; interepithelial lymphocytes are not necessarily increased in number (Figure 12.4). Studies suggest that the mucosa slowly reverts to normal after antibiotic therapy.

Giardial Infestation

Giardial infestation is a not uncommon cause of travellers' diarrhoea, and is also found in children who fail to thrive; heavy infestation can produce steatorrhoea and other evidence of malabsorption. There is a well-recognized association with variable hypogammaglobulinaemia and more especially with IgA deficiency, which should always be looked for[5]. On biopsy the mucosa can appear histologically normal in mild infestation, though giardia can be seen in spaces between individual villi (Figure 12.5). These do not always show the expected 'owl eyes' appearance of double nuclei and can present as sickle forms (Figure 12.6)[6] and a PAS stain can be helpful. No biopsy should be reported as normal until they have been deliberately looked for. More severe infestations, especially when there is associated hypogammaglobulinaemia, show varying degrees of mucosal flattening and some authors have described giardia within the tissues[7]. Recent very careful morphometric quantitative studies[8] using a Weibel graticule have shown a significant loss of villous surface area in patients with giardiasis and malabsorption, and suggest that histological and functional impairment correlate, are maximal soon after infestation, and improve on treatment.

Whipple's Disease

Whipple's disease is now recognized to be of bacillary origin. The bacilli are best recognized by transmission electron micrography[9] and in suspected cases a part of the biopsy should be fixed in buffered glutaraldehyde though formaldehyde-fixed material can also be used (Figure 12.7). The condition is usually found in males over 50 years, who present with loss of weight and polyarthralgia and are found to have steatorrhoea; generalized manifestations including systemic lymphadenopathy are common.

On biopsy the jejunal mucosa may show a normal villous pattern but partial shortening and thickening of villi is more common. At light microscopic level the lamina propria of villi and basal layer contains very numerous macrophages with granular eosinophilic cytoplasm (Figure 12.8). The contained material stains deeply with PAS (Figure 12.9), is diastase-resistant and does not stain either for lipids or mucosubstances, though small numbers of lipid-containing macrophages can also be present. The overlying enterocytes are not distorted or crowded together and there is no conspicuous increase in crypt zone activity. Electron microscopically bacilliform bodies can be seen immediately beneath the villous epithelial basement membrane, but are less frequent nearer to the muscularis mucosae; they are also visible within macrophages. Biopsy appearances may gradually improve after tetracycline treatment.

Other Inflammatory Disorders

These can be divided into those which are generalized and can be sampled using blind biopsy and those which are localized and, in the absence of direct visual endoscopy, are biopsied only by chance or, if more generalized, are found in the ileum rather than the jejunum. In this group are Crohn's disease, tuberculosis, Yersinial infections, typhoid, schistosomiasis and eosinophilic enteritis. Some also occur in the large bowel, can be electively sampled there and appearances in the small bowel can be anticipated from descriptions of resected specimens[10]. They virtually never occur in 'blind' biopsy material and are not described here.

There are a number of more generalized disorders rarely seen in biopsy material which are briefly described.

Though not uncommon in tropical countries *cholera* presents as an acute disease in epidemic form, is readily diagnosed without biopsy and demands urgent treatment. Biopsy studies are said to show either a normal mucosa or enterocyte necrosis and shedding along villous tips with an increase in lymphocytes and plasma cells in the lamina propria[11] and electron microscopic studies show diagnostic 'blebs' in surface and crypt cells. I have not seen biopsy material, which is not normally taken in this condition.

Interest in enteric *clostridial infections* has greatly increased with detailed description of antibiotic-associated colitis (see page 118). Various strains of *Clostridia* have long been recognized as associated with acute forms of jejunitis in adults, including the so-called Darm-brand enteritis in Germany, Pig Bel in New Guinea and acute jejunitis in Scandinavia[10]. In all of these there is acute necrosis of apical villus mucosa with marked oedema and congestion of the lamina propria. There may be an associated ischaemic factor but experimental work[12] suggests a direct toxic effect such as is seen in the large bowel in *Cl. difficile* infection in antibiotic-associated colitis. I have not personally seen any biopsy material.

Giardiasis has already been separately described (page 78). It is the most common infestation seen in biopsy material and has a recognized association with immune deficiency states. Other infestations include *ascariasis*, in which the small bowel mucosa is unaltered; *capillariasis*[13] in which the worm *Capillaria philippinensis* can sometimes be seen in the biopsy accompanied by a mild degree of mucosal flattening; *coccidiosis*, in which there is variable villous flattening with trophozoites often visible within individual enterocytes[14]; *hookworm infestations*, which are not usually associated with mucosal abnormalities when allowance is made for the wider range of mucosal normality present in Asiatics; and infestations by *Strongyloides stercoralis*, in which the mucosa can be flattened and the female worm is sometimes visible.

The Problem of Duodenitis

It is easy to biopsy the first and often the second part of the duodenum under direct vision using a fibreoptic gastroscope. This permits two separate patterns of investigation.

First, in patients with upper abdominal symptoms suggesting non-ulcer dyspepsia it is practicable to take duodenal as well as gastric biopsies. These, like gastric biopsies in this condition, may be normal or show varying degrees of mucosal damage and inflammatory change. Second, in patients with clinical evidence of malabsorption or steatorrhoea thought to be associated with a degree of mucosal flattening which is diffuse, such as g.i.e., changes should be present in the duodenum as well as the jejunum and duodenal biopsy may be preferable for diagnosis. In some patients, however, duodenitis and malabsorption may coexist and the changes present may represent a combination of two disorders.

Duodenitis: Patients with dyspepsia in the absence of duodenal ulcer may have a normal biopsy but it is more common to see mucosal changes[15]. These consist of varying degrees of villous flattening with increased crypt mitotic activity and an increase in lymphocytes and plasma cells in the lamina propria which may also contain polymorphs (Figures 12.10 and 12.12). These variations have been substantiated by careful morphological[16,17] and autoradiographic[18] studies, but some inflammatory changes can be found in subjects used as controls and, as in gastritis, are more common, in my experience, in people in older age groups. There is reasonable evidence[18] that duodenitis when severe may be followed by erosion and ulceration, but we do not yet know how commonly mild inflammatory changes with some degree of villous flattening can be found in patients who are symptomless, and how far these are reversible.

Duodenal biopsy in g.i.e: In uncomplicated g.i.e. (or other disorders causing generalized mucosal flattening) duodenal biopsy will show the same changes as jejunal biopsies. Because villous fusion is more common in the duodenum slight changes may be more difficult to interpret but there is not usually a problem (Figure 12.12). Children and adolescents without symptoms of dyspepsia are not likely to have coincident duodenitis, but young adults with g.i.e. may also have duodenitis and in them duodenal biopsies should be used with care for the diagnosis of g.i.e., since one does not know how much of any change present is simply the result of the duodenitis.

References

1. Snodgrass, D.R., Ferguson, A., Allan, F., Angus, K.W. and Mitchell, B. (1979). Small intestinal morphology and epithelial cell kinetics in lamb rotavirus infections. *Gastroenterology*, **76**, 477

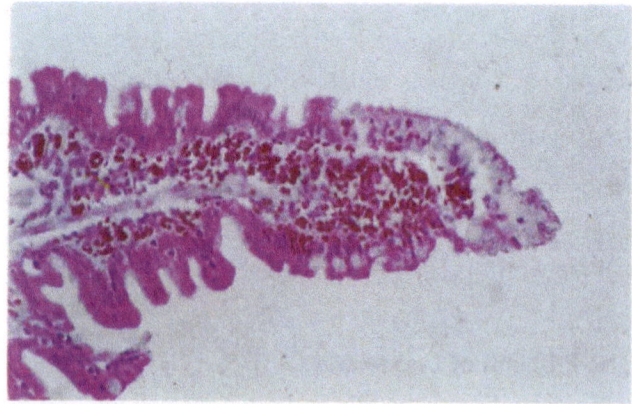

Figure 12.1 Caucasian child with probable viral diarrhoea. Individual villi were not shortened or thickened but there is obvious enterocyte degeneration at the villous tips.   H & E × 250

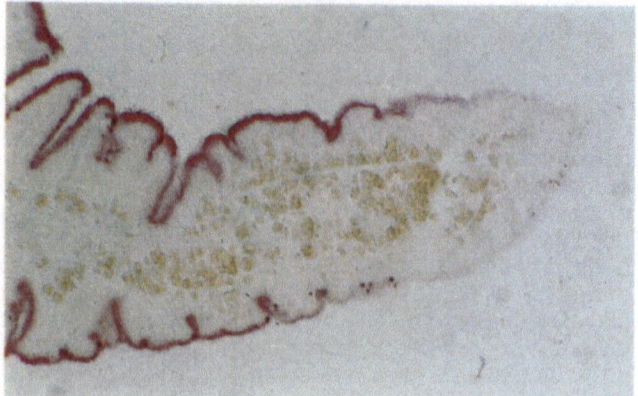

Figure 12.2 Step section from biopsy depicted in Figure 12.1. The enterocyte degeneration is confirmed by the loss of alkaline phosphatase.   Alkaline phosphatase technique × 250

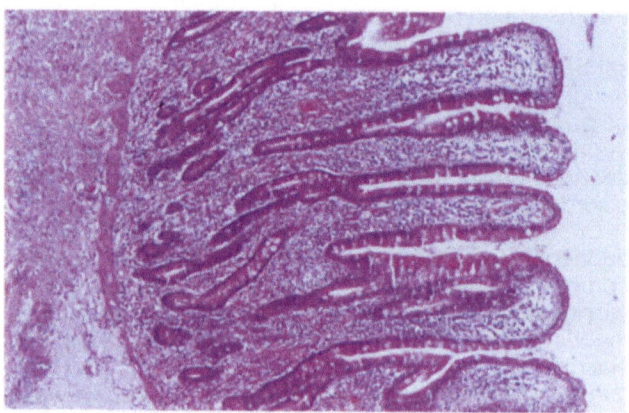

Figure 12.3 Caucasian child with proven *E. coli* infection. The villi are not obviously shortened but are slightly thicker than normal and the tips show some blunting. There is marked increased cellularity in the lamina propria which includes some polymorphs.   H & E × 125

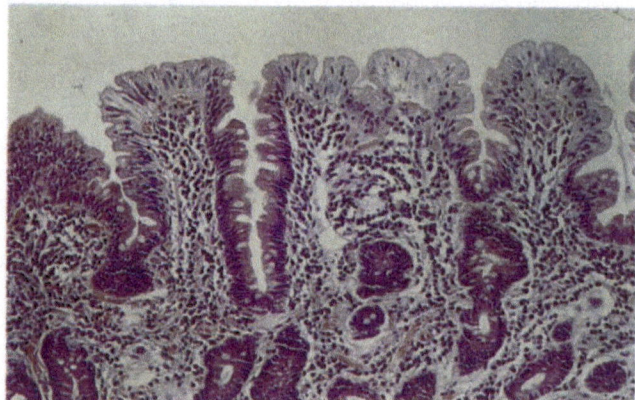

Figure 12.4 Tropical sprue. Some villous flattening is present but intra-epithelial lymphocytes are not increased in numbers. There is conspicuous oedema and a heavy rather superficial inflammatory cellular infiltrate.   H & E × 250

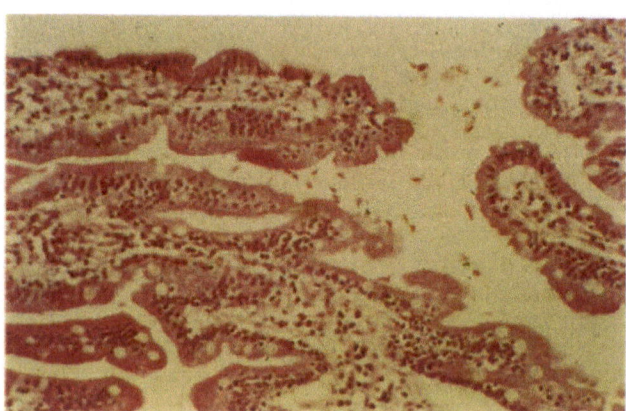

Figure 12.5 Giardiasis. In this poorly orientated biopsy the villi shown appear normal but numerous giardia can be seen in intervillous spaces.   H & E × 125

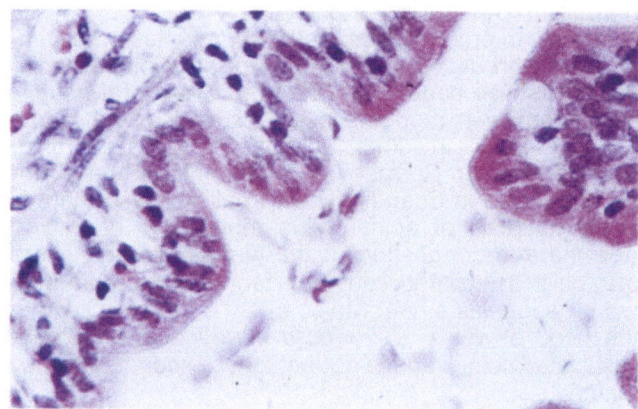

Figure 12.6 Jejunum: giardiasis. A high-power view shows giardia present in an intervillous space.   H & E × 250

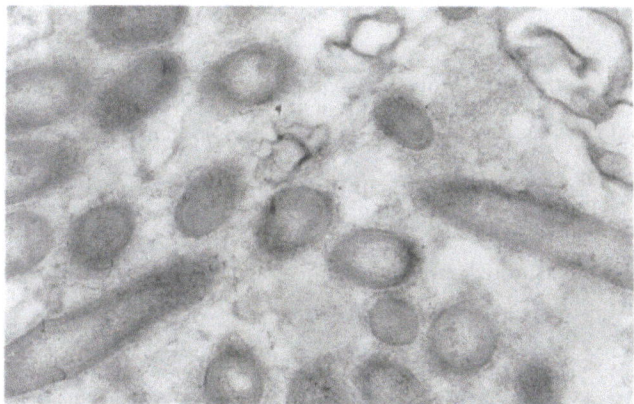

Figure 12.7 Whipple's disease. Electron micrograph of bacilli in longitudinal and cross-section. × 8000

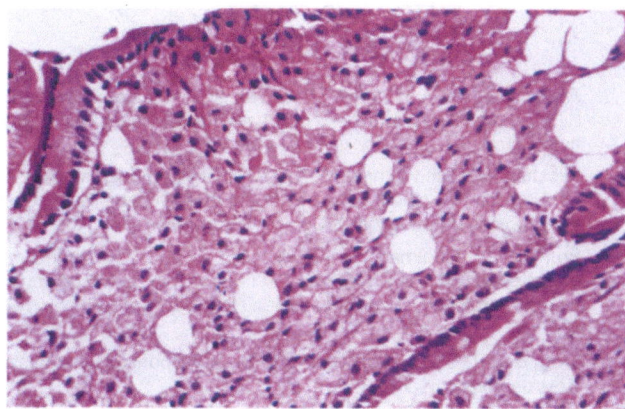

Figure 12.8 Whipple's disease. High-power view of villus showing macrophages with granular eosinophilic cytoplasm. Note the normal enterocytes. H & E × 250

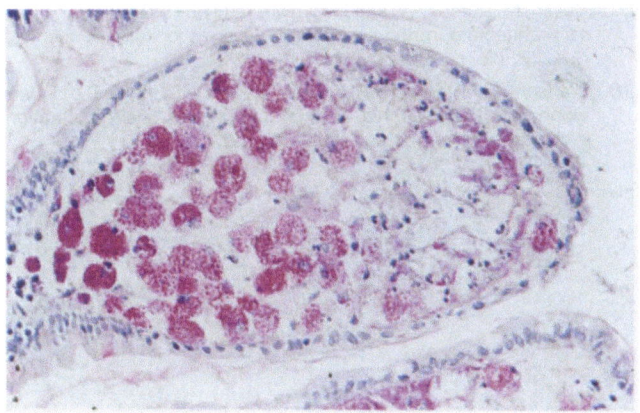

Figure 12.9 Whipple's disease. PAS-positive material in macrophages. Diastase–PAS × 320

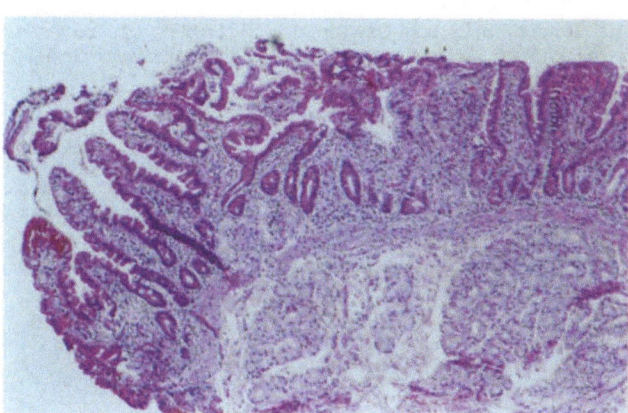

Figure 12.10 Duodenal biopsy in clinical non-ulcer dyspepsia. Some villi are shortened and flattened but many are normal and I would hesitate to diagnose duodenitis on this biopsy. H & E × 80

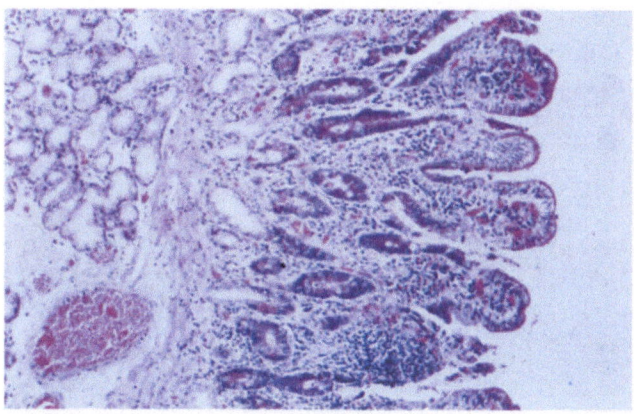

Figure 12.11 Duodenal biopsy in clinical non-ulcer dyspepsia. There is some shortening and flattening of all villi and an increased cellular infiltrate in the lamina propria. A diagnosis of duodenitis can be made. H & E × 125

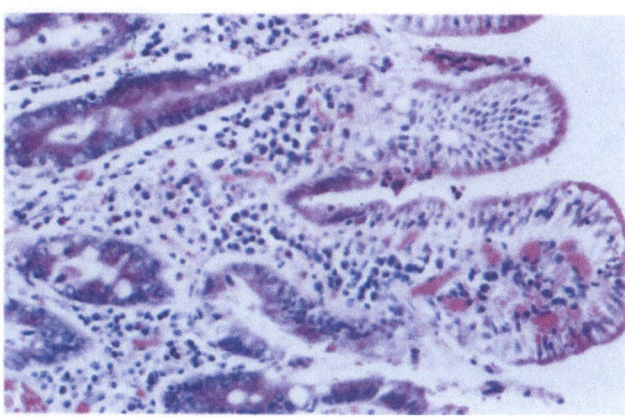

Figure 12.12 Higher power view of Figure 12.11. The increased cellular infiltrate is well shown but there is little distortion of enterocytes. H & E × 200

2. Agus, S. G., Dolin, R., Wyatt, R. G., Tousimis, A. J. and Northrop, R. S. (1973). Acute infectious non-bacterial gastroenteritis: intestinal histopathology. *Ann. Intern. Med.*, **79**, 18

3. Klipstein, F. A. and Schenk, E. A. (1975). Enterotoxigenic intestinal bacteria in tropical sprue. II. Effect of the bacteria and their enterotoxins on intestinal structure. *Gastroenterology*, **68**, 642

4. Brunser, O., Eidelman, S. and Klipstein, F. A. (1970). Intestinal morphology of rural Haitians: a comparison between overt tropical sprue and asymptomatic subjects. *Gastroenterology*, **58**, 655

5. Kraft, S. C. (1979). The intestinal immune response in giardiasis. *Gastroenterology*, **76**, 877

6. Hartong, W. A., Gourley, W. K. and Arvanitakis, C. (1979). Giardiasis: clinical spectrum and functional–structural abnormalities of the small intestinal mucosa. *Gastroenterology*, **79**, 61

7. Saha, T. K. and Ghosh, T. K. (1977). Invasion of small intestinal mucosa by *Giardia lamblia* in man. *Gastroenterology*, **72**, 402

8. Wright, S. G. and Tomkins, A. M. (1978). Quantitative histology in giardiasis. *J. Clin. Pathol.*, **31**, 712

9. Dobbins, W. O. III and Kawarishi, H. (1981). Bacillary characteristics in Whipple's disease: an electron microscopic study. *Gastroenterology*, **80**, 1468

10. Morson, B. C. and Dawson, I. M. P. (1979). *Gastrointestinal Pathology*, 2nd edn, Chap. 20. (Oxford: Blackwell Scientific Publications)

11. Asakura, H., Morita, A., Morishita, T., Tsuchiya, M., Fukumi, H., Ohashi, M., Uylangco, C. and Castro, A. (1973). Pathological findings from intestinal biopsy specimens in human cholera. *Am. J. Dig. Dis.*, **18**, 271

12. Arbuckle, J. R. B. (1972). The attachment of *Clostridium welchii (Cl. perfringens)* type C to intestinal villi of pigs. *J. Pathol.*, **106**, 65

13. Whalen, G. E., Rosenberg, E. G., Strickland, G. T., Gutman, R. A., Cross, J. H., Watten, R. H., Uylangco, C. and Dizon, J. J. (1969). Intestinal capillariasis: a new disease in man. *Lancet*, **1**, 13

14. Trier, J. S., Moxey, P. C., Schimmel, E. M., and Robles, E. (1974). Chronic intestinal coccidiomycosis in man: intestinal morphology and response to treatment. *Gastroenterology*, **66**, 923

15. Whitehead, R., Roca, M., Mekle, D. D., Skinner, J. and Truelove, S. C. (1975). The histological classification of duodenitis in fibre optic biopsy specimens. *Digestion*, **13**, 129

16. Hasan, M. and Ferguson, A. (1981). Measurements of intestinal villi in non-specific and ulcer-associated duodenitis – correlation between area of microdissected villus and villus epithelial cell count. *J. Clin. Pathol.*, **34**, 1181

17. Hasan, M., Sircus, W. and Ferguson, A. (1981). Duodenal mucosal architecture in non-specific and ulcer-associated duodenitis. *Gut*, **22**, 637

18. Bransom, C. J., Boxer, M. E., Palmer, K. R., Clark, J. C., Underwood, J. C. E. and Duthie, H. L. (1971). Mucosal cell proliferation in duodenal ulcer and duodenitis. *Gut*, **22**, 277

Disorders which affect the lymphoid tissues of the small intestine can be diffuse or localized; only the former are likely to be sampled on biopsy, and it is principally these that are discussed here.

Within the normal lamina propria are numbers of lymphocytes which can be shown to include both B and T cells. Lymphocytes emigrate onto the mucosal surface where they are thought to sample antigenic material. Some at least of those that are stimulated immigrate back into the lamina propria. Emigrating and immigrating cells can be seen as interepithelial lymphocytes in normal villi but cannot be distinguished one from another. Recent studies indicate that the majority are T cells.

Once returned, any B cells stimulated are likely to proliferate to form clones of plasma cells which will secrete specific antibody: it is also probable that antigens cross the enterocyte barrier and stimulate appropriate B lymphocytes within the lamina propria.

The IgA formed enters enterocytes as a monomer, unites with secretory piece within the enterocyte and passes out as a dimeric antibody onto the mucosal surface. IgM probably does the same but to a lesser extent. IgG is absorbed into the plasma and does not appear on the mucosal surface. Antibodies within plasma cells are readily identified using fluorescent or peroxidase techniques. It is likely that T cells which have immigrated proliferate and form some at least of the aggregates of lymphoid cells normally seen in lamina propria and submucosa.

There are also macrophages in the lamina propria, readily demonstrable using an acid phosphatase technique (Figure 13.1).

It is well known that diffuse disorders affecting lymphocytes and plasma cells occur in small intestinal mucosa and can be recognized in biopsy material. Problems in terminology have arisen in the diffuse lymphoma group in that what may well be the same tumours are described as being malignant histiocytosis of the intestine with a presumed origin from a monocyte/macrophage cell or as immunoblastic sarcomas with a presumed origin from an immune competent cell. It is usually sufficient on biopsy material to recognize the cells concerned as malignant.

Diffuse Immunodeficiency States

The majority of patients with inherited or acquired defects in cellular or humoral immunity do not have clinical evidence of malabsorption and have histologically normal intestinal biopsies. In many with humoral immune defects detailed differential counts of plasma cells using antisera to IgA, IgG and IgM will show an absolute diminution in all types of cell. Patients with defects in cellular immunity often have diminished numbers of lymphocytes[1]. A small group already referred to as hypogammaglobulinaemic sprue (page 74) have combined gluten-induced enteropathy (g.i.e.) and IgA deficiency with a flat mucosa, while others may have associated giardial infestation (page 78) which, if severe, may itself lead to mucosal flattening with infiltration of the lamina propria by eosinophils and histiocytes. Some patients with immune deficiency syndromes also have nodular lymphoid hyperplasia (not to be confused with multiple lymphomatous polyposis – see below) and this can occasionally be biopsied. Appearances are of follicles, usually with clearly defined hyperplastic germinal centres, in the lamina propria (Figure 13.2). The mucosa immediately over a follicle may appear flattened (Figure 13.2) but this is a local phenomenon and adjacent villi are not affected. Sometimes the noules do not have germinal centres (Figure 13.3). Nodular lymphoid hyperplasia can also occur in the absence of immunologial defect[2] but appears always to be a reactive process. In my view morphometry, especially the counting of absolute numbers of lymphocytes and differential counts of plasma cells using immunocytochemical techniques, has a definite place in biopsies from patients with suspected immunological defect.

Multiple Lymphomatous Polyposis

This condition, which is rare but well described[3], is not to be confused with nodular lymphoid hyperplasia. It commonly involves small and large bowel and affects an older age group, usually those over 50 years; there is no regular association with giardiasis though there may be dysgammaglobulinaemia. On biopsy small nodules without germinal centres, consisting of lymphocytes and histiocytes, are found in the lamina propria and not uncommonly infiltrate the muscularis mucosae (Figure 13.4). Generalized diffuse lymphosarcomatous change or a localized lymphoma can follow. There is no primary mucosal disturbance and the lymphoid nodules, though they commonly project as polyps, rarely ulcerate the overlying epithelium.

Immunoproliferative Small Intestinal Disease (α-Heavy Chain Disease)

This condition is widespread in Middle Eastern countries but is also found in South Africa and elsewhere. Young adults, usually male, present with diarrhoea, abdominal pain and fever and are found to have malabsorption. Examination of serum shows the presence of free Fc portions of IgA consisting of parts of the heavy chain.

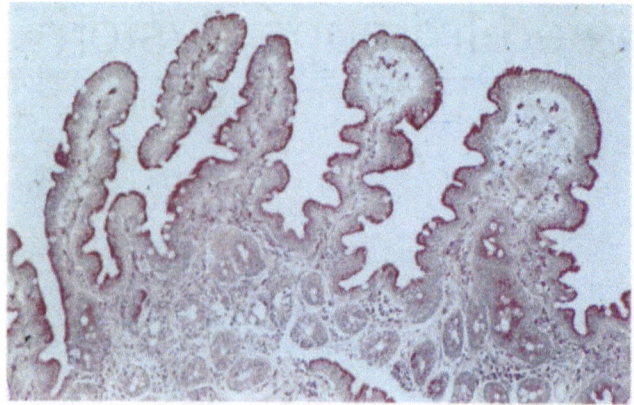

Figure 13.1   Normal biopsy, acid phosphatase technique. Phagolysosomes within enterocytes and macrophages in the lamina propria are both well delineated.   ×80

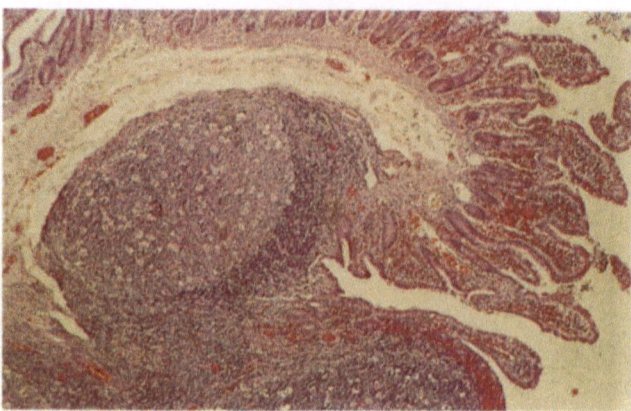

Figure 13.2   Nodular lymphoid hyperplasia in a resected specimen. Germinal centres are conspicuous and the mucosa overlying the nodule is flattened. H & E × 32

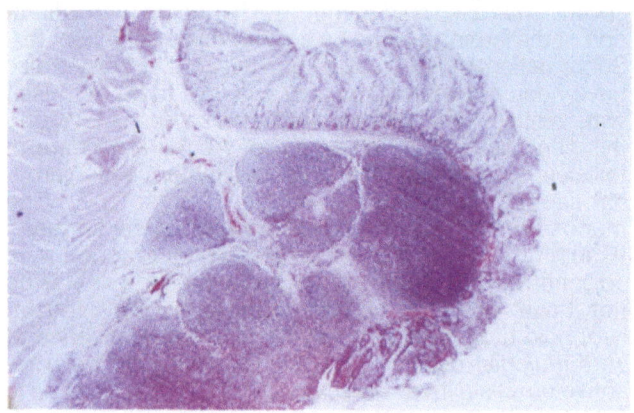

Figure 13.3   Nodular lymphoid hyperplasia in a resected specimen. Germinal centres were not present in this example.   H & E × 20

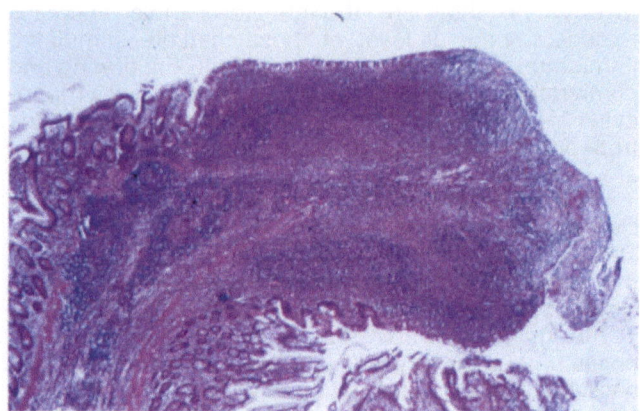

Figure 13.4   Multiple lymphomatous polyposis. This nodule, which had no germinal centre, has infiltrated the muscularis. The cells are lymphocytes and histiocytes.   H & E × 32

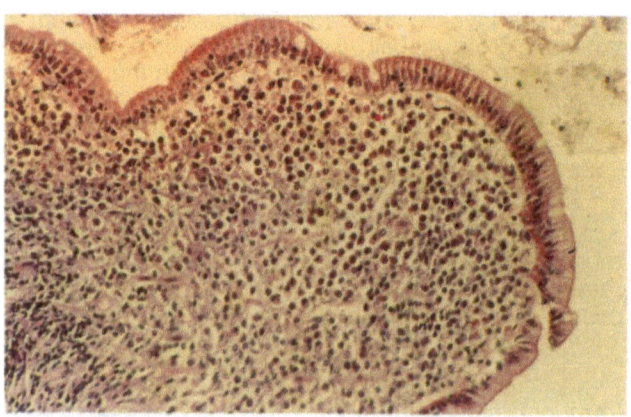

Figure 13.5   Immunoproliferative small intestinal disease. The lamina propria contains numerous plasma cells and there is some villous flattening but surface enterocytes are normal.   H & E × 125

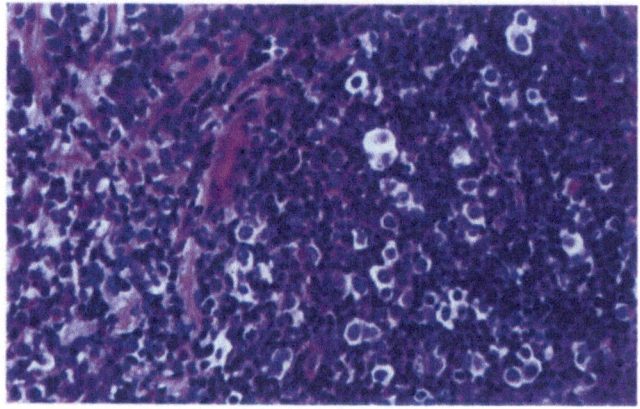

Figure 13.6   Immunoproliferative small intestinal disease. Plasma cells, lymphocytes and histiocytes are all present. Subsequent laparotomy revealed immunoblastic sarcoma in three separate sites.   H & E × 320

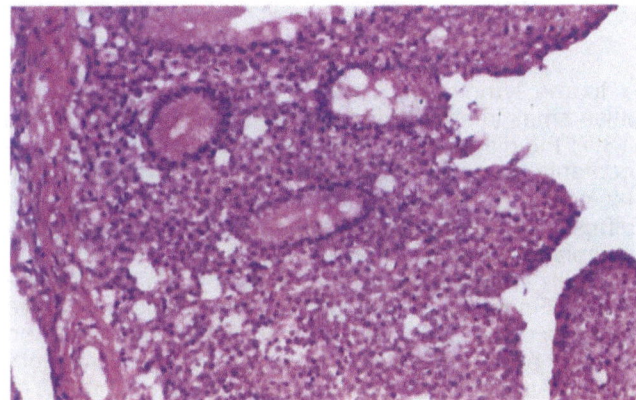

Figure 13.7 Immunoproliferative small intestinal disease; immunoblastic sarcoma. Plasmacytoid cells in the lamina propria show pleomorphism which was diffuse through a considerable length of jejunum. H & E × 125

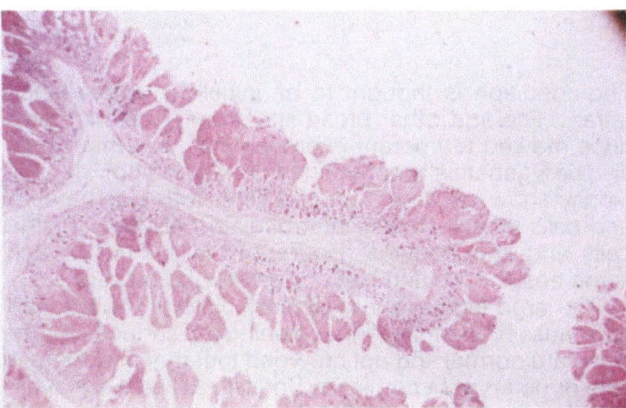

Figure 13.8 Waldenstrom's macroglobulinaemia. Enlarged histiocytes containing eosinophilic material are clearly shown. Appearances can mimic Whipple's disease but the material is not PAS-positive. H & E × 20

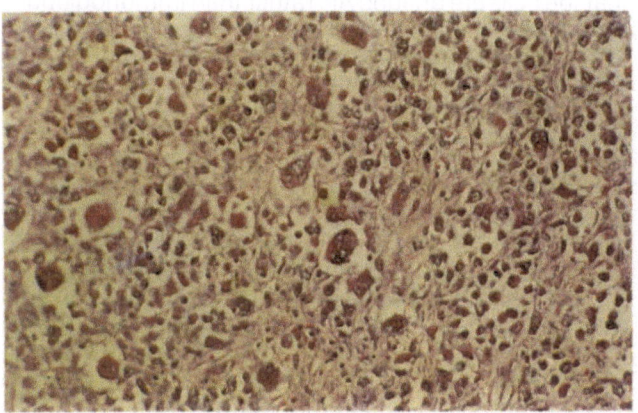

Figure 13.9 Diffuse immunoblastic lymphoma. Tumour cells are pleomorphic and giant cell forms are numerous. H & E × 250

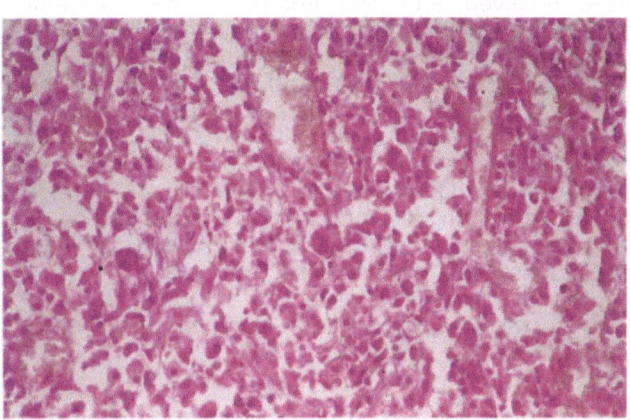

Figure 13.10 Malignant lymphoma in gluten-induced enteropathy. Appearances here are those of immunoblastic sarcoma, as in Figure 13.9, including the presence of tumour giant cells. H & E × 250

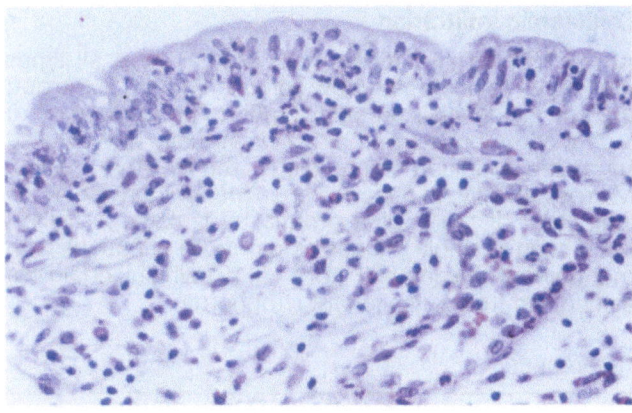

Figure 13.11 So-called 'early' or prelymphoma in g.i.e. The mucosa is flattened and the surface enterocytes crowded as in g.i.e., but in addition there are single histiocytes lying below and infiltrating surface epithelium. This patient subsequently developed a diffuse lymphoma. H & E × 250

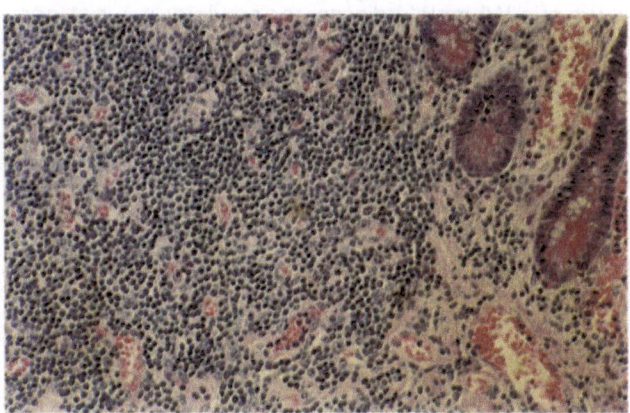

Figure 13.12 Leukaemic infiltration. This patient was diagnosed on this biopsy as having a malignant lymphoma. Subsequent haematological studies showed him to have a monocytoid leukaemia and a careful restudy of the biopsy showed monocytoid cells in the more general lymphocytic cell picture. See also Figure 14.5. H & E × 125

The condition is thought to be initially infective since tetracycline and other broad-spectrum antibiotics produce marked temporary improvement[4], but there may also be a genetically determined predisposition[5]. Jejunal biopsy shows a lamina propria filled with plasma cells and cells which appear intermediate between plasma cells and lymphocytes (Figures 13.5 and 13.6) and some eosinophils and histiocytes may be present.

The large increase in cellularity distorts the villi and can cause broadening and flattening but surface enterocytes are normal and not crowded together and there is little or no crypt hyperplasia. Specific antisera are available for detecting heavy chains and these may be of value. This is the commonly seen picture; some workers recognize a second pattern with diffuse follicular lymphoid hyperplasia and fewer plasma cells[6] and there is good reason for preferring the title immunoproliferative small intestinal disease to that of α-chain disease.

Some patients respond initially to broad-spectrum antibiotics though little is recorded as to changes in subsequent biopsies. Many, however, including some who have received antibiotic treatment, will eventually develop malignant lymphomas which may be diffuse or localized; the latter can be single or multiple[6]. These are generally described as immunoblastic sarcomas (Figure 13.7) and are thought to derive from the B cells which give rise to the original abnormal plasma cells. One group of workers[6] believes that when the original disorder has the pattern of a diffuse follicular lymphoid hyperplasia the neoplasm which develops will be an undifferentiated lymphosarcoma. All of the ones which I have seen are to me suggestive of immunoblastic sarcoma.

Recently occasional patients have been described with γ- rather than α-heavy chain disease[7]; biopsy appearances are identical.

Monoclonal IgM Gammopathy (Waldenstrom's Macroglobulinaemia)

Intestinal changes in this gammopathy are rare but are very distinctive when they do occur[8]. The small intestinal mucosa presents a slightly nodular appearance. Microscopically the principal feature is the large number of histiocytes in the lamina propria. These have a fine foamy cytoplasm which contains structureless eosinophilic material (Figure 13.8) which can superficially mimic Whipple's disease or amyloid; it is not normally PAS-positive, does not have the ultrastructural appearances of amyloid or show any bacterial forms and does not stain with Congo red. It is probably macroglobulin. The deposits produce secondary distortion of villus architecture but there is no primary damage.

Diffuse Intestinal Lymphomas

Most primary and nearly all secondary lymphomas in the small intestine form discrete tumours which are unlikely to be biopsied. Diffuse lymphomas occur particularly in association with coeliac syndromes, including g.i.e. and idiopathic steatorrhoea and also in some inflammatory bowel conditions including Crohn's disease[9]. Their incidence in immunoproliferative small intestinal disease and in multiple lymphomatous polyposis has already been discussed. There is also some evidence[10] that isolated single cells or small groups of abnormal cells can be found in biopsies long before overt lymphoma appears. The diffuse lesion has been defined by different workers as immunoblastic lymphoma[11,12] or malignant histiocytosis of the intestine[13,14].

In the lymphoma associated with immunoproliferative small intestinal disease already described (Figure 13.7) the diagnosis of immunoblastic lymphoma is acceptable. Tumours are usually multiple but discrete, but, by courtesy of colleagues in Baghdad, I have seen diffuse examples sampled by biopsy. The lamina propria is replaced by a pleomorphic lymphoma in which plasma cells are present and tumour giant cells often numerous (Figure 13.9). Such growths can be (and have been) mistaken for Hodgkin's disease; but this condition is in my experience rare in the bowel and the giant cells are not typical Reed–Sternberg cells. In some, but not all, examples, α-chain production can be demonstrated immunocytochemically[12].

Localized and diffuse lymphomas are also associated with g.i.e. and with idiopathic steatorrhoea. These appear to be diffuse malignant histiocytomas of the intestine[13,14] rather than immunoblastic since individual tumour cells contain lysozyme, many contain C3 element of complement and some contain all major classes of heavy chain and both light chains, which suggests that the cells are phagocytic rather than immunoglobulin synthesizers. Nevertheless, as with the immunoblastic lymphomas, plasma cells are present as are giant cells and I am not certain that the distinction is not more one of terminology than of pattern (Figure 13.10). In biopsies one should look particularly for evidence of phagocytosis, but in practice the important thing is to determine whether or not some form of malignant lymphoid tumour is present.

Some very interesting studies are now available on possible early lesions[10]: they have made use of studies on 'normal' or 'uninvolved' mucosa in patients who have had proven 'lymphoma' elsewhere, and on earlier biopsies from patients who have subsequently developed the disease. Significant findings are the presence of small groups of apparently normal histiocytes lying almost immediately beneath the surface epithelium and sometimes infiltrating into it (Figure 13.11); occasionally there are small crypt abscesses associated with gland destruction by the histiocytes. I have looked for and found these changes myself, but I have not studied enough material to be certain of their significance.

There is also some evidence that diffuse malignant histiocytosis is related to ulcerative jejunitis[13].

Leukaemic Infiltration

About 15% of all patients with leukaemia of all types who come to necropsy show some infiltration in the gut: the true incidence is probably higher. The jejunum is not a very common site and biopsy is virtually never called for as the condition can be diagnosed by other means. Microscopically, in resected specimens, there is diffuse infiltration of the lamina propria by leukaemic cells: I have seen a single jejunal biopsy from a patient with monocytoid leukaemia (Figure 13.12) which I could not distinguish from a malignant lymphoma.

References

1. Eidelman, S. (1976). Intestinal lesions in immune deficiency. *Hum. Pathol.*, **7**, 427

2. Matuchansky, C., Duprey, F., Briaud, M., Babin, P., Touchard, G., Block, P., Le Normand, Y. and Morichau-Beauchaut, M. (1982). Diffuse nodular lymphoid hyperplasia of the adult small intestine without detectable systemic or digestive immunodeficiency. *Gastroenterol. Clin. Biol.*, **6**, 239 (French: English summary)

Continued on page 90

Isolated and Localized Lesions

Hamartomatous polyps, neoplasms, developmental anomalies and vascular disorders all occur in the small intestine but are localized and therefore not normally subject to biopsy. They are, however, important in two ways. First, it is now possible to biopsy localized lesions in the first and second part of the duodenum under direct vision. I have now seen biopsies from two patterns of endocrine cell tumour (Figures 14.1 and 14.2), mucosal spread from a carcinoma of pancreas (Figure 14.3), and a carcinoma at the ampulla of Vater in a patient with gluten-induced enteropathy (g.i.e.) (Figure 14.4), and this list will increase as small intestinal biopsy instrumentation improves.

Second, a blind biopsy may by chance sample the edge of a localized lesion. It is not likely to be diagnostic under these conditions, but it is important to remember that villous flattening with inflammatory change is a common finding at the margin of local lesions of whatever aetiology. The presence of unusual mononuclear cells may alert one to the possibility of a leukaemic infiltrate (Figure 14.5), while progressive flattening proceeding to ulceration or pseudopyloric metaplasia may suggest the possibility of an ischaemic lesion (Figure 14.6). The adverse prognostic significance of subepithelial histiocytes in g.i.e. has already been mentioned (page 86 and Figure 13.11).

Other Generalized Disorders

Amyloid Disease

Jejunal biopsy is not used for the routine diagnosis of amyloid disease but amyloid can occasionally be seen in biopsies taken from other disease conditions. It is usually found in the coats of small and medium-sized arteries in the submucosa, when this is included in the biopsy (Figure 14.7): I have only once seen it in lamina proprial vessels, but it can be present in the muscularis mucosae.

Systemic Sclerosis

The changes in this disorder are usually confined to the submucosa and muscularis propria, but jejunal biopsy can show oedema of lamina propria which progresses slowly to fibrosis and collagenization. It is very doubtful if these changes could ever be diagnostic in a mucosal biopsy.

Systemic Mast Cell Disease

Malabsorption with subtotal villous flattening and an increase in number of mast cells in the lamina propria has been described[1,2]. I have never seen a biopsy from this condition.

Mucoviscidosis

There has been much debate as to whether, in small or large intestinal biopsies, there is any qualitative or quantitative difference in the mucosa from normal and whether abnormalities in secreted mucin are histochemically detectable[3]. All studies, including our own, have shown that the only histological change is an enlargement of individual goblet cells, not always sufficient to be diagnostic, and an increased volume of histochemically normal mucin between individual villi. Studies on the ileal mucosa in resected specimens from patients with meconium ileus confirm these views (Figure 14.8).

Lymphangiectasia

Patients with lymphangiectasia present with diarrhoea, steatorrhoea and evidence of protein loss which in turn may produce ascites and oedema. The serum albumin is low. The condition is readily diagnosed on biopsy (Figure 14.9). Villi are often distorted by the presence within the lamina propria of dilated lymphatics, and there may be concomitant oedema. The muscularis mucosae may show the pigment of 'brown bowel' syndrome (see below).

'Brown Bowel' Syndrome

It is now well recognized that many patients with malabsorption or protein loss from whatever cause may, at laparotomy, show a curious golden-brown colouration of the bowel wall[4]. This is due to the presence of pigment granules, which have the histochemical properties and autofluorescence of lipofuscin and lie within smooth muscle cells of the muscularis propria (Figures 14.10 and 14.11). In some but not all patients this pigment can also be seen in the muscularis mucosae. When found there, usually as an incidental observation, it is an indication for the administration of a high-protein diet and vitamin supplements.

Endometriosis

Endometriosis occasionally involves the small intestine and can produce obstruction necessitating operation. I have never seen it in a biopsy but the illustration (Figure 14.12) from a resected specimen indicates that if biopsy of small bowel lesions under direct vision is further developed such a lesion may occasionally be encountered.

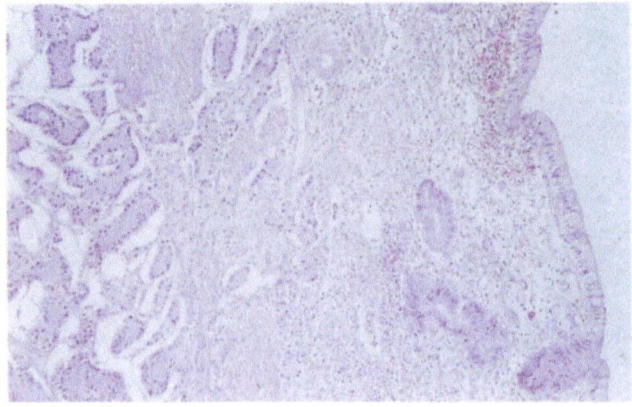

Figure 14.1 Endocrine cell tumour in duodenum. There was marked overlying mucosal flattening, the reason for which was not determined. H & E × 100

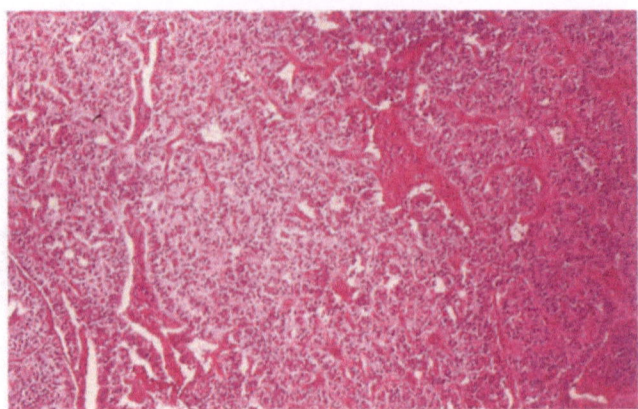

Figure 14.2 Endocrine cell tumour in duodenum. The ribbon pattern suggests a possible origin from pancreatic rest. H & E × 100

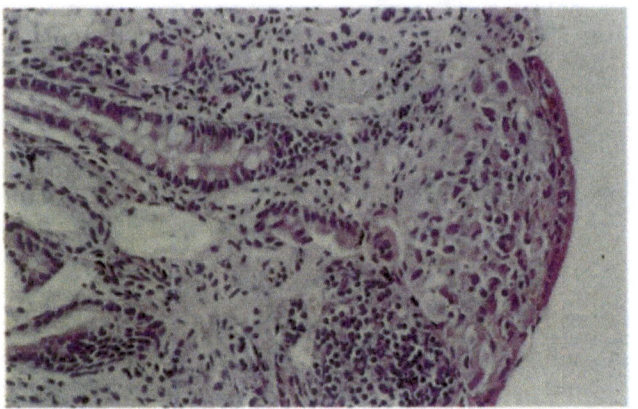

Figure 14.3 Secondary carcinoma of pancreas producing a duodenal mucosal nodule which was biopsied. The carcinoma cells lie immediately beneath the mucosa. H & E × 320

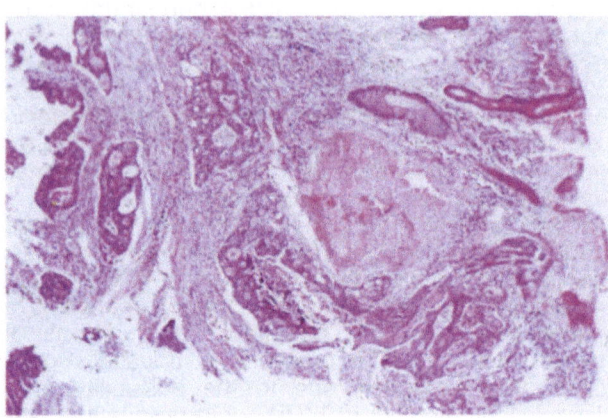

Figure 14.4 Carcinoma of duodenum in g.i.e. The growth lay near the ampulla of Vater and clinically caused jaundice in a patient with g.i.e. H & E × 65

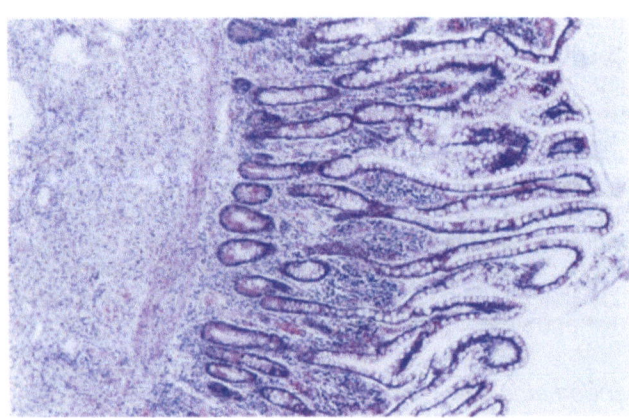

Figure 14.5 Monocytoid leukaemia. This jejunal biopsy came from a young man thought clinically to have immuno-proliferative small bowel disease. Histology suggested a lymphoma or a leukaemic infiltrate; the latter proved to be correct. See also Figure 13.12. H & E × 80

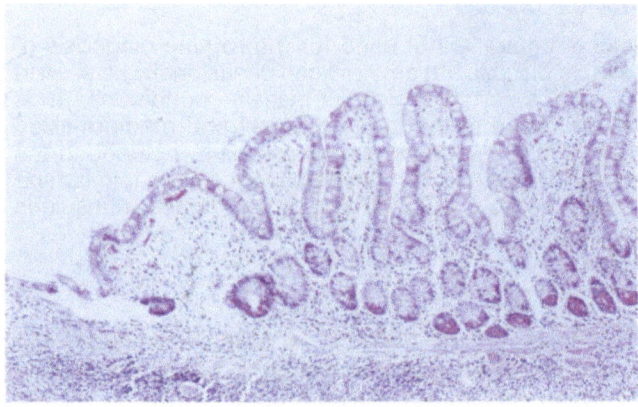

Figure 14.6 Ischaemic ulceration in lower duodenum. The relatively normal mucosa at the right-hand side tails away to an ulcer on the left, which is becoming covered by a single layer of regenerative epithelium. This biopsy was taken from the ulcer edge under direct vision. H & E × 80

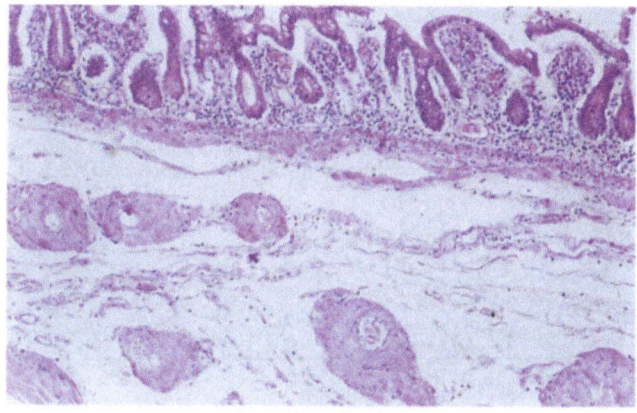

Figure 14.7 Amyloid. This was an unexpected finding in a jejunal biopsy for malabsorption in a middle-aged woman. The walls of submucosal arteries show heavy deposits of extracellular amyloid.   H & E × 125

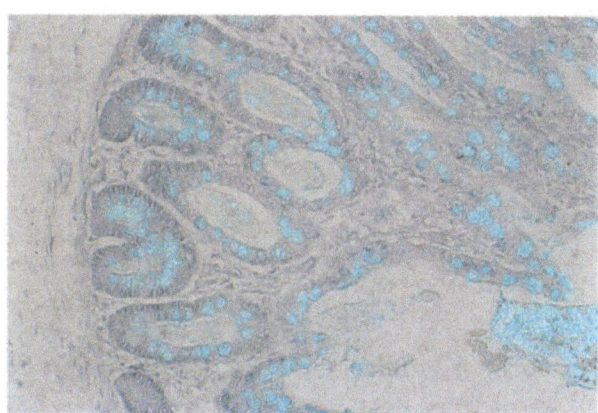

Figure 14.8 Ileum in mucoviscidosis. The enlarged goblet cells, which are slightly increased in number, contain histochemically normal sialomucin.   Alcian blue pH 2.5 × 100

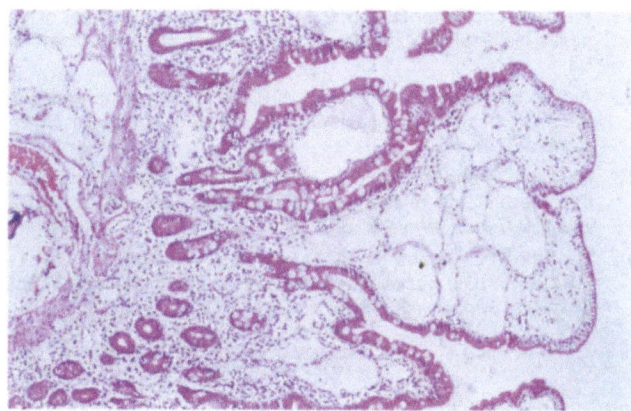

Figure 14.9 Lymphangiectasia. Jejunal villi are distorted due to marked dilation of lymphatics in the lamina propria. Similar dilation is just visible in the submucosa and can also be present in mesenteric lymph nodes.   H & E × 65

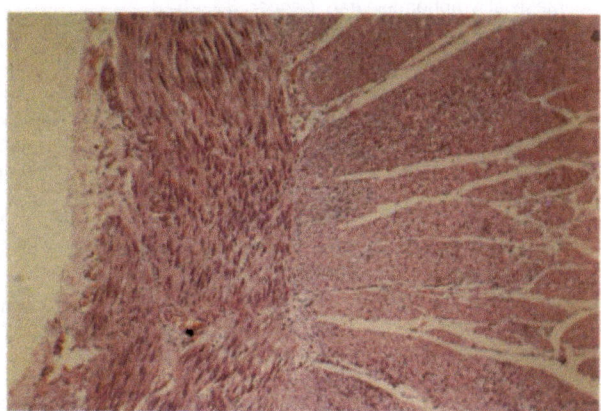

Figure 14.10 Brown bowel syndrome, resected specimen. The altered smooth muscle fibres are clearly seen especially in the longitudinal muscle (right).   H & E × 80

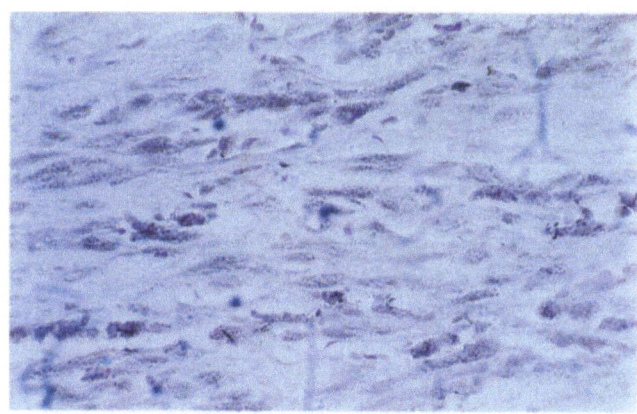

Figure 14.11 Higher-power view of Figure 14.10. Granules of pigment can be seen within individual muscle cells.   H & E × 250

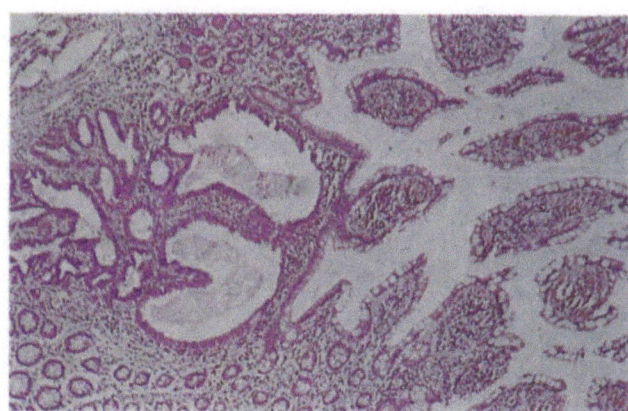

Figure 14.12 Endometriosis. An island of endometrial glands can be seen in this ileal specimen. Later resection confirmed the presence of more generalized endometriosis.   H & E × 200

References

1. Scott, B.B., Hardy, G.J. and Losowsky, M.S. (1975). Involvement of the small intestine in systemic mast cell disease. *Gut,* **16,** 918

2. Ammann, R.W., Vetter, D., Deyhle, P., Tschen, H., Sulser, H. and Schmid, M. (1976). Gastrointestinal involvement in systemic mastocytosis. *Gut,* **17,** 107

3. Johansen, P.G. and Kay, R. (1969). Histochemistry of the rectal mucosa in cystic fibrosis of the pancreas. *J. Pathol.,* **99**, 299

4. Foster, C.S. (1979). The brown-bowel syndrome: a possible smooth muscle mitochondrial myopathy? *Histopathology,* **3**, 1

References to Chapter 13 – continued

3. Sheahan, D.G., Martin, F., Baginsky, S., Mallory, G.K. and Zamcheck, N. (1971). Multiple lymphomatous polyposis of the gastrointestinal tract. *Cancer,* **28**, 408

4. Russell, R.M., Abadi, P. and Ismail-Beigi, F. (1977). Role of bacterial overgrowth in the malabsorption syndrome of primary small intestinal lymphoma in Iran. *Cancer,* **39**, 2579

5. Nikbin, B., Banisadre, M., Ala, F. and Mojtabai, A. (1979). HLA AW19, B12 in immunoproliferative small intestinal disease. *Gut,* **20**, 226

6. Nassar, V.H., Salem, P.A., Shahid, M.J., Alami, S.Y., Balikian, J.B., Salem, A.A. and Nasrallah, S.M. (1978). 'Mediterranean abdominal lymphoma' or immunoproliferative small intestinal disease. Part II. Pathological aspects. *Cancer,* **41**, 1340

7. Bender, S.W., Danon, F., Preud'homme, J.L., Posselt, H.G., Roettger, P. and Seligmann, M. (1978). Gamma heavy chain disease simulating alpha chain disease. *Gut,* **19**, 1148

8. Bedine, M.S., Yardley, J.H., Elliott, H.L., Banwell, J.G. and Hendrix, T.R. (1973). Intestinal involvement in Waldenstrom's macroglobulinaemia. *Gastroenterology,* **65**, 308

9. Lewin, K.J., Ranchod, N. and Dorfmann, R.F. (1978). Lymphomas of the gastrointestinal tract. A study of 117 cases presenting with gastrointestinal disease. *Cancer,* **42**, 693

10. Isaacson, P. (1980). Malignant histiocytosis of the intestine: the early histological lesion. *Gut,* **21**, 381

11. Henry, K. and Farrer-Brown, G. (1977). Primary lymphomas of the gastrointestinal tract. 1. Plasma cell tumours. *Histopathology,* **1**, 53

12. Al-Saleem, T. and Zardawi, I.M. (1979). Primary lymphomas of the small intestine in Iraq: a pathological study of 145 cases. *Histopathology,* **3**, 89

13. Isaacson, P. and Wright, D.H. (1978). Malignant histiocytosis of the intestine. Its relationship to malabsorption and ulcerative jejunitis. *Hum. Pathol.,* **9**, 661

14. Isaacson, P., Wright, D.H., Judd, M.A. and Mepham, B.L. (1979). Primary gastrointestinal lymphomas. A classification of 66 cases. *Cancer,* **43**, 1805

The normal large intestine presents a haustrated appearance, but the mucosa covering it appears, on superficial inspection, to have a smooth surface, giving a 'fold and furrow' effect (Figure 15.1), which is greatly exaggerated in diverticular disease. Longitudinal sections show a further series of corrugations sometimes called innominate grooves, or, more classically, palmettes or antheniums[1] (Figure 15.2), with tall straight central crypts abutted on either side by shorter ones which curve outward. The cause of these is unknown. The normal mucosa consists of straight unbranched tubules at right angles to the lumen and opening onto the luminal surface (Figure 15.3). At the base of each tubule is a crypt zone in which undifferentiated stem cells mature as they grow upwards (Figure 15.4) and differentiate into goblet and absorptive cells; the former are more numerous in the deeper part of the crypt, the latter towards the surface. A fibroblastic sheath surrounds the crypt zone. Detailed histochemical studies have shown that in the right and transverse colons sialomucins predominate in the lower one-third of the mucosa (Figure 15.5), while in the descending and sigmoid colons and the rectum the pattern reverses and sulphomucins predominate in the lower third with sialo- and sulphomucins present equally in the upper two-thirds (Figure 15.6) and in surface goblet cells[1-4]. Endocrine cells, some argentaffin, some argyrophil, and others which do not stain with either technique, are present also at the bases of crypts; occasional Paneth cells are normally present in the caecum and ascending colon but not elsewhere.

The lamina propria contains plasma cells, lymphocytes and occasional eosinophils; techniques for cholinesterase also demonstrate fine nerve fibrils within it (Figure 15.7). Immunocytochemical studies combined with differential plasma cell counts show that the normal ratio of IgA : IgG : IgM-containing plasma cells is 100 : 16 : 9 (Figure 15.8). Immunological techniques are also available for demonstrating the precise hormonal content of many endocrine cells (Figure 10.11) as well as other substances such as fibrolectin.

The muscularis mucosae is well formed. The submucosa contains collagen, elastic and reticulin fibres, blood vessels and lymphatics and a variable but usually small amount of adipose tissue. Ganglion cells and nerve fibres are present in the submucosal plexus and are readily demonstrated using histochemical esterase techniques (Figures 15.9 and 15.10). These techniques are invaluable in Hirschsprung's disease.

Aggregates of lymphocytes, with or without germinal follicles, are present in lamina propria, muscularis and submucosa, often bridging the muscularis and so lying within all three compartments (Figure 15.11). In children they can enlarge sufficiently to be visible endoscopically as yellowish-white nodules 1-2 mm in diameter[5].

The normal anal canal is lined partly by cloacal, partly by ectodermal epithelium and can be divided into three zones. The lowest zone extends from the anal verge, where the true skin ends, to the mucocutaneous junction which is approximately Hilton's 'white line' and is lined by squamous epithelium in which some skin appendages are present. The middle zone extends upwards to the dentate (pectinate) line and is lined by modified squamous epithelium without skin appendages. The uppermost zone is lined by epithelium transitional between squamous and columnar, which often has a cuboidal structure and is sometimes called cloacogenic; it blends with the columnar and glandular epithelium of the rectum. Anal ducts, which drain the anal glands lying in the submucosa and sometimes within the internal sphincter itself, open into the canal just above the dentate line (Figure 15.12). The various paterns of epithelium already described intermingle in this zone.

Large Intestinal Biopsies

Large intestinal biopsies fall naturally into three groups, all of which are taken under some form of direct vision. The most common is still the relatively large, usually single biopsy taken through a proctoscope or a sigmoidoscope from a visible localized lesion or a more generalized inflammation such as a polyp or a generally reddened eroded or ulcerated mucosa. It has the advantage, when properly taken, of adequate depth which includes some submucosa, is usually easy to orientate and can be placed on filter paper by the clinician. With the development of colonoscopes and fibreoptics, small multiple biopsies from the colon as far proximal as the caecum can be taken under direct vision. They are more superficial, often consisting of mucosa only which is sometimes not full thickness, and are best orientated in the laboratory. They permit a wider range of biopsy diagnosis. Certain storage disorders in children can be diagnosed by appropriate histochemical studies on myenteric or, less readily, submucosal ganglion cells[6], demanding a full-thickness biopsy (see page 150). Until recently similar biopsies were needed in Hirschsprung's disease but some success is now claimed for mucosal punch biopsies and a cholinesterase technique for this condition[7] is described on page 146. They should be sent to the laboratory, unfixed, wrapped in gauze moistened in saline to prevent dehydration during transport.

Besides their value in pure diagnosis, large intestinal biopsies have a major role in continuing patient surveillance. They can be used to assess activity and response to treatment in ulcerative colitis, to reveal dysplasia in patients with long-standing colitis and to study the possible recurrence of familial adenomas after fulguration,

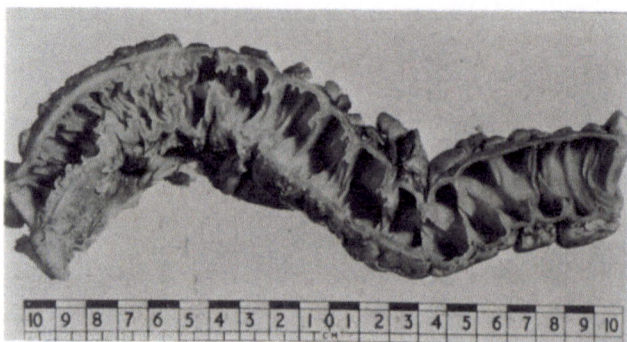

Figure 15.1 Descending colon in diverticular disease. Normal haustration is visible on the right, becoming increased as the zone of diverticular disease is approached on the left

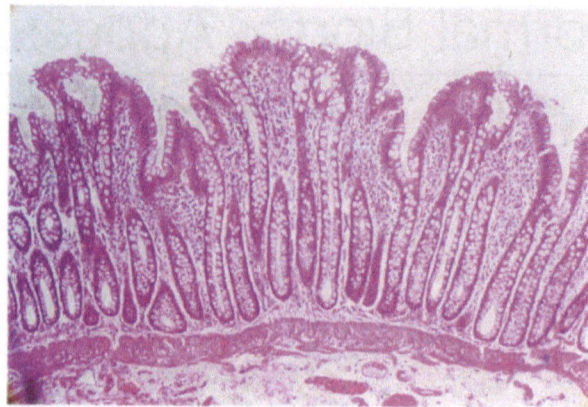

Figure 15.2 Normal rectal mucosa showing the innominate grooves. H & E × 80

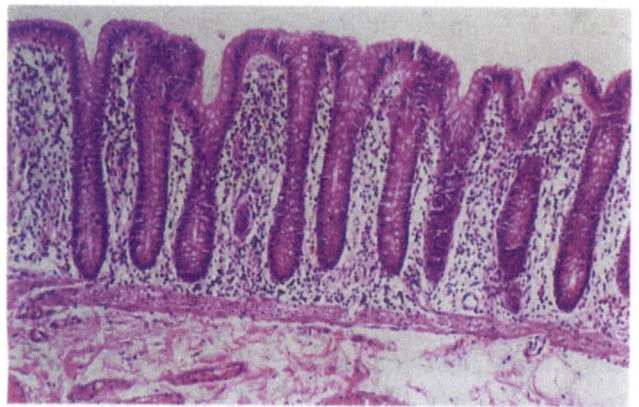

Figure 15.3 Normal large bowel mucosa. Tubules are straight and unbranched and goblet and absorptive cells can be clearly distinguished. H & E × 80

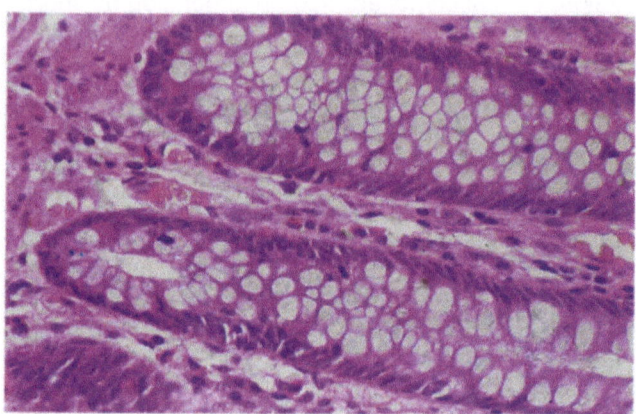

Figure 15.4 Normal crypt zone. There is only slight evidence of activity and goblet cells predominate. H & E × 320

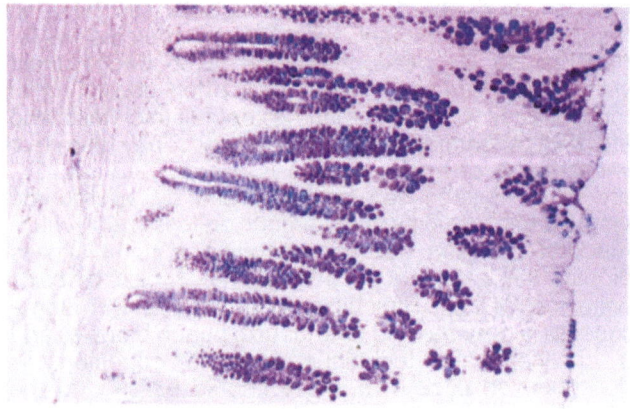

Figure 15.5 Normal ascending colon. Sialomucins (blue) predominate in the lower one-third of the mucosa with sulphomucins (brown) mainly in the upper two-thirds. High iron diamine (HID); Alcian blue (AB) × 125

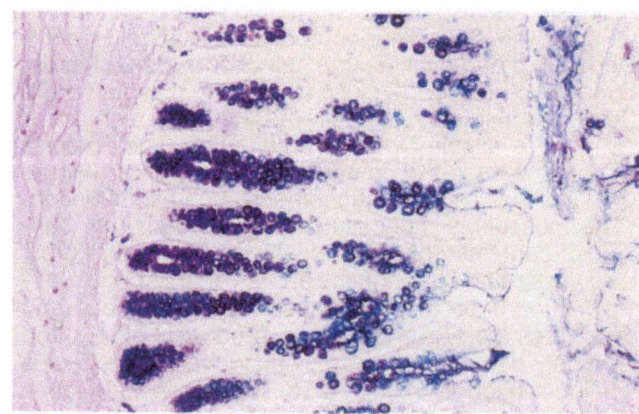

Figure 15.6 Normal sigmoid colon. Sulphomucins (brown) predominate in the lower part of the crypt, with both sulpho- and sialomucins in equal amounts in the upper part. HID-AB technique × 125

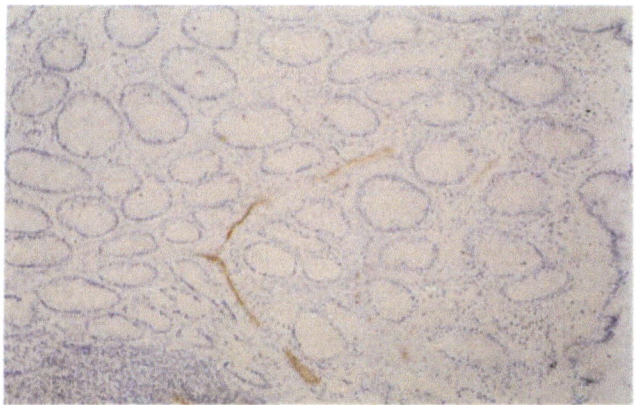

Figure 15.7 Normal rectum. Fine nerve fibres are present within the lamina propria. Cholinesterase technique × 320

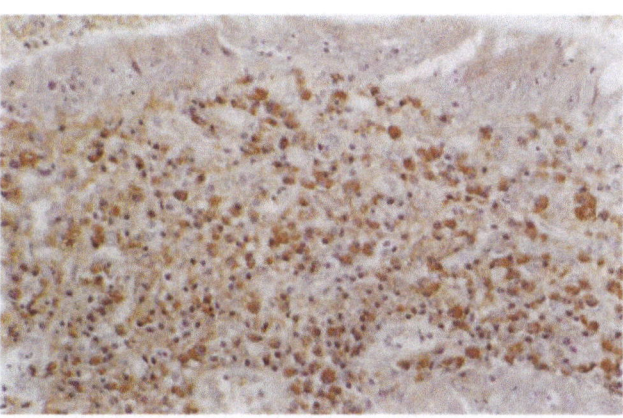

Figure 15.8 Normal rectum. Distribution of IgA-containing plasma cells in lamina propria. Peroxidase-antiperoxidase (PAP) technique × 320

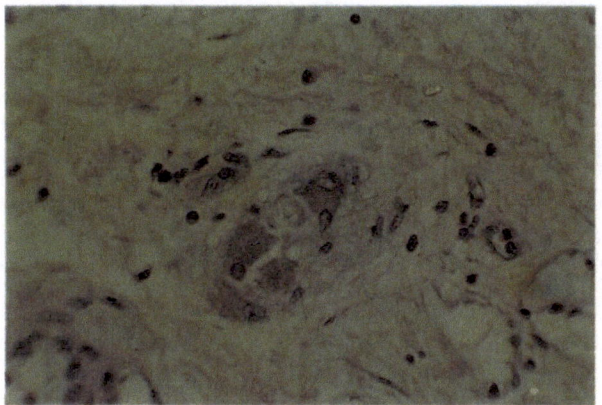

Figure 15.9 Normal ganglion cell in submucosal plexus. H & E × 320

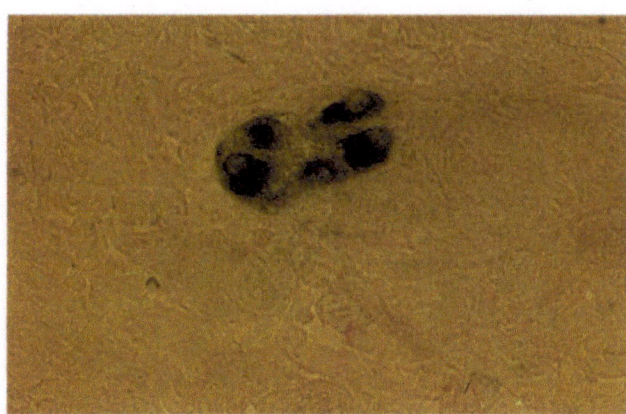

Figure 15.10 Normal ganglion cells, myenteric plexus. Indoxyl esterase technique × 320

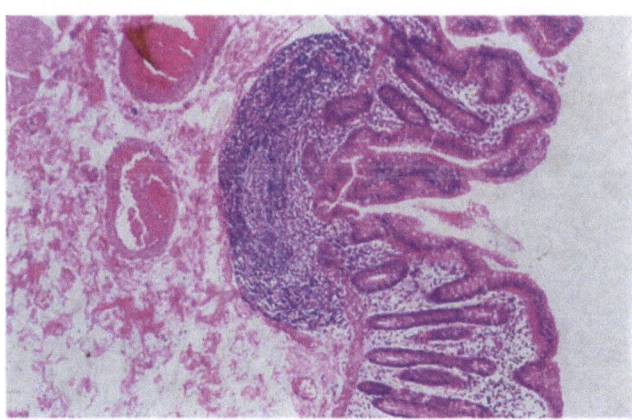

Figure 15.11 Normal rectum. Lymphoid aggregate lying astride the muscularis mucosae. H & E × 65

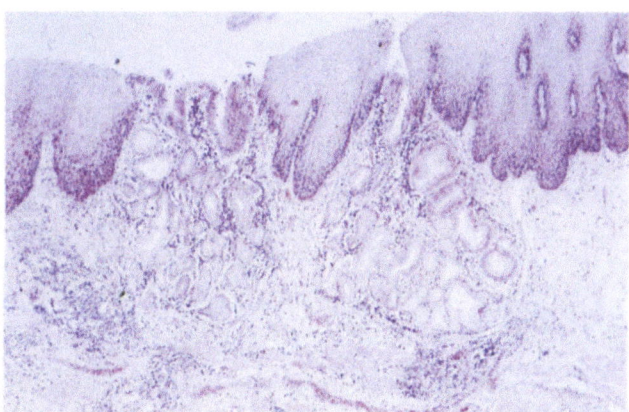

Figure 15.12 Normal anal cloacogenic zone. There is a mixture of squamous, columnar and basaloid epithelium with anal glands and a small ductule is just visible at the top of the right-hand group of glands. H & E × 65

to name but three examples. Every pathologist needs to be proficient in their interpretation and this section forms the greatest single part of the book.

Special Techniques of Value

Techniques for Mucosubstances

These include PAS with diastase for neutral, Alcian blue at pH 2.5 for acid non-sulphated (sialomucins) and Alcian blue at pH 0.5–1.0 for acid sulphated (sulpho-mucin) mucosubstances. The use of a high iron diamine technique allows sialomucins and sulphomucins to be demonstrated simultaneously. I have found these and more elaborate techniques valuable in attempting to differentiate acute colitis from acute Crohn's disease in patients with indeterminate colitis and in research, but not routine studies on dysplasia and the potential malignancy of different patterns of adenoma. Most routine biopsies can be interpreted without them.

Techniques for Esterases in Ganglion Cells and Nerve Fibres

Many pathologists, myself included, believe that cholin-esterase techniques are invaluable for detecting ganglion cells or their absence, and the presence of thickened nerve trunks in the lamina propria in suspected Hirschsprung's disease. The latter can be demonstrated in punch biopsies which do not include the myenteric plexus. Material should be received unfixed (see above). I have not found other enzyme techniques of diagnostic value.

Techniques for Investigation of Storage Disorders

This, though a specialized study, can be undertaken by any laboratory prepared to perform the special stains required[6]. Histochemical studies are more informative when linked with appropriate electron microscopy and in my view are best done in specialized centres. Special arrangements for transport of unfixed material will be necessary.

Immunocytochemical Techniques

It is practicable to localize IgA, IgG and IgM-containing plasma cells and to identify some at least of the hormones contained in endocrine cell granules, provided that reliable antisera are available. I do not find them of use routinely; the special instances in which they can be helpful are commented on in the text. Some laboratories prefer unfixed or specially fixed material and individual arrangements must be made.

References

1. Filipe, M. I. and Branfoot, A. C. (1974). Abnormal patterns of mucus secretion in apparently normal mucosa of large intestine with carcinoma. *Cancer*, **34**, 282

2. Filipe, M. I. and Branfoot, A. C. (1976). Mucin histochemistry of the colon. *Curr. Top. Pathol.*, **63**, 143

3. Lev, R. and Orlic, D. (1974). Histochemical and radioautographic studies of normal human fetal colon. *Histochemistry*, **39**, 301

4. Culling, C. F. A., Reid, P. E. and Dunn, W. L. (1976). A new histochemical method for the identification and visualization of both side chain acylated and non-acylated sialic acids. *J. Histochem. Cytochem.*, **24**, 1225

5. Riddlesberger, M. M. Jr and Lebenthal, E. (1980). Nodular colonic mucosa of childhood; normal or pathological? *Gastroenterology*, **79**, 265

6. Brett, E. M. and Lake, B. D. (1975). Reassessment of rectal approach to neuropathology in childhood. Review of 307 biopsies over 11 years. *Arch. Dis. Child.*, **50**, 753

7. Patrick, W. J. A, Besley, G. T. N. and Smith, I. I. (1980). Histochemical diagnosis of Hirschsprung's disease and a comparison of the histochemical and biochemical activity of acetyl-cholinesterase in rectal mucosal biopsies. *J. Clin. Pathol.*, **33**, 336

16

Large Intestine and Anal Canal: Patterns of Non-infective Inflammatory Bowel Disease

In this group are included Crohn's disease, ulcerative colitis and the mild non-specific proctocolitis from which it has to be distinguished, and those examples of colitis indeterminate in which acute ulcerative lesions cannot, on biopsy, be fitted into any definite category.

Crohn's Disease

This condition – first called regional ileitis since ileum and appendix are the sites most commonly involved, and later regional enteritis because of increasing recognition of large bowel involvement – is of undetermined aetiology. It is becoming increasingly common, has a high morbidity rate, shortens life expectancy and carries a slightly increased risk of carcinoma. The peak age incidence lies between 20 and 29, with a second smaller peak between 50 and 59 and a third from 70 to 79[1]. About 70% of all patients present with small intestinal disease which may later involve the large bowel; in some 30% the disease presents primarily either in small and large bowel simultaneously or in the large intestine alone[2]. Anal fissures or fistulae are not uncommon and should always suggest the possibility of large bowel lesions.

Macroscopic Appearances

Lesions can be single or multiple; when multiple they are usually discontinuous with skip zones of normal bowel between them. The disease involves the full thickness of the bowel wall including the serosa and often the local mesenteric lymph nodes[3]; fissures and mucosal ulceration are characteristic features and as might be expected with serosal involvement, adhesions and fistula formation are common, especially after resections.

Microscopic Appearances

Many pathologists looking at biopsy material prefer not to know the clinical history; my own belief is that the differential diagnosis can at times be so difficult that every available item of information, including particu-

larly the 'clinical sense' of a good physician, must be taken into consideration at some stage.

The earliest lesions visible endoscopically and likely to be biopsied are oedema, which is located in the submucosa and imparts rigidity to the bowel, small ulcers located on mucosal folds (Figure 16.1) and sometimes small erythematous mucosal plaques which bleed readily[4]. Fissuring ulceration is common but a cobblestone pattern is rarer and is usually seen in later lesions[2,5,6] (Figure 16.2). The earliest microscopic lesions probably develop in the aggregates of lymphoid tissue normally present in the lamina propria; these become hyperplastic and swollen, leading to erosion of the overlying mucosa and so to fissure formation (Figure 16.3). Biopsy material taken at this stage usually includes some normal mucosa, in which there is no increased vascularity and no diminution in goblet cells (Figure 16.4). Mucosal fissures are initially small and a whole or a part of one can be included in a biopsy (Figure 16.5). The lamina propria forming the fissure wall often shows a non-specific granulation tissue reaction (Figure 16.6), sometimes containing giant cells (Figure 16.7) and sometimes with ill-defined but recognizable sarcoid-like granulomas (Figure 16.8). Occasionally a biopsy of apparently normal mucosa adjacent to a zone of Crohn's disease can show surface erosion with doubtful (Figure 16.9) or more definite (Figure 16.10) granulomas. When present these features are sufficient for a diagnosis of Crohn's disease, provided that tuberculosis can be excluded. Others, which are less significant, are the presence of crypt abscesses and Paneth cell metaplasia, both of which are less common in Crohn's disease than in ulcerative colitis; the relative lack of vascularity; and the presence of submucosal oedema. Occasionally acute arteritis may be present as part of the disease. The aggregates of lymphocytes and the transmural inflammation which are such well-known features of Crohn's disease are not normally appreciable in biopsies. When repeat biopsies are requested one may occasionally see old hyalinizing granulomas (Figure 16.11).

Special Investigations

Various workers have studied the value or otherwise of special investigations in Crohn's disease; their opinions can be summarized as follows:

There is some evidence that a high granuloma count

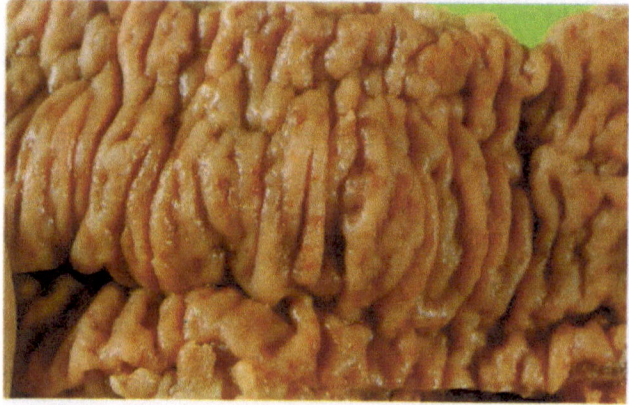

Figure 16.1   Early Crohn's disease. Small ulcers are present on oedematous mucosal folds

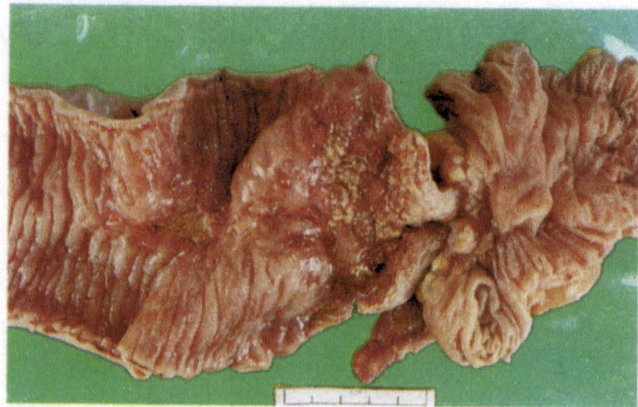

Figure 16.2   Crohn's disease in the caecal region showing fissuring ulceration and some cobblestoning

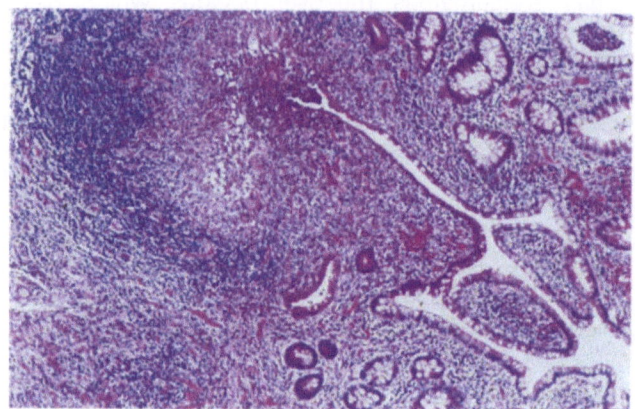

Figure 16.3   Crohn's disease. Early fissure formation at the bottom of a crypt with early granuloma formation.   H & E × 320

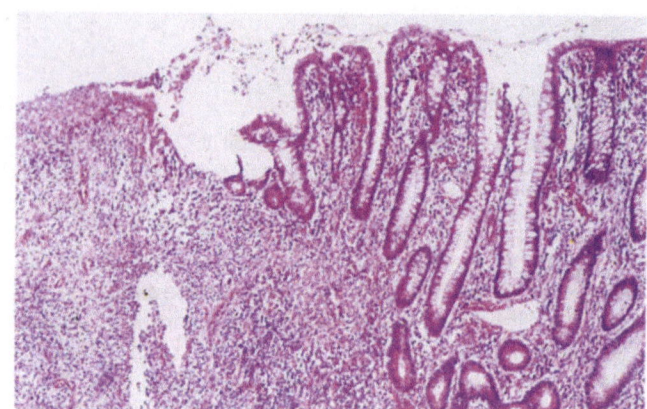

Figure 16.4   Crohn's disease. Early ulceration. The biopsy includes some intact mucosa in which there is no increased vascularity and in which goblet cells are present.   H & E × 250

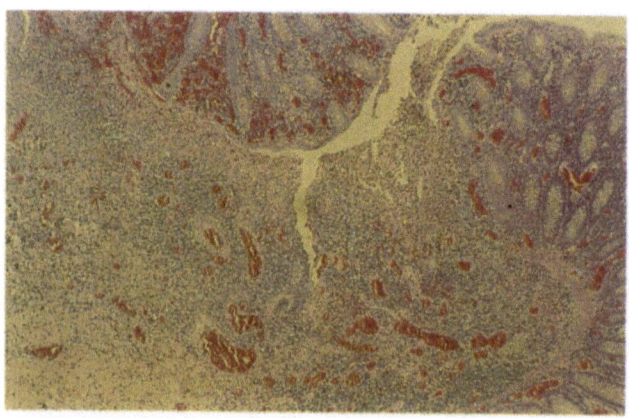

Figure 16.5   Crohn's disease. Early mucosal fissuring, which appears as a split in the submucosa; the whole is included in one biopsy.   H & E × 125

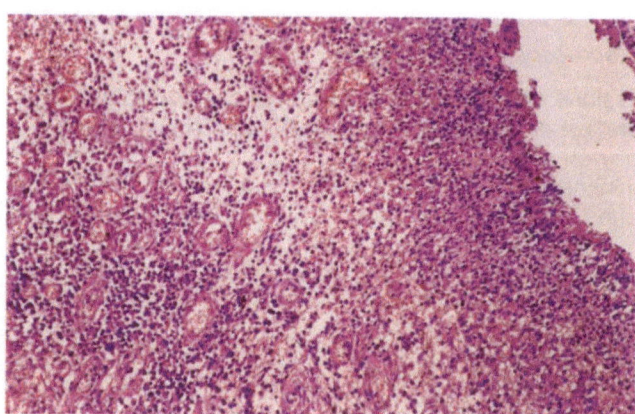

Figure 16.6   Crohn's disease, fissure wall. A non-specific granulation tissue reaction with marked chronic inflammation is present.   H & E × 250

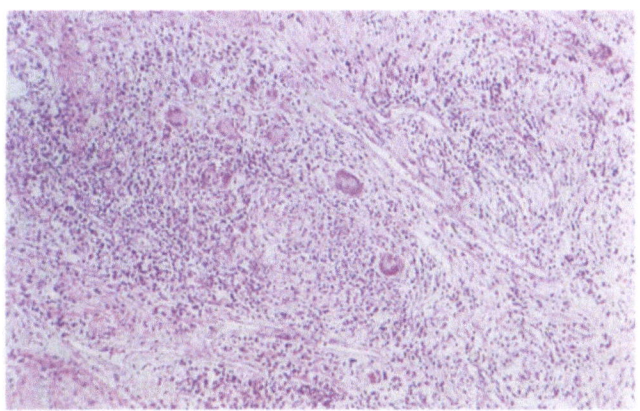

Figure 16.7   Crohn's disease, fissure wall. This is a fissure of longer standing which has extended down to the muscle. Giant cells are present.   H & E × 125

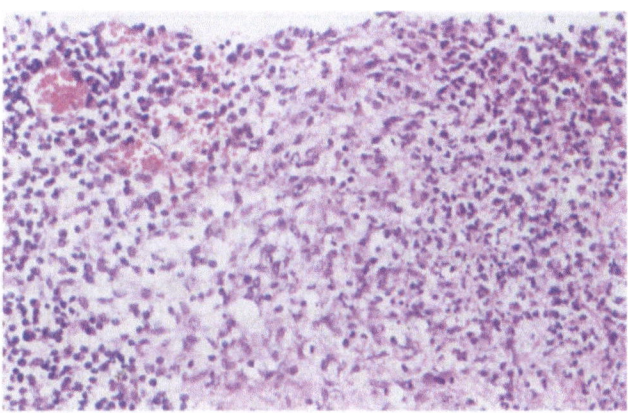

Figure 16.8   Crohn's disease, fissure wall. No giant cells are present here, but there is an ill-defined granuloma. These are often the only evidence which points to Crohn's disease in early lesions.   H & E × 320

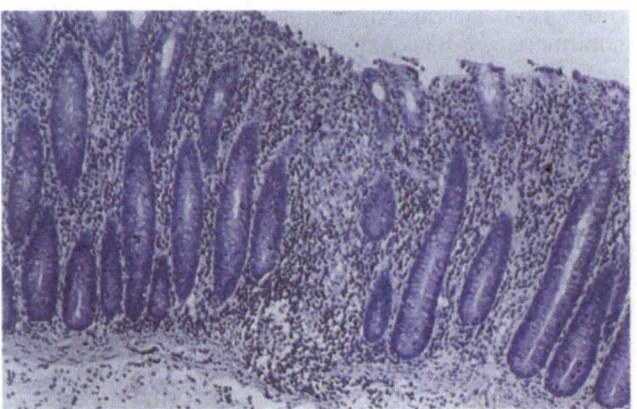

Figure 16.9   Rectal biopsy from suspected Crohn's disease. In the centre there is some gland drop-out and a suggestion of an ill-formed granuloma. H & E × 125

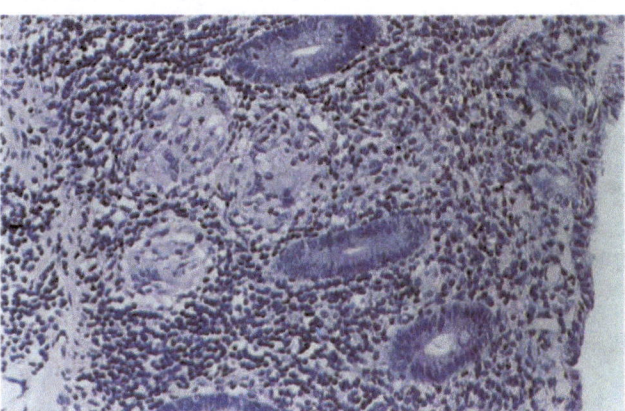

Figure 16.10   Rectal biopsy, proven Crohn's disease of colon. Small definitive granulomas are present in the mucosa well away from the affected zone.   H & E × 320

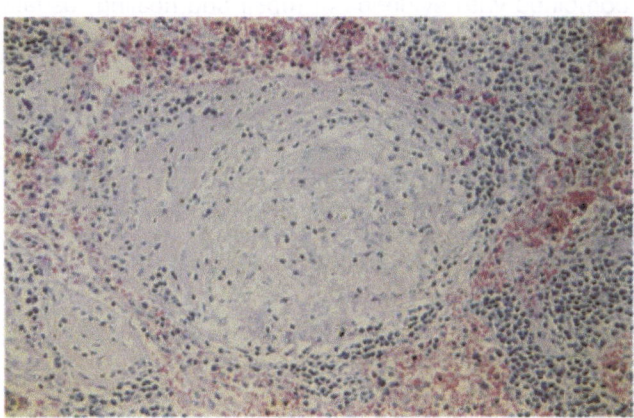

Figure 16.11   Crohn's disease. Old hyalinized granuloma.   H & E × 320

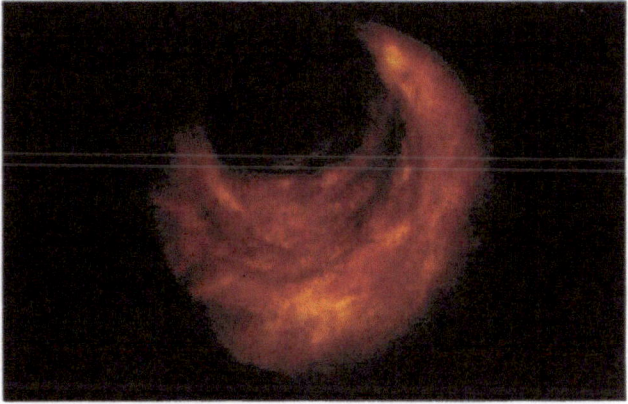

Figure 16.12   Ulcerative colitis. Endoscopic appearance in the early stages, showing velvety red mucosa

is related to a better prognosis[7] though I do not know how far this study, which was made on resected specimens, is reproducible on biopsy material. Histochemical studies on mucins indicate that goblet cell mucin and goblet cells themselves may be slightly reduced in acute Crohn's disease but not to the extent seen in ulcerative colitis, while enzyme studies have not proved helpful[8,9]; neither have immunological studies for identifying lysozyme[10]. Claims have been made that plasma cells containing IgA[11] and IgE[12] may be increased in number in Crohn's disease and in ulcerative colitis but counts are not of value in separating the two conditions.

Rectal Biopsies in Crohn's Disease

There have also been a number of studies on the value of rectal biopsy in the diagnosis and prognosis of Crohn's disease situated in other regions of the large bowel. In one study a single rectal biopsy was positive in only 54/349 biopsies, and in 53 of these the disease had already been diagnosed on other grounds[13]. If two biopsies are taken, part of each is serially sectioned and granulomas carefully searched for, the pick-up rate rises and the investigation probably becomes worthwhile as a routine[14]. There is also some evidence that when the degree of histological abnormality is considerable, and particularly if unsuspected ulceration or fissuring is present, the prognosis is poor[15].

The slight but proven tendency to malignancy[16] is discussed in Chapter 20.

Ulcerative Colitis

Ulcerative colitis is a disease of exacerbations and remissions, which make it difficult to assess the stage of the disease and the effects of treatment. The ages of maximal incidence show a first peak at 20–29 for men, 30–39 for women, and a second peak at 70–79 for both sexes; the middle-age peak seen additionally in Crohn's disease does not occur[1]. Like Crohn's disease, it is of undetermined aetiology, is becoming more common, has a high morbidity and shortens life expectancy; operative treatment is more successful but the cancer risk is much greater in long-standing disease[2]. The inflammation begins in the rectum and spreads proximally on a continuous basis, so that skip areas do not occur. It involves mucosa and superficial submucosa only, though a fulminating form involving all coats of the transverse colon is well known. Fissuring ulceration is not a feature, and fistulae and adhesions are not complications since the serosa is uninvolved. In many patients the disease progresses from an acute through a chronic active to a quiescent phase and these changes can be reflected in mucosal biopsy appearances[17,18]; the quiescent phase can be reactivated if relapse occurs and is always susceptible to dysplastic mucosal changes. Serial biopsies at selected time intervals can be helpful in judging the progress of the disease and in assessing the response to treatment (see below).

Early Active Ulcerative Colitis

The earliest endoscopic change is a marked congestion of the mucosa which appears red and velvety (Figure 16.12) and often shows small surface erosions or ulcers (Figure 16.13). Biopsy at this stage shows a combination of mucosal erosion or ulceration, loss of gland elements and a striking vascularity of the lamina propria (Figure 16.14). Crypt abscesses, consisting of collections of polymorphs within dilated glands which later rupture (Figure 16.15), are common but by no means confined to ulcerative colitis; neutrophil polymorphs are rare in the lamina propria but plasma cells, lymphocytes and eosinophils are all present. There is often conspicuous replacement of gland elements by vascular granulation tissue (Figure 16.16) and in the epithelium which remains goblet cells are reduced in number and in mucin content (Figure 16.14). These changes are normally limited by the muscularis mucosae, but crypt abscesses may rupture through the muscle and lamina proprial inflammation extend into the submucosa. Inflammatory changes then spread longitudinally, usually involving only the superficial submucosa but lifting up the overlying mucosa to form the beginning of an inflammatory or 'pseudo' polyp (Figures 16.17 and 16.18), in which reparative mucosal hyperplasia often occurs later (Figure 16.19). In fulminating colitis in the transverse colon the inflammatory changes extend into the deep submucosa and muscularis propria and perforation becomes a likely complication, but these changes are not likely to be seen in biopsy material.

Chronic Active Ulcerative Colitis

The histological separation of an acute from a chronic active phase is by no means hard and fast, and some workers separate only into active and quiescent forms. The term 'chronic active' may be used to designate a lesion in which the active disease already described is combined with evidence of repair and healing, usually with mucosal regeneration. Crypt abscesses become less common, there is some hyperplasia of lymphoid aggregates with a heavy mononuclear cell infiltrate in the lamina propria (Figure 16.20). Reparative hyperplasia of gland elements leads to further polyp formation (Figure 16.19) and to irregular branching of tubules (Figure 16.20) and Paneth cells begin to appear in the crypt zones (Figure 16.21). Like crypt abscesses, they are not confined to ulcerative colitis but are much less common in Crohn's disease.

Quiescent Ulcerative Colitis

In the quiescent phase the mucosa is thinner than normal and gland elements are reduced in number (Figure 16.22). Aggregates of lymphocytes and an increased number of mononuclear cells are still present in the lamina propria and sometimes in the superficial mucosa, but there is no longer excessive vascular dilatation. Since the disease is superficial, fibrosis and consequent stricture formation are not features but contraction of the muscle coats occurs, simulating fibrotic narrowing and causing actual shortening of the bowel. The thickened contracted circular coat is clearly visible in resected specimens but not in biopsy material. Dysplastic precancerous changes can be present in long-standing colitis and are discussed in Chapter 20.

Apart from the fulminating lesion in the transverse colon there are few pathological complications. Herniation of mucosa into the submucosa[19], and colitis cystica profunda in the form of diffuse mucus-containing cysts in the submucosa[20] are both well recognized.

Special Investigations

As in Crohn's disease, histochemical and other specialized studies have not proved of great value on biopsy material[21]. The presence or relative absence of goblet cells containing mucin in Crohn's disease and ulcerative colitis respectively can usually be detected in conventionally processed material or at most requires a simple PAS stain[22]. Claims that eosinophil counts in rectal biopsies are of value in prognosis[23] have not yet been fully substantiated. The value of sequential biopsies in this and other inflammatory conditions is discussed later in this chapter.

Idiopathic (Non-specific) Proctitis and Proctocolitis

Clinical observations show that there is a group of patients who present with symptoms suggestive of ulcerative colitis and who have a proctitis extending as far as the rectosigmoid junction who do not necessarily progress to full-blown ulcerative colitis[24]. The histological changes are similar to, but less severe than, those seen in ulcerative colitis, mucus depletion and an inflammatory infiltrate, which often contains polymorphs, in the lamina propria being the most common (Figures 16.23 and 16.24); they cannot, in my view, be conclusively separated on rectal biopsy alone. Separation may be possible if the 'normal' mucosa in the transverse or descending colon is sampled[24] for in those patients who will subsequently develop colitis, mild inflammatory changes can be detected histologically even when the colon is macroscopically normal (Figure 16.25).

The Differential Diagnosis of Inflammatory Bowel Disease

Any pathologist of experience who is honest will admit to studying resected specimens and biopsy material on which he or she has been unable to decide whether the inflammatory changes present indicate ulcerative colitis, Crohn's disease or some other disorder including ischaemic bowel disease or antibiotic-associated colitis. Careful study of a number of sections, or perhaps a repeat biopsy, usually allow the last two conditions to be distinguished, but the distinction between colitis and Crohn's disease can at times be impossible even on a resected specimen. Many books[2] present tables of the features to look for and I include one here (Table 16.1). Ashley Price has done considerable service in recognizing this difficulty and has coined the term colitis indeterminate to cover such patients[25]; he and Basil Morson have stressed the value of sequential biopsies in all patients with inflammatory bowel disease.

Table 16.1   Endoscopic and microscopic differentiation of Crohn's disease from ulcerative colitis

	Crohn's disease	Ulcerative colitis
Endoscopic features	Disease discontinuous. Rectum not always involved. Fissures often visible. Inflammatory polyps not common.	Disease continuous. Rectum always involved. No fissuring, except in fulminating disease. Inflammatory polyps common and extensive.
Microscopic features	Vascular dilatation not a feature. Severe mucosal and submucosal oedema. Inflammation transmural. Crypt abscesses not common. Mucus secretion relatively normal. Paneth cell metaplasia rare. Sarcoid type granulomas in 50% of biopsies. Fissuring may be seen in biopsies. Precancerous epithelial change very rare.	Marked vascular dilatation present. Little oedema present. Inflammation in mucosa and superficial submucosa. Crypt abscesses common. Mucus secretion much reduced. Paneth cell metaplasia common. Granulomas not present. Fissuring not present if not fulminating. Precancerous epithelial change sometimes seen.
Anal lesions	Common and often contain sarcoid type granulomas.	Less common and usually non-specific.

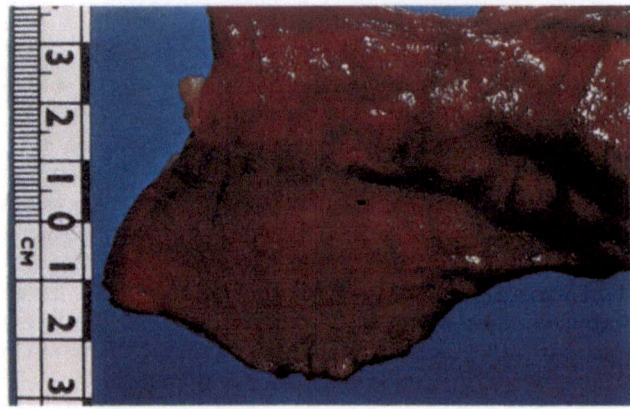

Figure 16.13   Ulcerative colitis (U.C.) early stage, showing velvety mucosa with early erosion and ulceration

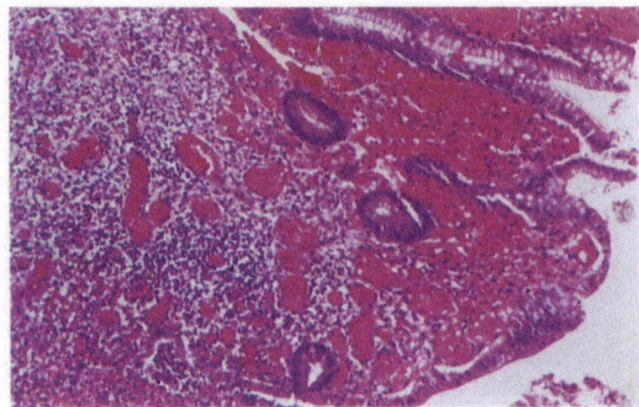

Figure 16.14   U.C., early active phase. Note the very marked degree of congestion and the loss of gland elements. Goblet cells are reduced in number.   H & E × 320

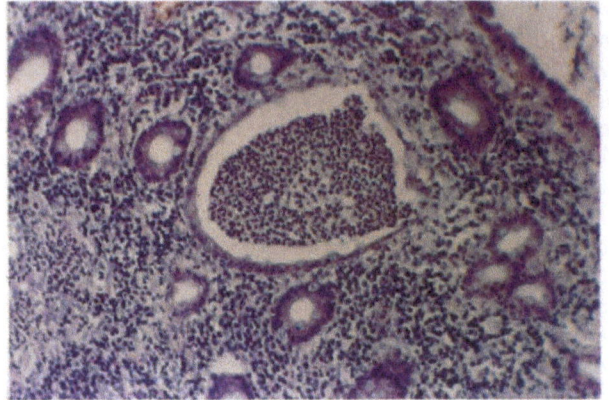

Figure 16.15   U.C., early active phase. A crypt abscess.   H & E × 320

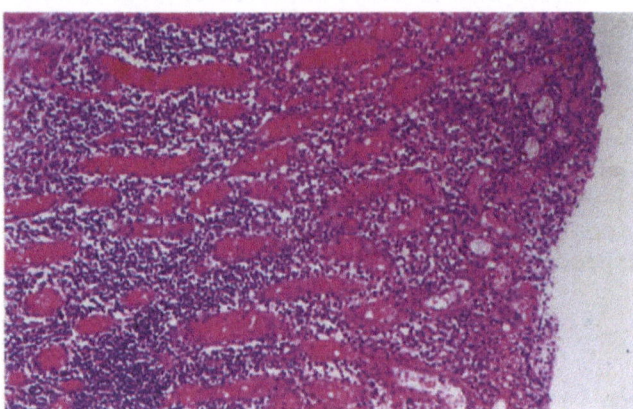

Figure 16.16   U.C., early active phase. Gland elements are replaced by vascular granulation tissue with marked round cell infiltration.   H & E × 250

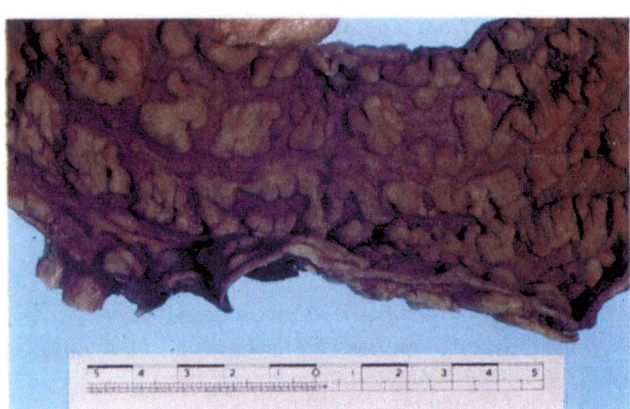

Figure 16.17   U.C., early active phase. Mucosal ulceration with the beginnings of undermining to form inflammatory polyps. Resected specimen.

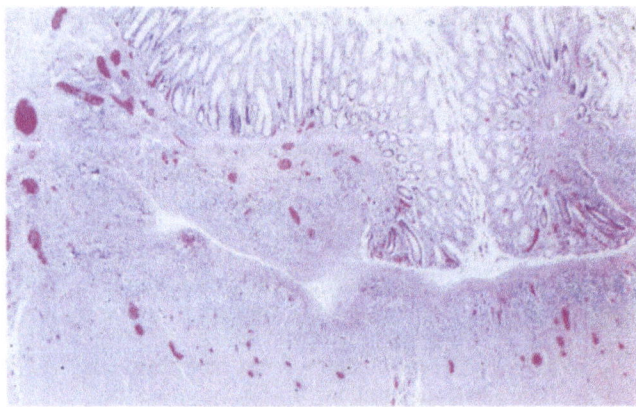

Figure 16.18   U.C., early active phase. A small ulcer is becoming undermined producing an appearance which superficially resembles fissuring. Further splitting will raise the mucosa and superficial submucosa away from the deeper mucosa to form one pattern of inflammatory polyp.   H & E × 65

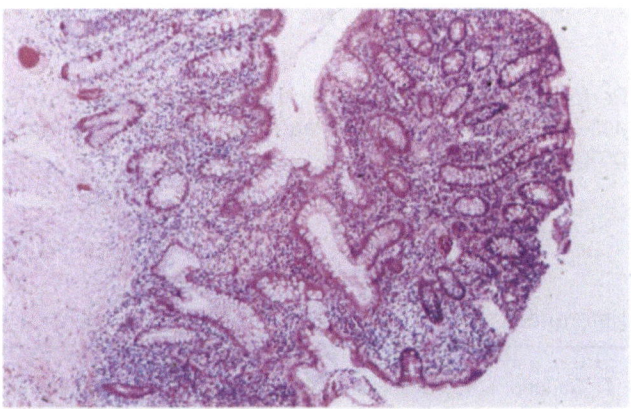

Figure 16.19   U.C., early active phase. A reparative type of polyp; the result of mucosal hyperplasia.   H & E × 100

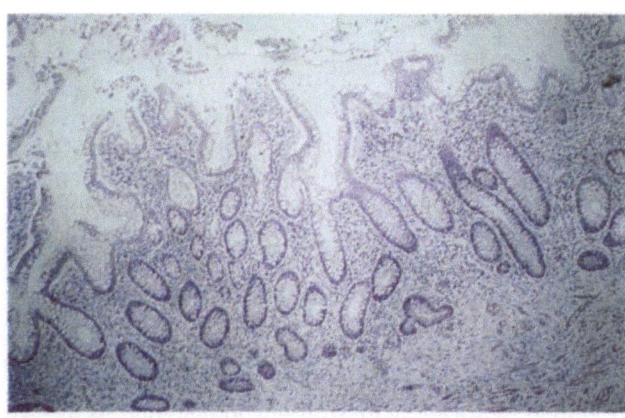

Figure 16.20   U.C., chronic active phase. There has been regeneration of damaged mucosa with irregular branching of tubules and a marked round cell infiltrate in the lamina propria. Paneth cells are present in the deeper glands.   H & E × 100

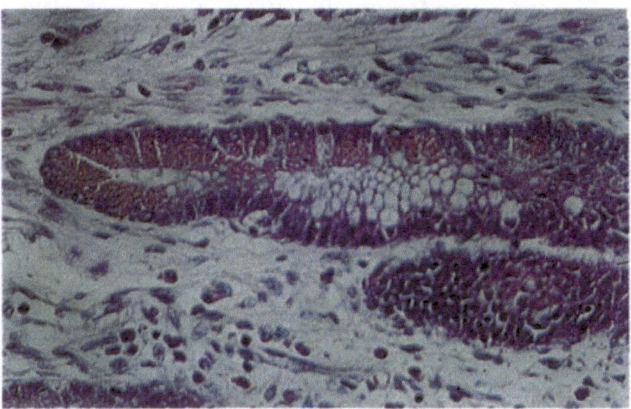

Figure 16.21   U.C., chronic active phase. Paneth cells in deep gland elements.   H & E × 320

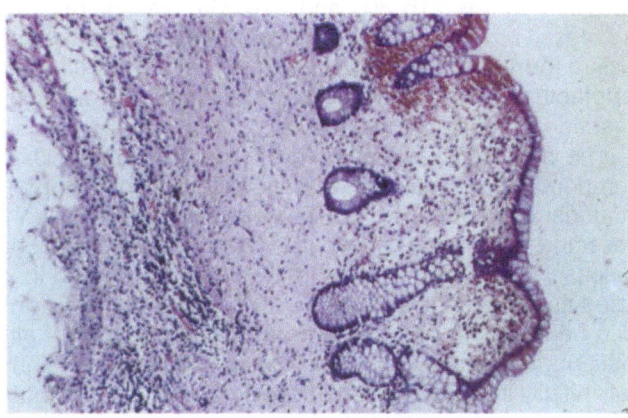

Figure 16.22   U.C., quiescent phase. The mucosa is thinnned and gland elements are reduced in number. There are still increased numbers of mononuclear cells in the lamina propria, but there is now no appreciable vascular dilatation.   H & E × 100

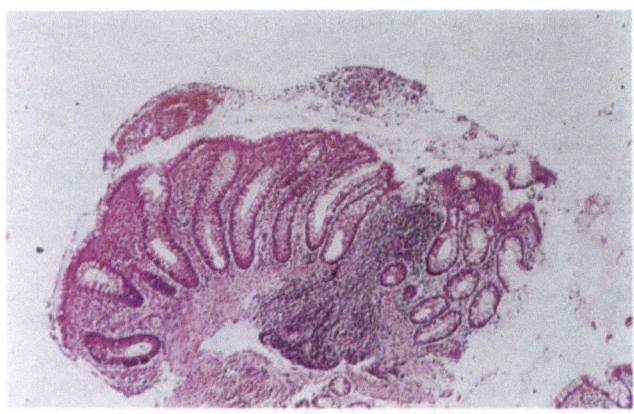

Figure 16.23   Non-specific proctitis. There is slight irregularity and some drop-out of gland elements with an increased number of mononuclear cells in the lamina propria. It is impossible to tell on this biopsy whether this is U.C. or non-specific inflammation.   H & E × 32

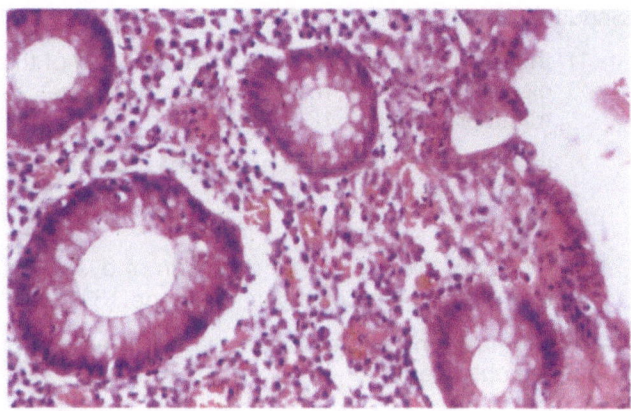

Figure 16.24   Non-specific proctitis. There is surface erosion and a few polymorphs are present in the lamina propria which are rare in U.C.   H & E × 320

Colitis Indeterminate

The problem of distinguishing Crohn's disease from ulcerative colitis usually arises in patients with severe and acute symptoms, often accompanied by dilatation of the transverse colon suggesting fulminating ulcerative colitis. Macroscopically there is mucosal oedema, ulceration often with 'cobblestoning' and sometimes with fissuring (Figure 16.26). The rectum may appear to be spared and there may be an appearance of discontinuous lesions because the degree of involvement, though in fact total, varies greatly in severity. In biopsy material the differentiation can be quite impossible on a single sample. The single factor which I have found most helpful is a detailed study of fissures if any are present. In Crohn's disease the fissures tend to be lined by recognizable granulation tissue, there may be a suggestion of true granuloma formation and a careful search of serial sections may reveal distorted giant cells (Figures 16.27–16.29). In the fissures of fulminating colitis (Figures 16.30 and 16.31) vascularity is increased but there is little or no tendency to granulation tissue formation; the tissues seem to have been almost artefactually torn apart with no distinct histological reaction to the tear itself.

The most reliable means to a certain diagnosis is a temporal one. Enquiry for, and study of, previous biopsy material is helpful and further biopsies taken from unresected bowel at a later date will often reveal which disease is present. 'Colitis indeterminate' should be used as a 'holding' diagnosis until a more firm decision can be made. In my own experience about 15% of all patients with acute colitis who come to urgent resection fall initially into the indeterminate group; of these about 20% will remain unclassified (some because no further material becomes available), while of the remainder about two-thirds behave as, and later show histological evidence suggestive of, Crohn's disease while one-third appear to have ulcerative colitis.

The Value of Sequential Biopsies

Sequential biopsies are useful in the following ways:

(1) they allow one to follow the natural course of the disease and its response or otherwise to treatment (Figures 16.32–16.35);

(2) they may provide, in patients with colitis indeterminate, a means of making a differential diagnosis;

(3) they may allow the early detection of dysplastic and premalignant changes (see page 131).

To gain the maximum information the following points should be observed:

(1) biopsies should always be taken as nearly as possible from the same site; carefully labelled multiple biopsies are more likely to be helpful than single ones;

(2) they should be interpreted by the same pathologist and, ideally, examined by clinician and pathologist together.

Performed thus they are both an invaluable form of assessment and a way of learning more of the natural progress of the disease.

References

1. Garland, C. F., Lilienfeld, A. M., Mendeloff, A. I., Markowitz, J. A., Terrell, K. B. and Garland, F. C. (1981). Incidence rates of ulcerative colitis and Crohn's disease in 15 areas of the United States. *Gastroenterology*, **81**, 1115

2. Morson, B. C. and Dawson, I. M. P. (1979). *Gastrointestinal Pathology*. 2nd edn., Chapters 20 and 33. (Oxford: Blackwell)

3. Kraft, S. C. (1978). The regional lymph nodes in regional enteritis. *Gastroenterology*, **75**, 319

4. Watier, A., Devroede, G., Perey, B., Haddad, H., Madarnas, P. and Grand-Maison, P. (1980). Small erythematous mucosal plaques; an endoscopic sign of Crohn's disease. *Gut*, **21**, 835

5. Lockhart-Mummery, H. E. and Morson, B. C. (1960). Crohn's disease (regional enteritis) of the large intestine and its distinction from ulcerative colitis. *Gut*, **1**, 87

6. Price, A. B. and Morson, B. C. (1975). Inflammatory bowel disease; the surgical pathology of Crohn's disease and ulcerative colitis. *Hum. Pathol.*, **6**, 7

7. Chambers, T. J. and Morson, B. C. (1979). The granuloma in Crohn's disease. *Gut*, **20**, 269

8. Dawson, I. M. P. (1972). The histochemistry of Crohn's disease. *Clin. Gastroenterol.*, **1**, 309

9. Dawson, I. M. P. (1972). The value for diagnosis and research of special investigations on rectal biopsies in Crohn's disease. *Br. J. Surg.*, **59**, 806

10. Klockars, M., Reitamo, S., Reitamo, J. J. and Moller, C. (1977). Immunohistochemical identification of lysozyme in intestinal lesions in ulcerative colitis and Crohn's disease. *Gut*, **18**, 377

11. Skinner, J. M. and Whitehead, R. (1974). The plasma cells in inflammatory disease of the colon: a quantitative study. *J. Clin. Pathol.*, **27**, 643

12. O'Donoghue, D. P. and Kumar, P. (1979). Rectal IgE cells in inflammatory bowel disease. *Gut*, **20**, 149

13. Hill, R. B., Kent, T. H. and Hansen, R. N. (1979). Clinical usefulness of rectal biopsy in Crohn's disease. *Gastroenterology*, **77**, 938

14. Surawicz, C. M., Meisel, J. L., Ylvisaker, T., Saunders, D. R. and Rubin, C. E. (1981). Rectal biopsy in the diagnosis of Crohn's disease; value of multiple biopsies and serial sectioning. *Gastroenterology*, **80**, 66

15. Ward, M. and Webb, J. N. (1977). Rectal biopsy as a prognostic guide in Crohn's disease. *J. Clin. Pathol.*, **30**, 126

16. Gyde, S. N., Prior, P., Macartney, J. C., Thompson, H., Waterhouse, J. A. and Allen, R. N. (1980). Malignancy in Crohn's disease. *Gut*, **21**, 1024

17. Morson, B. C. (1972). Rectal biopsy in inflammatory bowel disease. *N. Engl. J. Med.*, **287**, 1337

18. Yardley, J. H. and Donowitz, M. (1977). Colo-rectal biopsy in inflammatory bowel disease. In *The Gastrointestinal Tract*. pp. 50–54. International Academy of Pathology (Baltimore: Williams & Wilkins)

19. Dyson, J. L. (1975). Herniation of mucosal epithelium into the submucosa in chronic ulcerative colitis. *J. Clin. Pathol.*, **28**, 189

20. Tedesco, F. J., Sumner, H. W. and Kassens, W. D. Jr. (1975). Colitis cystica profunda. *Am. J. Gastroenterol.*, **65**, 339

21. Dawson, I. M. P. (1981). The value of histochemistry in the diagnosis and prognosis of gastrointestinal diseases. In Stoward, P. J. and Polak, J. M. (eds.). *Histochemistry; the Widening Horizons.* pp. 127–162. (Chichester, John Wiley & Sons)

22. Filipe, M. I. and Dawson, I. M. P. (1970). The diagnostic value of mucosubstances in biopsies from patients with ulcerative colitis and Crohn's disease. *Gut,* **11**, 229

23. Heatley, R. V. and James, P. D. (1979). Eosinophils in the rectal mucosa. A simple method of predicting the outcome of ulcerative proctocolitis? *Gut,* **20**, 787

24. Das, K. M., Morecki, R., Nair, P. and Berkowitz, J. M. (1977). Idiopathic proctitis. I. The morphology of proximal colonic mucosa and its clinical significance. *Am. J. Dig. Dis.*, **22**, 524

25. Price, A. B. (1978). Overlap in the spectrum of non-specific inflammatory bowel disease – colitis indeterminate. *J. Clin. Pathol.*, **31**, 567

Figures 16.25–16.35 will be found overleaf.

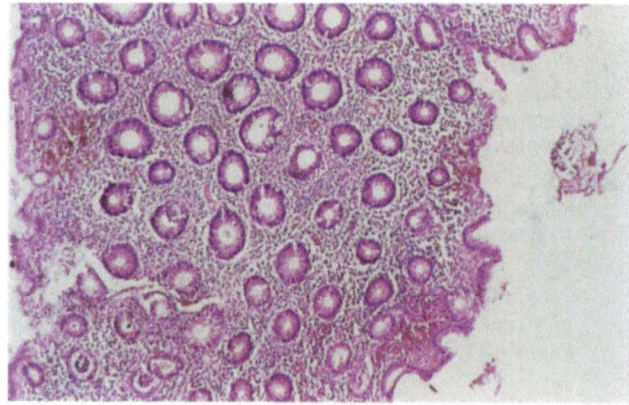

Figure 16.25 Transverse colonic biopsy in doubtful proctitis. There is early erosion and an inflammatory infiltrate in the lamina propria, suggesting that the rectal condition is U.C. rather than non-specific proctitis, though the fact that the biopsy is tangential makes diagnosis more difficult.   H & E × 320

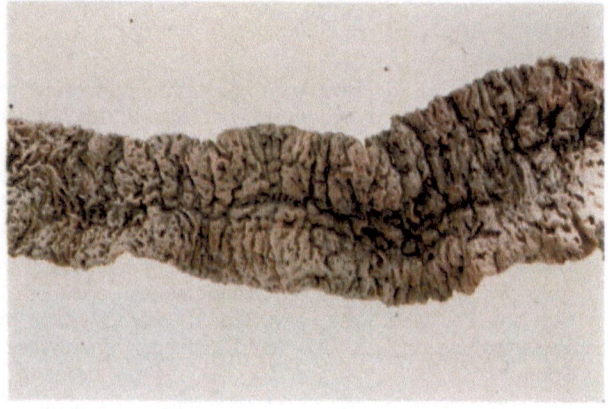

Figure 16.26 Colitis indeterminate (C.I.). Fissuring ulceration with cobblestoning and mucosal oedema

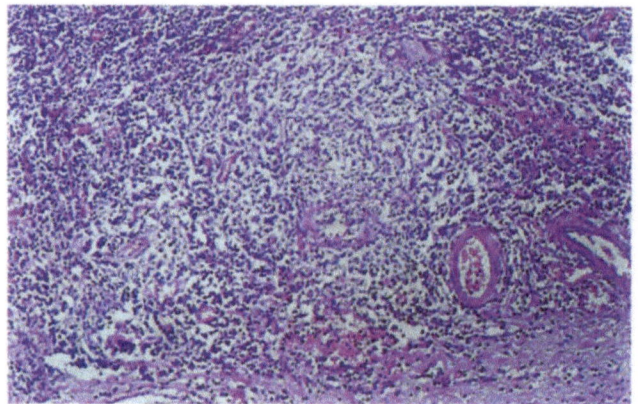

Figure 16.27 C.I. Granulation tissue response with a suggestion of granuloma formation, insufficient to justify a positive diagnosis of Crohn's disease.   H & E × 125

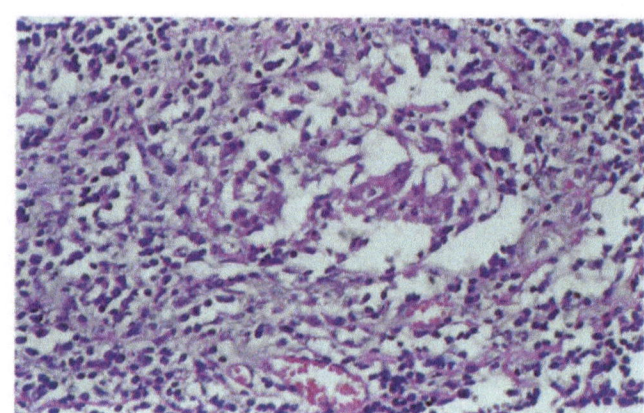

Figure 16.28 C.I. A more suggestive granuloma in a patient who later was confirmed as having Crohn's disease.   H & E × 250

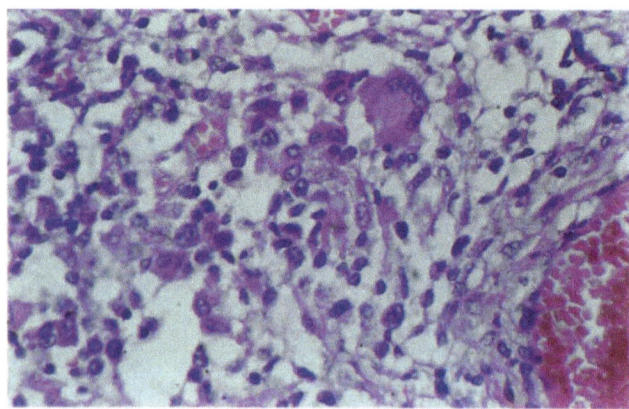

Figure 16.29 C.I. Granuloma with distorted giant cells. Many would regard this as sufficient evidence for a diagnosis of Crohn's disease.   H & E × 250

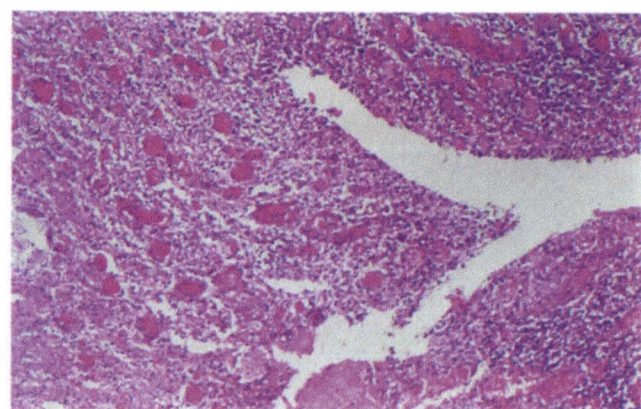

Figure 16.30 C.I. Fissuring is common but in this example there is marked vascularity and no granulomatous reaction. The tissue looks as if it had been torn apart to produce the fissure. Appearances are more suggestive of U.C. but no certain diagnosis is possible.   H & E × 125

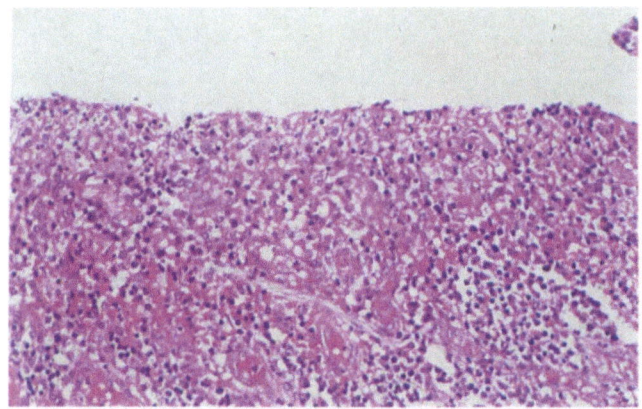

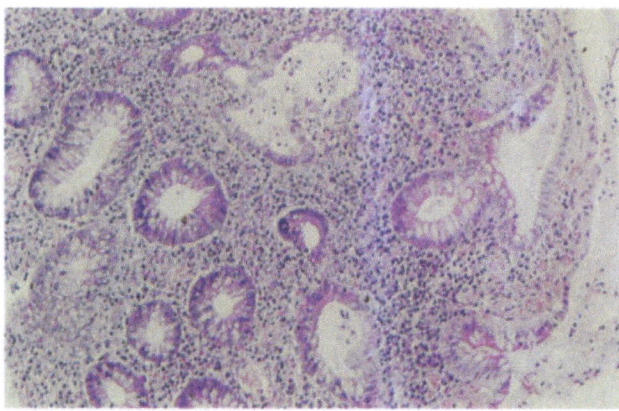

Figure 16.31 A higher-power view of the edge of the fissure in Figure 16.30. There is no real granulomatous or even granulation tissue reaction at the edge, which almost looks as if it had been artefactually produced.   H & E × 250

Figures 16.32–16.35 Sequential biopsies in U.C. Figure 16.32 (day 1) shows the early active phase with crypt abscesses and round cell infiltrate in lamina propria. Figure 16.33 (day 8) shows a similar appearance but without crypt abscesses. Figure 16.34 (day 15) shows the chronic active phase with gland drop-out but less inflammation. Figure 16.35 (day 25) shows evidence of healing with branching of glands in a relatively normal mucosa.   All H & E × 100

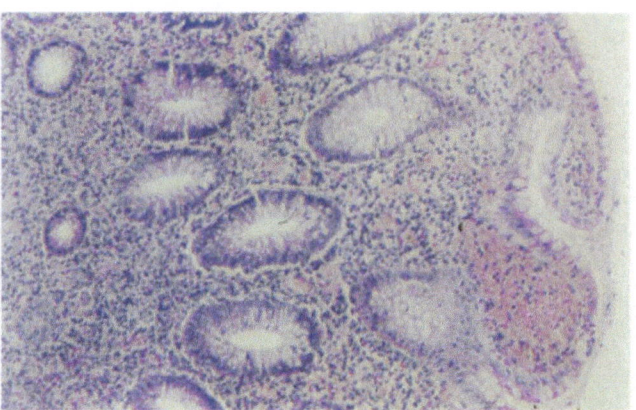

Figure 16.33

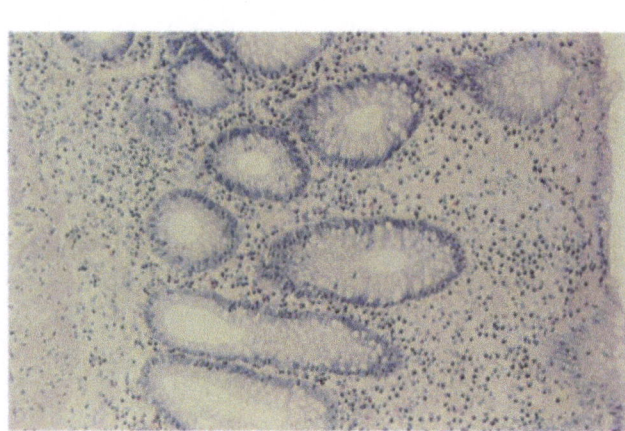

Figure 16.34

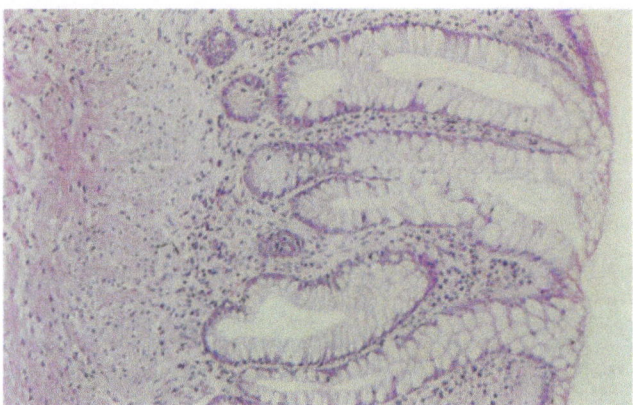

Figure 16.35

17

Large Intestine and Anal Canal: Patterns of Infective and Inflammatory Bowel Disease

Infective bowel disease can be caused by bacteria, viruses, protozoa and metazoa. Many of them involve both small and large intestine. They present clinically with diarrhoea, sometimes with blood, and are usually accompanied by colicky abdominal pain and sometimes, especially in young children, dehydration. All patients with persistent diarrhoea should be carefully investigated; stool cultures, appropriate viral studies and microscopic examination of stools for ova or parasites are obligatory. The majority will respond to appropriate treatment, so that colonoscopy and biopsy are not often performed unless diarrhoea persists. An interesting study on 74 patients referred to a Scottish infectious diseases department with non-specific diarrhoea allowed a provisional separation of infective diarrhoea from non-infective inflammatory bowel disease and other disorders on histological grounds[1] and illustrated the value of rectal biopsy in all patients with persistent diarrhoea.

Bacterial Diarrhoeas

Salmonella and Shigella Infections

These are the two common groups of responsible organisms in bacterial diarrhoeas though strains of *E. coli* can be causative on occasions. The common microscopic changes in the acute phase are surface mucosal erosion, sometimes with a fibrinous exudate, degeneration and sometimes regeneration in the superficial crypt zone, poorly formed crypt abscesses often with some crypt distension with mucin and a mixed acute and chronic inflammatory reaction, which includes some emigrating polymorphs, in the lamina propria[2,3] (Figure 17.1). Such changes, particularly the presence of polymorphs, are, even with a negative stool culture, distinct from those seen in chronic non-infective inflammatory bowel disease and suggest, though they do not prove, an infective origin. It must be remembered, however, that *Salmonella* infections can complicate chronic non-infective inflammatory bowel disease, especially after treatment with steroids. Repeat biopsy after appropriate treatment is often helpful diagnostically; there is likely to be marked improvement in infective disease, little in ulcerative colitis or Crohn's disease.

Campylobacter Infection

Infection of the large bowel by *Campylobacter jejuni*, an S-shaped Gram-negative organism, has become well recognized over the last few years[4-6]. Clinically, endoscopically and histologically the disease can mimic ulcerative colitis but a careful and extensive survey[5] which included a comparison with proven *Shigella* and *Salmonella* infections showed that the findings in all of these three types of infection were histologically similar. My own material confirms this. The presence of rupturing crypt abscesses and a mixed inflammatory cellular infiltrate in the lamina propria, along with considerable surface exudate in which polymorphs are present (Figures 17.2 and 17.3) are all common, but the changes seem to me more severe in *Campylobacter* infection, particularly in regard to crypt abscesses and polymorphs in the lamina propria.

Yersinial Infections

These are described in the small intestine. I have not seen a large intestinal example in biopsy or resected material aside from the appendix, but changes would presumably mimic those seen in the small intestine[7].

Tuberculosis

Large intestinal tuberculosis is rare in Britain[8]; it is usually seen in immigrants, involves the caecum or rectum and is secondary to open pulmonary tuberculosis. That said, I have now seen nine patients with colonic disease in the last 10 years, of whom three were indigenous Caucasians. Four had no evidence of pulmonary disease and in them the large bowel lesion was apparently primary. In all patients in whom a diagnosis of Crohn's disease is finally made, the possibility of tuberculosis should always be considered and as far as possible excluded.

Endoscopically there is usually clearly defined ulceration, often with an associated stricture (Figure 17.4). Sometimes small tubercles are visible in the adjacent mucosa.

Microscopically the principal features are a well-marked granulomatous reaction, sometimes but not

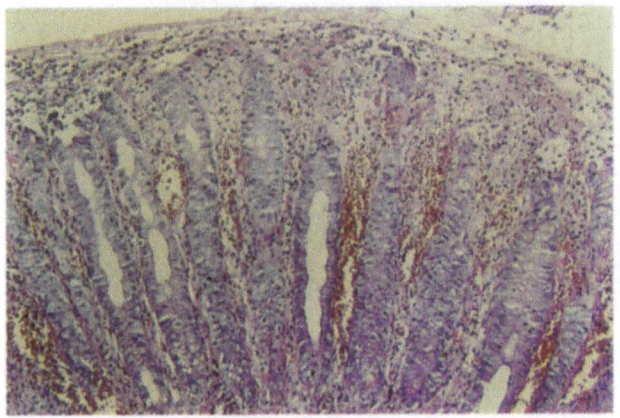

Figure 17.1 Bacterial diarrhoea (*Salmonella*). There is surface mucosal erosion with a fibrinous exudate and polymorphs in the lamina propria. Some crypt regeneration is beginning. H & E × 125

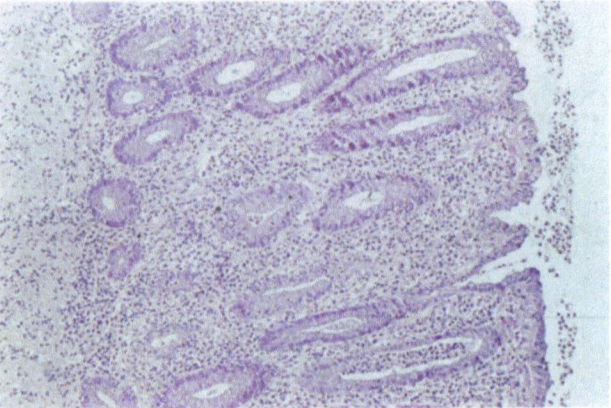

Figure 17.2 Bacterial diarrhoea (*Campylobacter*). There is a surface fibrino-purulent exudate with crypt abscesses and a mixed cellular infiltrate in the lamina propria. H & E × 125

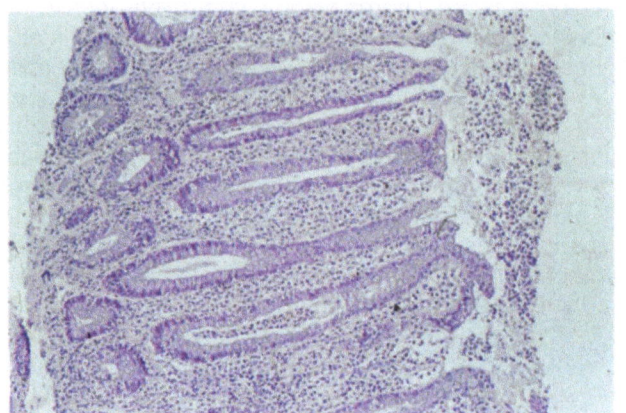

Figure 17.3 Bacterial diarrhoea (*Campylobacter*). A similar picture to Figure 17.2. H & E × 125

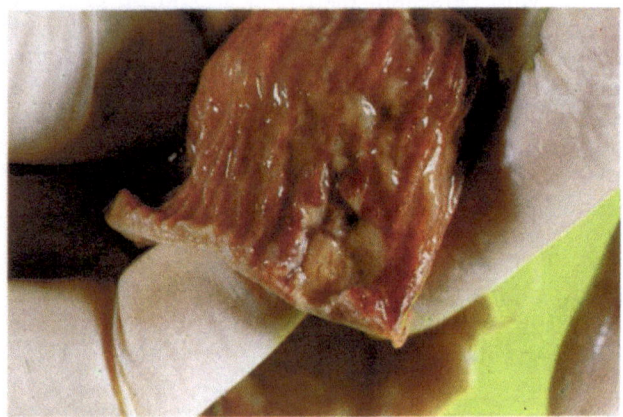

Figure 17.4 Colonic tuberculosis. Clearly defined tuberculous ulcers. Resected specimen

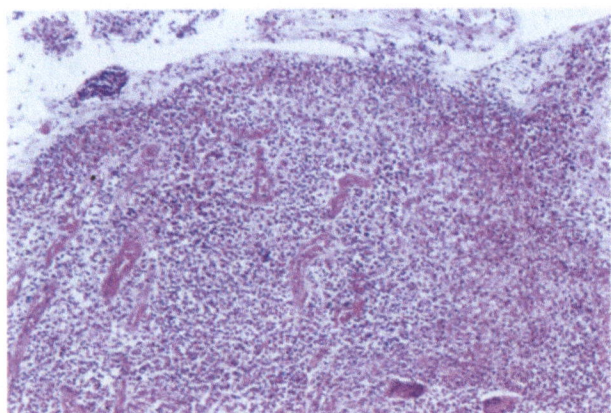

Figure 17.5 Tuberculosis. The mucosa has ulcerated and is largely replaced by granulation tissue, in which granulomas with giant cells but without caseation are present and have extended into the submucosa. H & E × 80

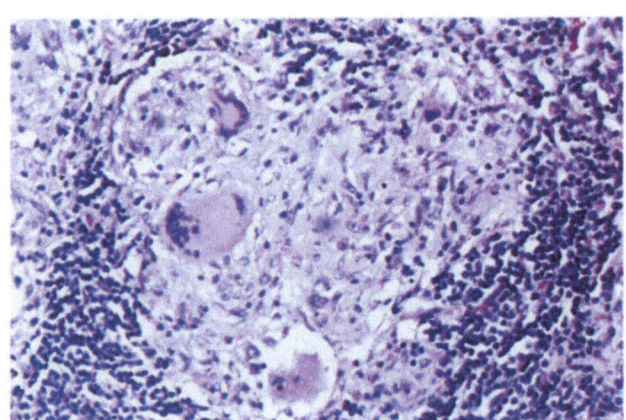

Figure 17.6 Tuberculosis. Higher-power view of a tuberculous granuloma. Without caseation these cannot definitely be distinguished histologically from Crohn's disease, but they are usually more florid and 'juicy' in appearance. H & E × 320

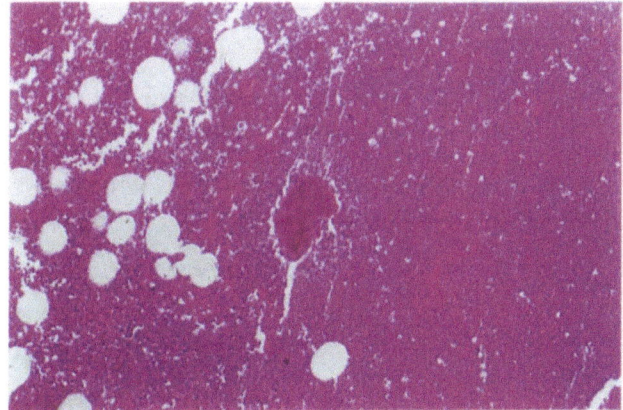

Figure 17.7 Perianal actinomycosis. A characteristic colony of actinomyces lies in the centre of purulent granulation tissue.   H & E × 80

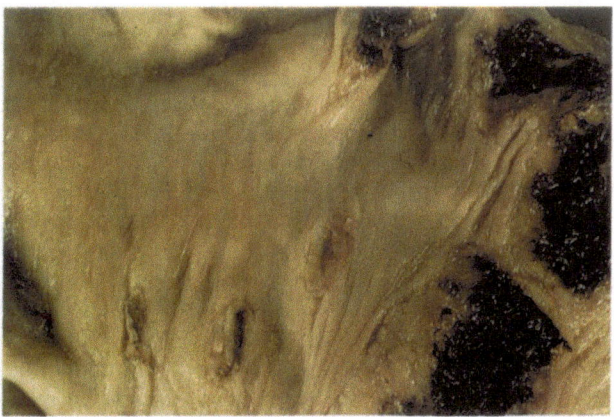

Figure 17.8 Amoebic colitis. The ulcers are discrete and the intervening mucosa appears normal. The larger ulcers (right) can have a haemorrhagic appearance. Resected specimen

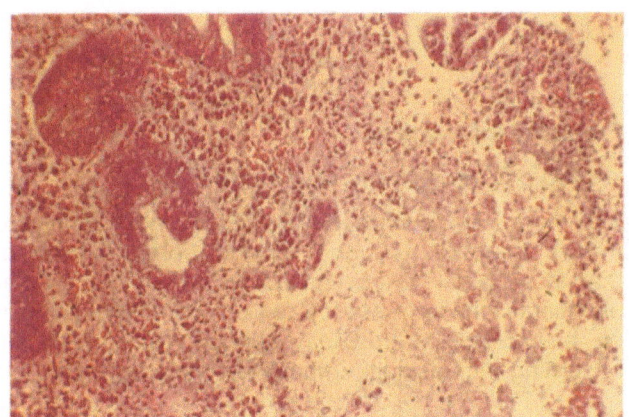

Figure 17.9 Amoebic dysentery. There is early mucosal erosion and eosinophils are present in the lamina propria. Some amoebae are present in the debris on the surface.   H & E × 250

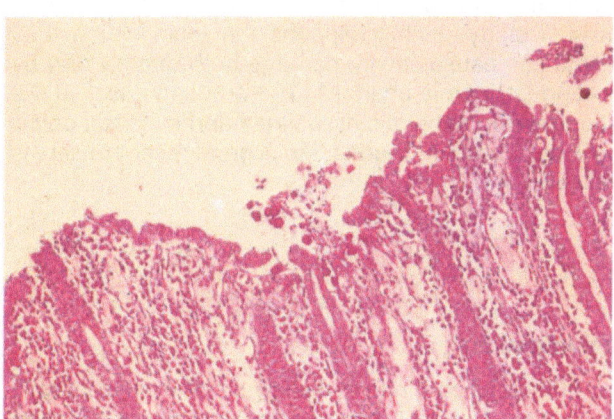

Figure 17.10 Amoebic dysentery. An early mucosal erosion with amoebae on the surface.   PAS stain × 250

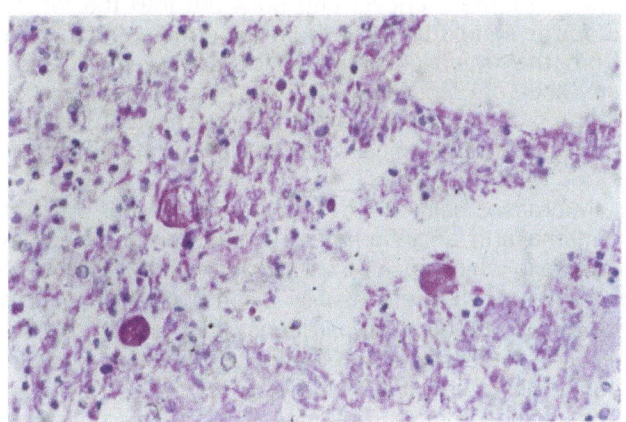

Figure 17.11 .Amoebic dysentery. Amoebae in surface debris. PAS technique × 320

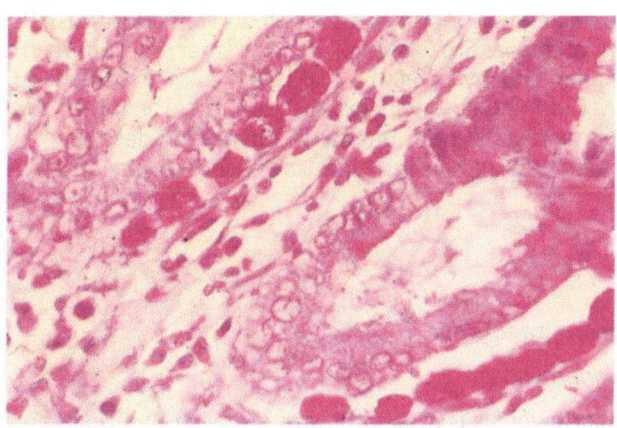

Figure 17.12 .Amoebic dysentery. Amoebae in tissues adjacent to glands.   PAS technique × 320

always with caseation and usually more florid than is seen in Crohn's disease; the tubercles often have a 'juicier' look (Figures 17.5 and 17.6). The submucosa is fibrotic rather than oedematous. Great stress is laid in some textbooks on the identification of tubercle bacilli in such lesions. I use a fluorochrome (auramine O or equivalent) for screening; if apparently positive material is found I confirm with a Ziehl-Nielsen stain, but I frankly believe that screening only with Ziehl-Nielsen is a waste of time; it is rarely if ever positive in non-caseating lesions and a negative result does not exclude a tuberculous infection.

Clostridial Infections

Clostridia are present in the normal intestinal flora of many people and cause no problems unless there is concomitant mucosal injury or alteration of normal large bowel ecology. If this happens the toxin which they liberate can cause severe damage both directly and by initiating ischaemic changes. The problem arises in the large bowel in antibiotic associated and neonatal colitis and is discussed in Chapter 18. A good recent review is available[9].

Viral Infections

Viral infections confined to the large bowel are probably uncommon; combined small and large bowel infection can be caused by adeno-, entero-, echo- and Coxsackie viruses, and there is not uncommonly a concomitant *E. coli* infection. Outbreaks and epidemics occur, particularly in institutions, in children below the age of 2 years and in old people; some of these can be associated with concurrent or pre-existing bronchiolitis. I know of no biopsy studies on purely large intestinal virally infected material in acute diarrhoea, though studies are available on the small bowel (see page 78), but changes are likely to be non-specific and mild; nuclear and cytoplasmic inclusions should be looked for. Cytomegalic inclusion disease rarely involves the gastrointestinal tract but cases have been described[10]. Lymphogranuloma venereum is described on page 111.

Fungal Infections

Actinomycosis

Actinomycosis is rare in the large bowel but reports are available[11]. There is spread to surrounding structures (retroperitoneal or perianal tissues). The most common infecting organism is the microaerophilic *Actinomyces israelii*, but some aerobic *Nocardia* can also be involved. Since *Actinomyces* are normal intestinal commensals, and since surrounding structures are almost always involved, it seems probable that invasion takes place

through the sites of minor mucosal injury. Caecum and lower rectum or anal canal are the commonest sites. Histologically the lesion is suppurative, with the formation of much granulation tissue, and characteristic colonies of branching filamentous organisms are present (Figure 17.7).

Other Fungal Infections

It is likely that patients with primary ulceration of the rectum or anus from other causes may acquire a secondary fungal infection, particularly if they have been treated with steroids or are immuno-compromised. I have not seen a biopsy example but, from a study of oesophageal lesions, one would expect to see demonstrable fungi with a relative absence of inflammatory response.

Protozoal Infestations

Amoebic Dysentery and Colitis

Infestation with *Entamoeba histolytica* is not confined to tropical countries though it is more common in them than in temperate ones; I have now seen it in a number of patients who have never travelled outside Britain even on a package-deal holiday, and it appears to be becoming increasingly common in male homosexuals (page 111). The life cycle is simple. Encysted amoebae are ingested in water or food and become active (vegetative) in the large bowel. They lodge on the mucosal surface, liberate enzymes which damage the surface mucosa producing erosion, burrow under the eroded mucosal edge and so penetrate down into the submucosa, producing a number of flask-shaped ulcers with relatively normal intervening mucosa (Figure 17.8). The amoebae multiply in the lesions, are shed into the lumen, encyst and pass out into the faeces. Biopsies should be taken from the edges of ulcers and from the mucosal debris which covers them, since amoebae are most easily found in the mucus adherent to the overhanging edge of an ulcer. They can easily be recognized histologically and there is no need for 'hot stool' examinations.

Microscopically there is mucosal erosion with oedema and an inflammatory reaction in the lamina propria in which eosinophils are often numerous (Figure 17.9). Amoebae are usually clearly visible in haematoxylin and eosin preparations (Figures 17.10 and 17.11); they also stain well with PAS (Figure 17.12) and can be detected using immunofluorescent techniques[12]. The distinction from *Entamoeba coli* is rarely a problem; *E. histolytica* has four, *E. coli* eight nuclei, but the easiest and best way is to look for ingested red cells (Figure 17.12). Rarely amoebae may be seen within small veins.

Metazoal Parasitic Infestations

Schistosomiasis

The symptoms of schistosomiasis are caused by a granulomatous reaction in various tissues to the ova of one of the three varieties of trematode, *S. mansoni, S. haematobium* or *S. japonica,* depending on the country of domicile. A larval stage of development occurs in certain water snails which liberate free-swimming larval forms called cerceriae. These penetrate the intact skin of those who wash or bathe in the water, migrate to the liver and there mature into adult worms. Fertilization takes place in portal veins and the females migrate into mesenteric veins and submucosal tributaries to lay their eggs. These pass out through the intestinal wall into the faeces, and, if they reach a suitable water supply, hatch out into larval forms which are then ingested by snails, so completing the cycle. Ova which become lodged in the mucosa or submucosa excite a granulomatous reaction which can be severe and extensive.

Endoscopically in the acute phase there is oedema, haemorrhage and mucosal ulceration followed by fibrosis, the development of strictures and sometimes reactive mucosal hyperplasia with polyp formation[13] (Figure 17.13).

Microscopically the ova are clearly recognizable and if well-preserved a precise diagnosis of the type is possible from the shape and position of the spine (Figure 17.14). A granulomatous reaction of epithelioid cells, giant cells, often with eosinophils and with an outer ring of fibrous tissue in later lesions (Figure 17.15) usually surrounds the ovum. Very occasionally a cross-section of a worm can be seen in biopsy (Figure 17.16).

Other Worm Infestations

Roundworms, hookworms, tapeworms and other varieties are found in the small intestine and segments of them or their ova may be detected in faecal material. They do not cause primary large bowel lesions.

Venereal Diseases

Homosexual practices in males bring their own organic complications in the rectum and anal canal. Lesions which histologically resemble self-induced proctitis or solitary ulcer syndrome, as well as amoebic infestation and shigella dysentery, are all described. The possibility, particularly in a young male, of a rectal or anal lesion being venereal must always be kept in mind.

Rectal and Anal Syphilis

The lesion most usually seen is a primary chancre, situated either at the anal margin or in the anal canal, less commonly in the rectum, where one may also see a thickened granular appearance[14]. Proctoscopically the ulcer edge is usually clearly defined and the ulcer itself is shallow with a yellowish-white base. Microscopically there is mucosal ulceration with a non-specific round cell reaction in which plasma cells predominate (Figure 17.17). It is sometimes possible to demonstrate spiro-chaetes in sections using a silver technique, but material taken fresh from the lesion is more appropriately examined using *Treponema* immobilization techniques.

Lymphogranuloma Venereum

This condition occurs in inguinal lymph nodes and occasionally in the rectum in male homosexuals[15]; it can affect the vagina in females and may spread thence to the rectum. The responsible organism is a chlamydia, which some would group with rickettsia, others with viruses; it is just visible microscopically. In the early phase there is a non-specific subacute proctocolitis which progresses to fibrosis and stricture formation and carries an increased risk of carcinoma. Biopsy findings are not distinctive and there is no accepted relationship between large bowel inflammation and *Chlamydia trachomatis* or *C. psittaci*[16].

Amoebiasis

The possibility of transmitting *Entamoeba histolytica* by sexual contact has already been mentioned[17]. The most florid example of amoebic proctitis which I have seen was caused in this way (Figure 17.18).

References

1. Dickinson, R. J., Gilmour, H. M. and McLelland, B. L. (1979). Rectal biopsy in patients presenting to an infectious disease unit with diarrhoeal disease. *Gut,* **20**, 141

2. Mandal, B. K. and Mani, V. (1976). Colonic involvement in salmonellosis. *Lancet,* **1**, 887

3. Radsel-Medvescek, A., Zargi, R., Acko, M. and Zajc-Satler, J. (1977). Colonic involvement in salmonellosis. *Lancet,* **1**, 601

4. Willoughby, C. P., Piris, J. and Truelove, S. C. (1979). Campylobacter colitis. *J. Clin. Pathol.,* **32**, 986

5. Price, A. B., Jewkes, J. and Sanderson, P. J. (1979). Acute diarrhoea, campylobacter colitis and the role of rectal biopsy. *J. Clin. Pathol.,* **32**, 990

6. Blaser, M. J., Parsons, R. B. and Wang, W.-L. W. (1980). Acute colitis caused by campylobacter fetus ss jejuni. *Gastroenterology,* **78**, 448

7. Gleason, T. H. and Patterson, S. D. (1982). The pathology of yersinial enterocolitica ileocolitis. *Am. J. Surg. Pathol.,* **6**, 347

8. Hawley, P. R., Wolfe, H. R. I. and Fullerton, J. M. (1968). Hypertrophic tuberculosis of the rectum. *Gut,* **9**, 461

9. Bartlett, J. G. (1981). *Clostridium difficile* and inflammatory bowel disease. *Gastroenterology,* **80**, 863

10. Levine, R. S., Warner, N. E. and Johnson, C. F. (1964). Cytomegalic inclusion disease in the gastrointestinal tract of adults. *Ann. Surg.,* **159**, 37

11. Udagawa, S. M., Portin, B. A. and Bernhoft, W. H. (1974). Actinomycosis of the colon and rectum: report of two cases. *Dis. Col. Rect.,* **17**, 687

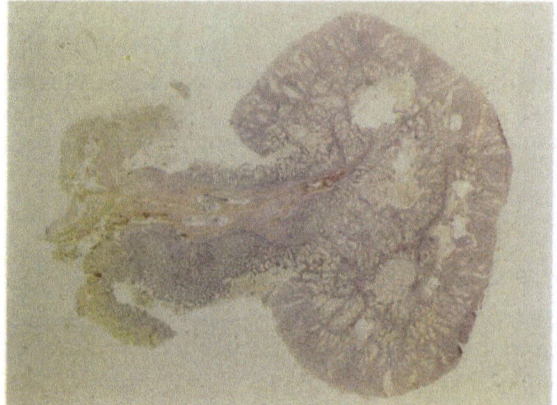

Figure 17.13   Schistosomal polyp. These polyps are the result of reactive mucosal hyperplasia following infestation with ova.   H & E × 20

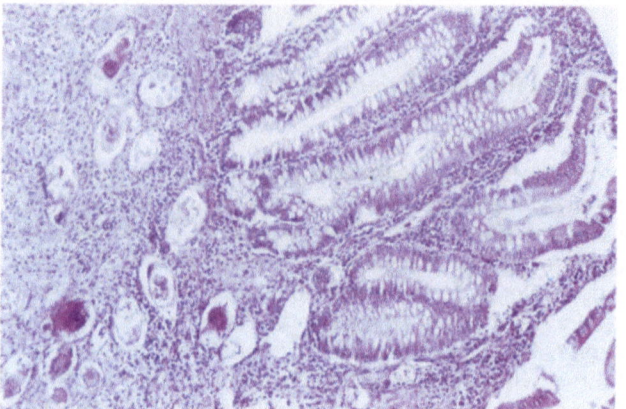

Figure 17.14   Rectal schistosomiasis. Numerous ova are present in the superficial submucosa, surrounded by an inflammatory reaction in which eosinophils are present.   H & E × 125

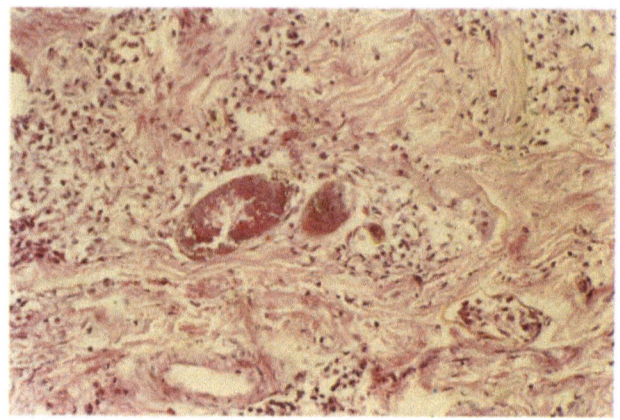

Figure 17.15   Schistosomiasis. In this later lesion there is little remaining inflammatory response and the two ova are surrounded by fibrous tissue. H & E × 320

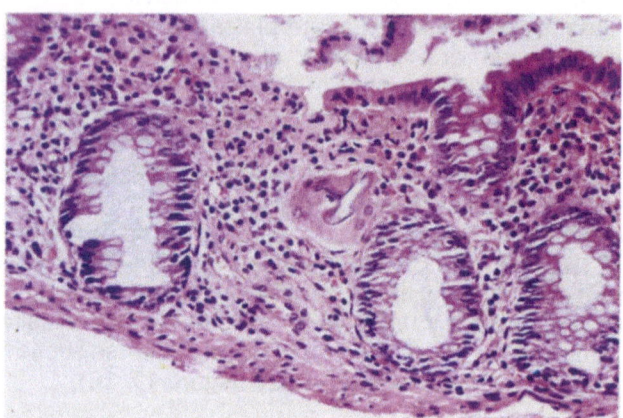

Figure 17.16   Schistosomiasis. Cross-section of a worm in a rectal biopsy – a rare finding!   H & E × 125

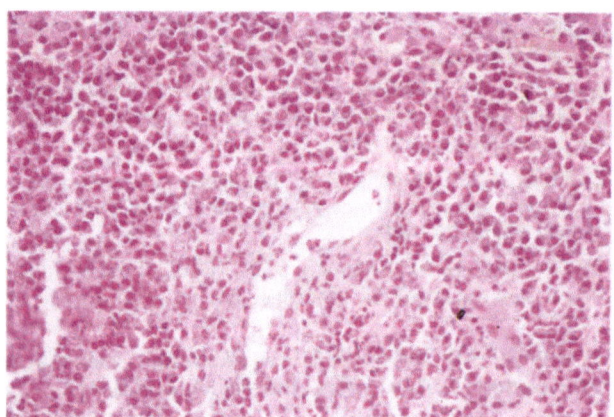

Figure 17.17   Syphilis. This anal biopsy from an ulcerated lesion clinically suggestive of chancre shows numerous plasma cells which should always arouse suspicion. *Treponema pallidum* was found in the surface exudate. H & E × 125

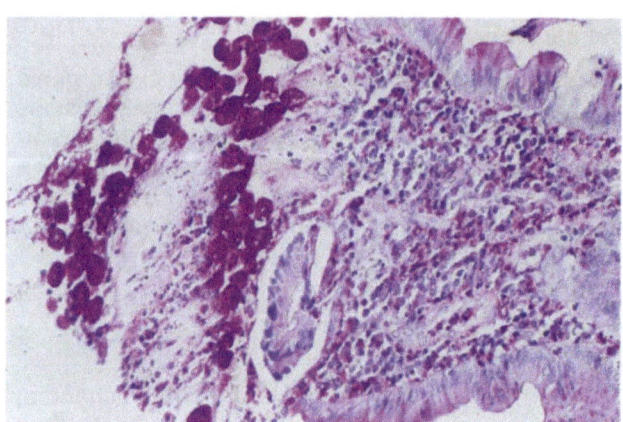

Figure 17.18   Amoebic infestation in a rectal biopsy from a male homosexual.   PAS technique × 125

12. Gilman, R., Islam, M., Paschi, S., Goleburn, J. and Ahmad, F. (1980). Comparison of conventional and immunofluorescent techniques for the detection of *Entamoeba histolytica* in rectal biopsies. *Gastroenterology,* **78**, 435

13. Tikriti, F. and Al-Saleem, T. (1976). Bilharzial polyposis of the rectum and sigmoid colon. *Br. J. Surg.,* **63**, 458

14. Akdamar, K., Martin, R. J. and Ichinose, H. (1977). Syphilitic proctitis. *Am. J. Dig. Dis.,* **22**, 701

15. Levine, J. S., Smith, P. D. and Brugge, W. R. (1980). Chronic proctitis in male homosexuals due to lymphogranuloma venereum. *Gastroenterology,* **79**, 563

16. Elliott, P. R., Forvey, T., Darovgar, S., Treharne, J. D. and Lennard-Jones, J. E. (1981). Chlamydiae and inflammatory bowel disease. *Gut,* **22**, 25

17. Burnham, W. R., Reeve, R. S. and Finch, R. G. (1980). *Entamoeba histolytica* infection in male homosexuals. *Gut,* **21**, 1097

Ischaemic bowel lesions are becoming increasingly common as people live to a greater age, and biopsy material from them is now often seen. It is important to realize that different causative factors may produce similar clinical patterns of presentation (usually severe diarrhoea with or without blood and varying degrees of dehydration, hypovolaemia and collapse) but with differing macroscopic and microscopic features in the early stages and requiring different regimes of treatment. They must be distinguished reliably from each other and from certain non-ischaemic lesions which may resemble them, and in this early biopsy plays a vital part[1].

The intestinal mucosa is the part of the bowel most sensitive to oxygen deprivation and therefore the earliest to show changes under adverse conditions. Its integrity depends on adequate replication of cells in the crypts to cover normal cell losses and make good damage from other causes, of which bacillary and viral infections are probably the most common. There is a constant and delicate balance between the potentially harmful bacterial or viral content of the lumen, whether by direct damage to the surface mucosa or by the production of toxins, and the ability of the mucosa to re-generate (Figure 18.1). Mucosal damage can thus be caused by an abnormal bacterial or viral content, either qualitative or quantitative or both, which overwhelms the normal defence mechanisms of the mucosa, or by a reduced blood supply in the presence of a normal bowel flora. In practice these two factors are associated in ischaemic bowel disease; the link is strengthened by the fact that many bacterial toxins, as well as a number of ingested drugs, appear to have a local vasoconstrictive effect.

Generalized ischaemia occurs in two main forms. In the first there is organic obstruction to the blood flow, usually arterial[1] but sometimes primarily venous as in intussusception or volvulus[2]. Arterial obstruction can result from external pressure or constriction of a major vessel, but is more commonly the result of athero-matous narrowing with or without a final thrombosis, or of necrotizing arteritis with thrombosis, or of embolism. The effects depend upon the vessel involved. In the small intestine the superior mesenteric artery divides to form a series of anastomosing arcades which provide a good collateral circulation until terminal end arteries pierce the muscularis mucosae to supply the mucosa. To produce pathological change any blockage must be either in the first 1–2 cm of the artery, before any major division has occurred, or in the terminal end arteries where it will lead to local ischaemia and ulceration[3]. Luminal narrowing in a large artery must involve at least 60% of the lumen to produce symptoms. In the large bowel the collateral anastomosis is less good, par-ticularly at the splenic flexure where the arterial distribu-tion changes from superior to inferior mesenteric, and ischaemic lesions are common at this site[4].

The second important form of ischaemia is that usually termed 'low-flow state'. The splanchnic circula-tion, through its vasoconstrictor action, plays a major role in blood pressure regulation. Such constriction, though it may be temporarily life-saving, can reduce the mucosal blood flow below acceptable levels. This can occur during shock, in severe haemorrhage, during operative procedures and following acute myocardial infarction[5,6]. All of these are more common in the elderly and all are aggravated by anaemia which is common in this age group.

Ischaemic lesions can be localized, when there is usually circumscribed mucosal ulceration – which can be seen on colonoscopy and biopsied, or generalized – when a variable length of bowel is involved. Biopsies, according to the stage of the disease at which they are taken, may show ischaemic mucosal necrosis, re-generation or repair with granulation tissue formation and sometimes fibrosis which can lead to stricture formation. The mucosa is always damaged first and worst; severe ischaemia or prolonged hypotension can also lead to necrosis of muscularis propria with the risks of perforation and peritonitis.

Ischaemic Colitis

The common clinical features of generalized ischaemic colitis are sudden onset of abdominal pain with severe diarrhoea, usually with the passage of much blood, and preceded or followed by collapse; it is often difficult to decide whether the collapse is the cause or the result of the bleeding. Treatment is resection as rapidly as possible and prognosis is poor. Many surgeons request rapid frozen section to exclude fulminating colitis or antibiotic associated disease.

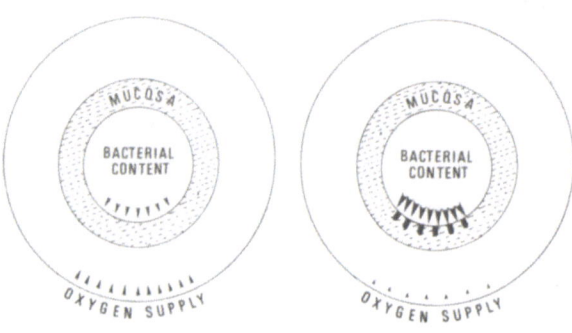

Figure 18.1   The diagram on the left shows the normal situation. The oxygen supply is adequate to maintain mucosal defences against the intraluminal bacteria which are normally present. If the oxygen supply is reduced or the bacterial content increased or altered in type, mucosal damage, as shown on the right, becomes probable

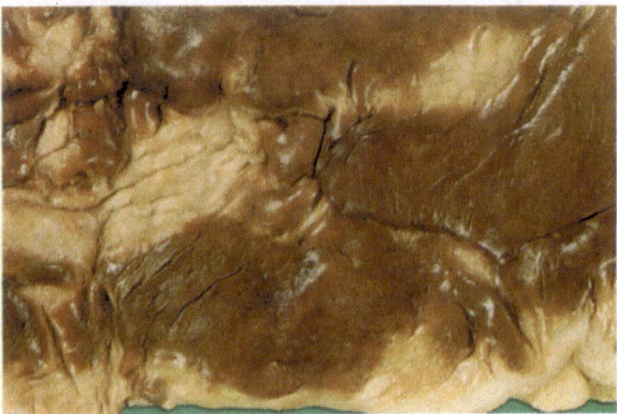

Figure 18.2   Ischaemic colitis (I.C.). Patchy mucosal congestion, oedema and haemorrhage occur. Resected specimen

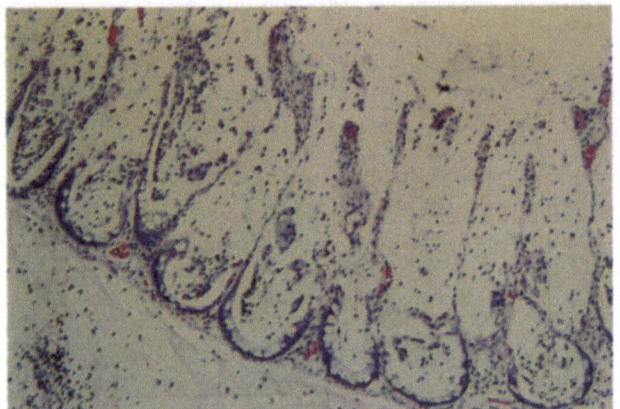

Figure 18.3   I.C., early mucosal damage. Epithelial cells have sloughed off from the upper part of the mucosa but some still remain intact at the base and regeneration is possible if the blood supply can be restored. There is submucosal oedema.   H & E × 100

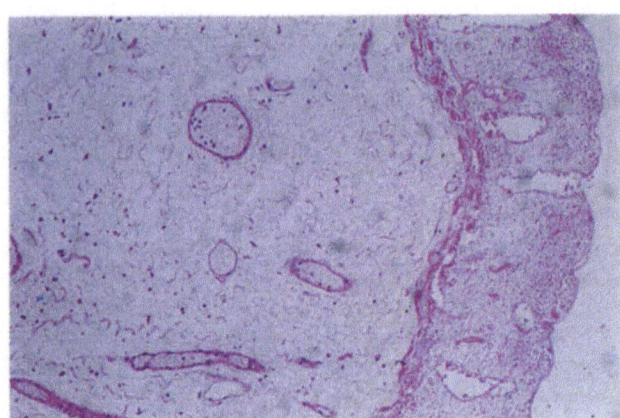

Figure 18.4   I.C. The mucosa is virtually completely necrotic over the whole length of the biopsy and there is very marked submucosal oedema. H & E × 65

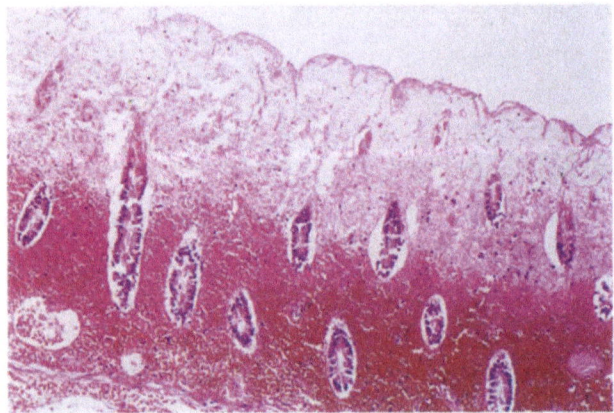

Figure 18.5   I.C. showing surface mucosal necrosis and haemorrhage in the deeper layers.   H & E × 100

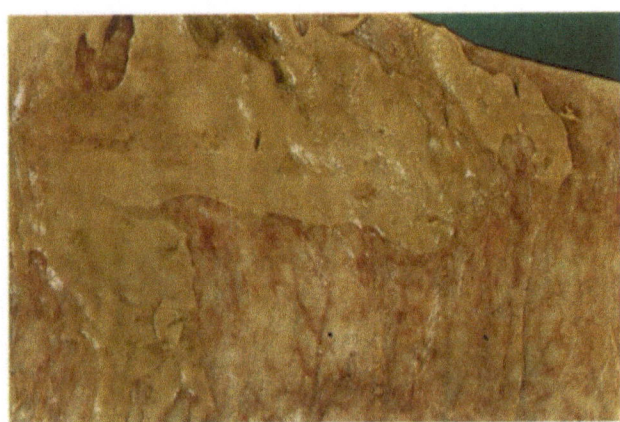

Figure 18.6   I.C. Surface coagulum, composed of desquamated mucosa, fibrin and debris. The mucosa has ulcerated and the surface without coagulum is in fact submucosa. Resected specimen

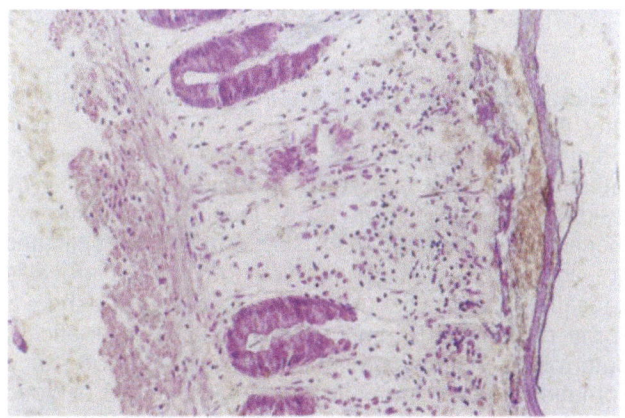

Figure 18.7 I.C. This biopsy shows clearly the outlines of dead cells and the intact muscularis mucosae. H & E × 100

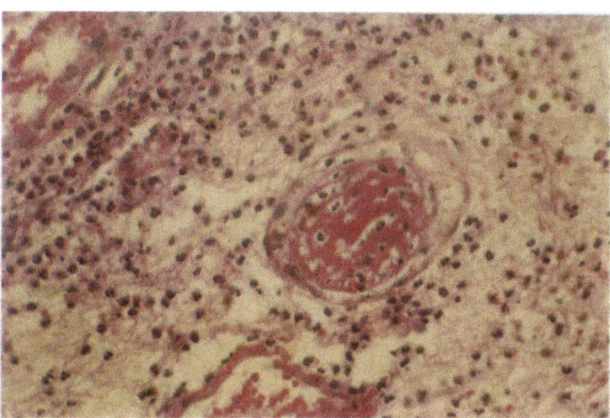

Figure 18.8 I.C. Fibrin thrombus in a small submucosal vessel. H & E × 320

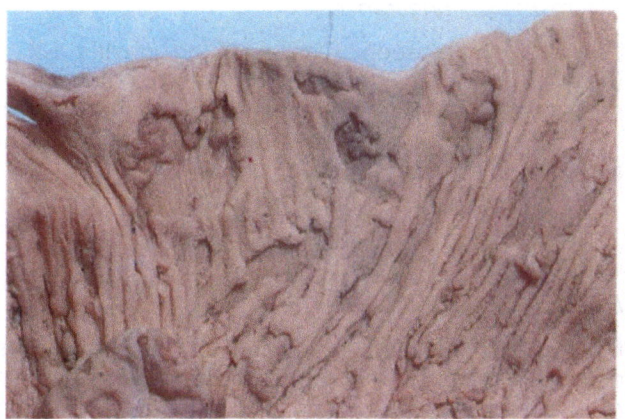

Figure 18.9 I.C. Healing ulcers. The mucosa has been undermined and there is an attempt at inflammatory type polyp formation as seen in ulcerative colitis. Resected specimen

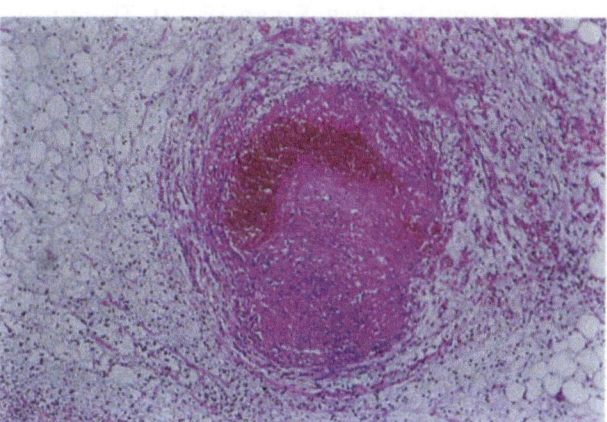

Figure 18.10 I.C. necrotizing arteritis with thrombosis as a cause of ischaemic colitis. H & E × 65

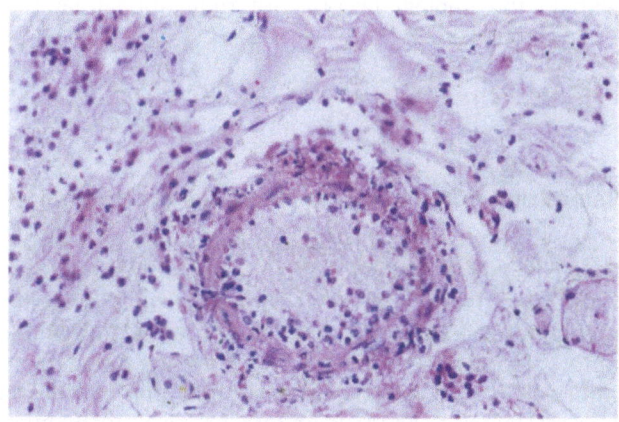

Figure 18.11 I.C. An early arteritic lesion in the submucosa. This may represent a secondary arteritis but should always prompt a consideration of a primary arteritis as a cause of the ischaemia. H & E × 100

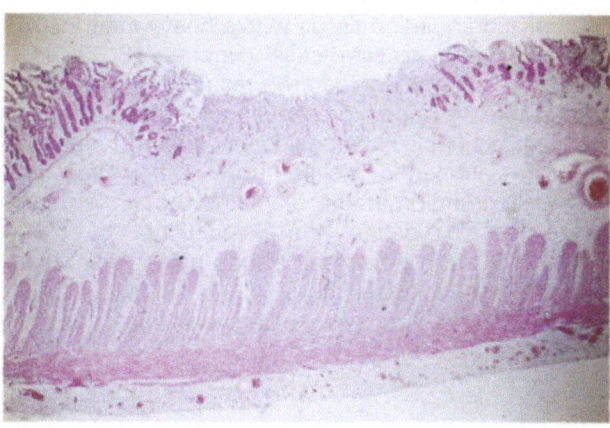

Figure 18.12 I.C. Healing phase. The small ulcer present has been repaired by granulation tissue without mucosal regeneration at this stage. H & E × 25

Macroscopic Appearances

The earliest visible colonoscopic evidence is conspicuous mucosal congestion and oedema with some haemorrhage. At laparotomy the outer surface of the bowel may appear normal, but is often congested and dusky in colour and may be obviously gangrenous (Figure 18.2).

Microscopic Appearances

Biopsy in the early stages characteristically shows marked submucosal oedema with ulceration and sloughing of surface mucosa; the deeper glands initially often remain more or less intact (Figures 18.3 and 18.4). Lesions are diffuse rather than multifocal as in antibiotic-associated colitis and all of the mucosa included in the biopsy is likely to be involved (compare Figures 18.3 and 18.4 with Figure 18.17). There may be a well defined haemorrhagic zone, usually confined to the deeper lamina propria (Figure 18.5).

The mucosal erosion or ulceration, and the associated bleeding, lead to the formation of a surface coagulum of debris, fibrin and sometimes polymorphs if secondary infection occurs (Figure 18.6). At this stage tubules appear swollen and expanded in their deeper parts while more superficially there may be coagulative necrosis so that the outlines of dead cells remain (Figure 18.7). Fibrin thrombi are often present in small vessels (Figure 18.8) but are the effect rather than the cause of ischaemic lesions. There is occasionally patchy undermining of mucosa with pseudopolyp formation reminiscent of fulminating ulcerative colitis (Figure 18.9) but the two conditions are not usually difficult to distinguish. If the submucosa is included a careful search should be made for intra-arterial thrombi containing red cells as well as fibrin in submucosal arteries, and for evidence of necrotizing arteritis (Figures 18.10 and 18.11), which can be a possible causative factor.

If the patient survives without operation mucosal regeneration begins and there is usually conspicuous submucosal granulation tissue with a heavy infiltrate of lymphocytes and plasma cells (Figures 18.12 and 18.13). A particular feature resulting from the haemorrhage is the presence of macrophages containing stainable haemosiderin, which helps to distinguish ischaemic colitis from other lesions. Occasional granulomatous reactions occur around included faecal material; these must not be misdiagnosed as Crohn's disease. Pseudo-pyloric glandular metaplasia also occurs (Figure 18.14). Biopsies from the edge of local ischaemic ulcers will show similar changes.

Antibiotic-associated Colitis

Extensive studies[7-9] have shown that the administration of broad-spectrum antibiotics may, in certain patients, disturb normal small and large bowel ecology and allow the unrestricted growth of anaerobic clostridia, particularly *Cl. difficile* in caecum and colon. The exotoxin which this organism liberates can directly damage intestinal mucosa and also produce ischaemic-type lesions, probably through a local vasoconstrictive mechanism. The antibiotics most commonly implicated are lincomycin and clindamycin but others are also causative. Lesions occur irrespective of age and there is some evidence that susceptibility may be genetically determined. Patients present with severe diarrhoea and sometimes dehydration, and though much loss of blood is rare they may be suspected clinically and endoscopically of having ischaemic colitis. Since the prognosis and treatment of these conditions are totally different accurate diagnosis, which is usually possible on biopsy when taken early, is vital.

Macroscopic Appearances

The early macroscopic lesion is diagnostic. Small (0.5–1.5 cm) yellow (paint-spot) raised patches are present on a congested mucosal background (Figures 18.15 and 18.16); later the patches become confluent and resemble ischaemic lesions.

Microscopic Appearances

Mushroom-like ('erupting volcano' or 'plateau') zones of exudate project into the lumen with intervening zones of relatively normal mucosa (Figure 18.17). The exudate is a mixture of fibrin, debris and polymorphs and appears to explode out from underlying glands, the lowermost layer of which remains relatively intact (Figure 18.18). The intervening mucosa may show some oedema of lamina propria but initially is not often eroded or ulcerated[8]. In later stages ulceration may become confluent and the picture become indistinguishable from ischaemic colitis. Fibrin thrombi are not seen in the earliest lesions but may appear later in mucosal capillaries[9,10].

Necrotizing Enterocolitis in Neonates and Infants

Lesions which resemble ischaemic colitis and others more closely resembling antibiotic-associated colitis are both seen in infants[11,12]; ischaemia and bacterial infection, especially clostridial, are probably interacting factors. Predisposing factors are exchange transfusion, umbilical artery or aortic catheterization, immaturity and perinatal hypoxia, all of which may cause interruption of the normal splanchnic blood supply. Thromboembolic occlusion of vessels is common, but is unlikely to be seen on biopsy, and the history suggests a primary ischaemic causation rather than a bacterial one. Ileum and colon can both be involved but only the latter is usually biopsied.

Macroscopically there is often severe mucosal and

submucosal oedema (Figure 18.19) which microscopically is associated with capillary dilatation and epithelial desquamation. A mushrooming appearance similar to that seen in antibiotic-associated colitis (Figure 18.20) has been the commonest finding in my own material and this suggests a clostridial rather than an ischaemic origin. It is, however, proper to point out that most if not all of these babies will have been given broad-spectrum antibiotics. A peculiarly severe form can be associated with Hirschsprung's disease in which there has been severe obstruction. When recovery occurs there is often extensive fibrosis with stricture formation, resembling that seen in congenital stenoses. Gas cysts may form in the submucosa, probably as a result of secondary bacterial infection in an ischaemic bowel (Figure 18.21).

Solitary Ulcers due to Drugs

These are included here since some are thought to result from the local lodging of a tablet or capsule in the intestinal mucosa with release of locally vasoconstrictive substances, causing local ischaemia. They are naturally more common in the small bowel, where they are not available for biopsy, but are also described in the large bowel in relation to naproxen, indomethacin and steroid therapy (Figures 18.22–18.24). Microscopically appearances do not differ appreciably from those seen in ischaemic colitis or local ischaemic ulceration.

Figures 18.13–18.24 will be found overleaf.

References

1. Alschibaja, T. and Morson, B. C. (1977). Ischaemic bowel disease. *J. Clin. Pathol.*, **30** Suppl. (Roy. Coll. Pathol.), **11**, 68

2. Grendell, J. H. and Ockner, R. K. (1982). Mesenteric venous thrombosis. *Gastroenterology*, **82**, 358

3. Whitehead, R. (1972). The pathology of intestinal ischaemia. *Clin. Gastroenterol.*, **1**, 613

4. Binns, J. C. and Isaacson, P. (1978). Age-related changes in the colonic blood supply: their relevance to ischaemic colitis. *Gut*, **19**, 384

5. Musa, B. U. (1965). Intestinal infarction without mesenteric occlusion. A report of 31 cases. *Ann. Intern. Med.*, **63**, 783

6. Delue, H. W. D. (1976). Necrotic colitis in the presence of normal vascularisation of the colon. *Arch. Chir. Neerl.*, **28**, 55

7. Tedesco, F. J., Anderson, C. B. and Ballinger, W. F. (1975). Drug-induced colitis mimicking an acute surgical condition of abdomen. *Arch. Surg.*, **110**, 481

8. Sumner, H. W. and Tedesco, F. J. (1975). Rectal biopsy in clindamycin-associated colitis. *Arch. Pathol.*, **99**, 237

9. Price, A. B. and Davies, D. R. (1977). Pseudomembranous colitis. *J. Clin. Pathol.*, **30**, 1

10. Bogomoletz, W. V. (1976). Fibrin thrombi: a cause of clindamycin-associated colitis. *Gut*, **17**, 483

11. de Sa, D. J. (1976). The spectrum of ischaemic bowel disease in the newborn. In Rosenberg, H. S. and Bolande, R. P. (eds.). *Perspectives in Pediatric Pathology*. Vol. 3, p. 273. (Chicago: Year Book Medical Publishers)

12. Tait, R. A. and Kealy, W. F. (1979). Neonatal necrotising enterocolitis. *J. Clin. Pathol.*, **32**, 1090

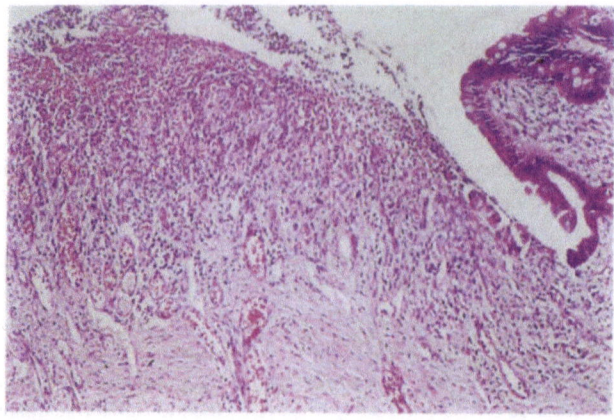

Figure 18.13   I.C. Healing phase. The ulcer base is formed of granulation tissue and re-epithelialization is beginning from the right-hand edge. Macrophages containing iron pigment were present at the edges.   H & E × 100

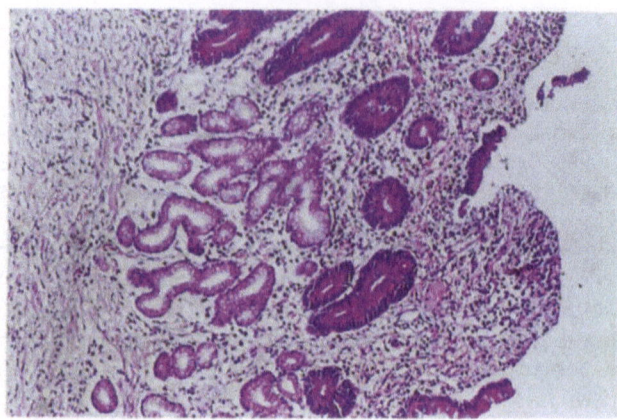

Figure 18.14   I.C. Healing phase. Pseudopyloric metaplasia.   H & E × 100

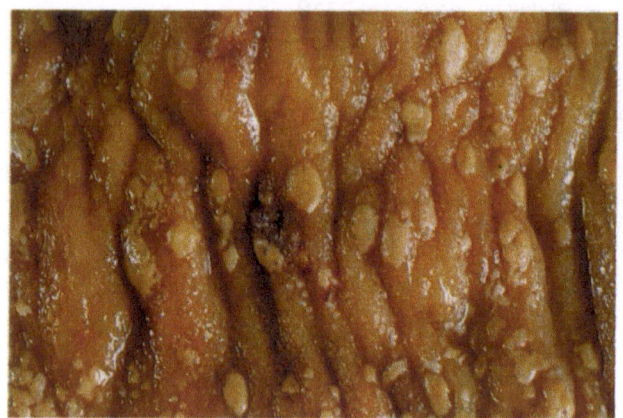

Figure 18.15   Antibiotic-associated colitis (A.A.C.). The early macroscopic lesion consists of small discrete raised spots against a mucosal background which is usually more congested than shown here.   Resected specimen

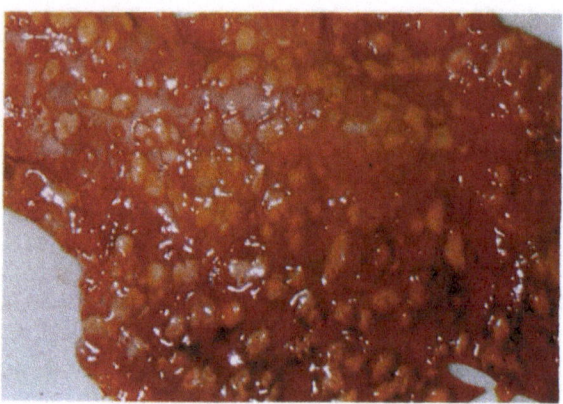

Figure 18.16   A.A.C. Slightly more advanced stage than that show in Figure 18.15. The mucosal congestion is more obvious and the patches are beginning to become confluent.   Resected specimen

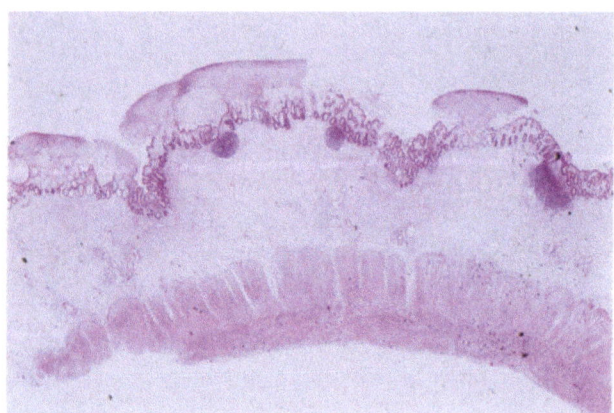

Figure 18.17   A.A.C. Typical mushroom-like (erupting volcano) lesions in A.A.C. These, which correspond to the 'paint spots' seen macroscopically (Figures 18.15 and 18.16) consist of superficial mucosal necrosis with exudate which is patchy, leaving zones of relative normal mucosa in between.   H & E × 25

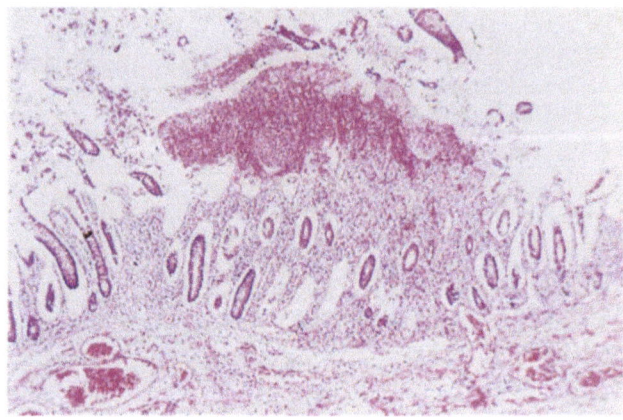

Figure 18.18   A.A.C. Higher-power view showing the surface exudate firmly attached to necrotic mucosa.   H & E × 80

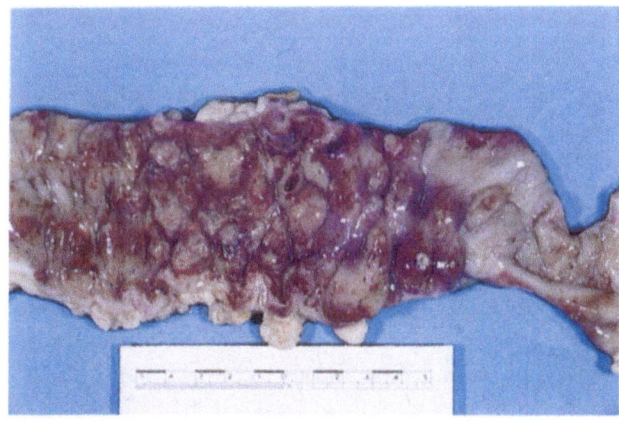

Figure 18.19 Necrotizing enterocolitis of infancy (N.E.I.). Resected specimen. Note the marked submucosal oedema with congestion and early haemorrhage

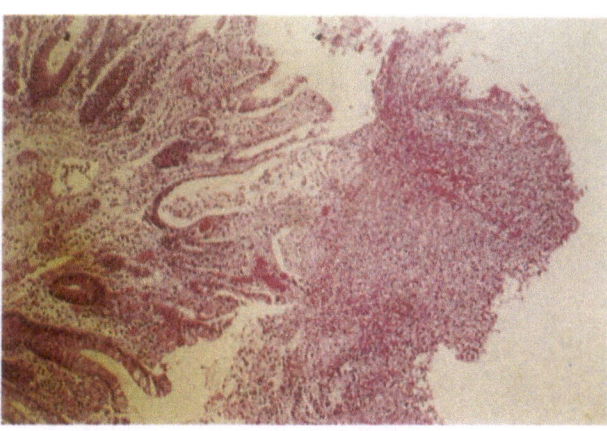

Figure 18.20 N.E.I. The mushrooming appearance is similar to that seen in antibiotic-associated colitis. H & E × 80

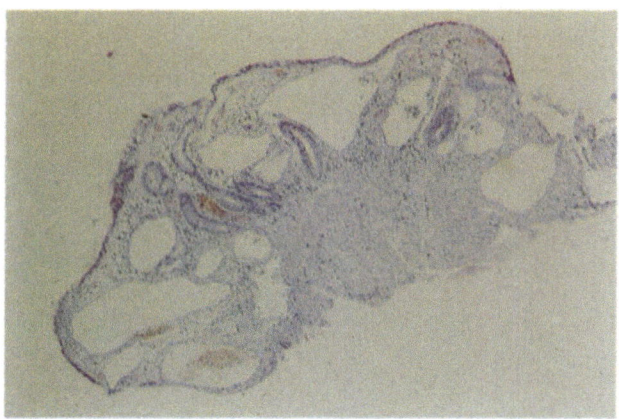

Figure 18.21 N.E.I. If recovery occurs in necrotizing enterocolitis gas cysts may form in the submucosa. H & E × 32

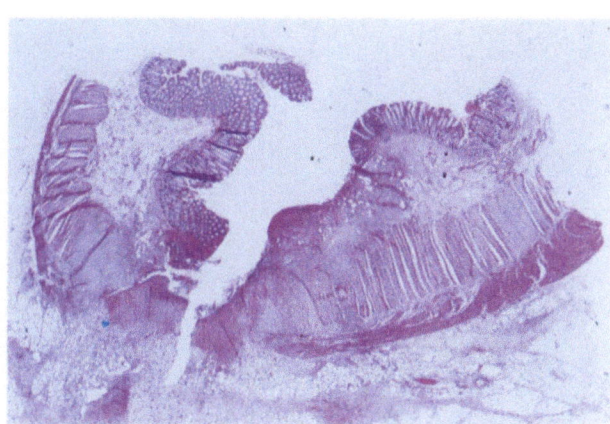

Figure 18.22 Naproxen ulcer. Appearances are those of acute non-specific ulceration. H & E × 25

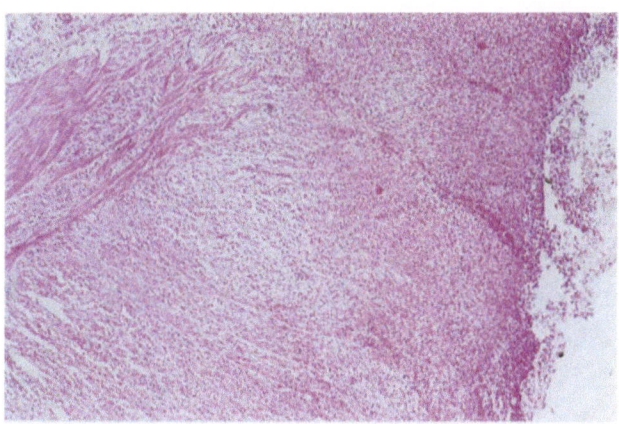

Figure 18.23 Naproxen ulcer. A higher-power view of Figure 18.22 to show the non-specific nature of the tissue reaction. H & E × 100

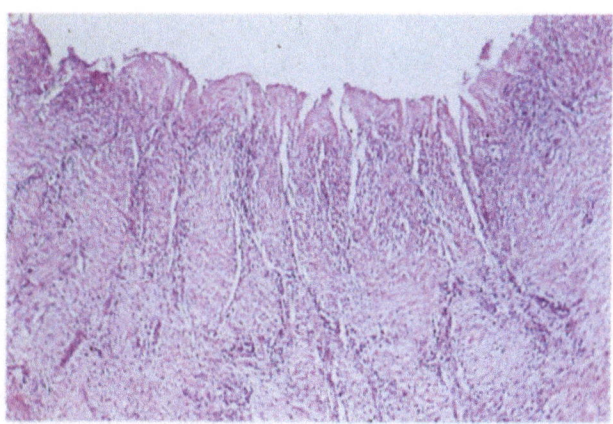

Figure 18.24 Steroid ulcer. The ulcerated zone has been replaced by granulation tissue which has become fibrosed. There was no attempt at epithelial regeneration at the time this biopsy was taken. It is impossible to say whether the steroids this woman was taking caused the ulcer, or merely delayed healing. H & E × 100

19

Large Intestine and Anal Canal: Polypoid Epithelial Lesions and Associated Dysplasias

Many large intestinal biopsies reach the laboratory with a one-word diagnosis of 'polyp'. Some are non-epithelial, others non-neoplastic; many are neoplastic and of epithelial origin. This chapter covers polypoid epithelial lesions of all types as they usually present to the pathologist. Polyps can be sessile or pedunculated; biopsies can merely sample the polyp or can include a stalk or adjacent normal epithelium and can be single or multiple. It is essential to see that every piece of material is blocked out in such a way that every fragment can be serially sectioned if need be. It is also important to orientate biopsies carefully and particularly to determine whether a stalk is present, and, if so, to ensure that it is included in the section.

Non-neoplastic Epithelial Polyps

These are of two kinds: those which are inflammatory proliferations of mucosa and granulation tissue have already been discussed (page 98). The remainder are malformations or hamartomas.

Peutz–Jeghers' Polyps

These have already been described on page 97; they are formed by a tree-like branching proliferation of the muscularis mucosae which carries with it a covering of epithelium normal to the part, including any specialized cells normally present. They are most common in the stomach and upper small bowel, usually present in childhood and are inherited, along with circumoral pigmentation, as an autosomal dominant, but single or multiple forms are occasionally seen in the large bowel. Endoscopically they have a lobulated outer surface, often a broad pedicle and are not often ulcerated (Figure 19.1). Microscopically the branching muscularis clothed in normal large bowel epithelium is usually unmistakeable (Figure 19.2). Buried epithelium, which appears to lie deep to muscularis, is common (Figure 19.2) and must not be interpreted as malignant; the best way of avoiding this is overall recognition of the type of polyp in a young patient with special stains to reveal the presence of endocrine cells in the buried epithelium; these are not usually a feature of carcinoma.

Juvenile Polyps

The common juvenile polyp may be single or be present in small numbers which often appear sequentially, usually with bleeding, sometimes with the passage of the polyp itself. They are probably hamartomas of the lamina propria. Endoscopically the outer surface is smooth rather than lobulated and is often ulcerated. There is frequently an attenuated pedicle which can undergo auto-amputation. The cut surface shows cystic spaces containing mucin (Figure 19.3). Microscopically there are cystic-dilated glands without mucosal hyperplasia, containing mucin and set in a plentiful stroma of oedematous lamina propria in which lymphocytes and plasma cells are increased in number. Surface epithelial erosion is common and polymorphs, indicating secondary infection, may be present (Figure 19.4).

Rare syndromes of multiple juvenile polyps have been described[1] in familial and non-familial forms which may also involve small bowel and stomach and form part of a juvenile polyp–metaplastic polyp–adenoma sequence[2]. Material from all patients with multiple juvenile polyps should be carefully examined for adenomatous changes.

Cronkhite–Canada Syndrome

In this rare syndrome, leakage of protein into the gastro-intestinal tract is associated with diarrhoea, malabsorption, electrolyte disturbances, skin pigmentation, alopecia and atrophy of the nails[3]. Lesions can be present in small and large bowel. In the latter they somewhat resemble juvenile polyposis to which some workers believe the condition is related[4], despite the differences in age and presentation. In the large bowel there is polypoidal mucosal proliferation without ulceration. Microscopically glands are dilated and contain mucus; there are sometimes crypt abscesses and the lamina propria is oedematous and contains an increased number of inflammatory cells (Figure 19.5).

Metaplastic (Hyperplastic) Polyps

Metaplastic polyps are probably the most frequently occurring polyp in humans and since they usually have no neoplastic potential it is important prognostically to

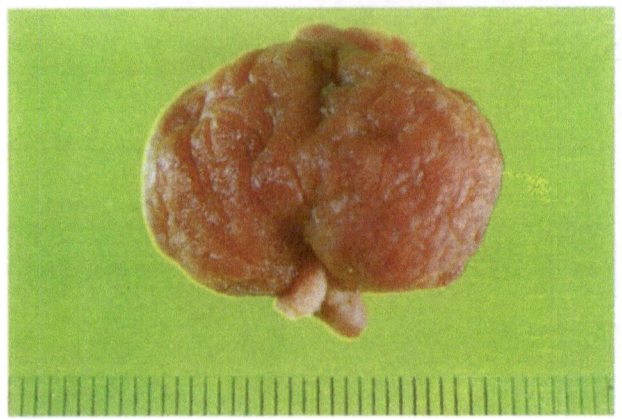

Figure 19.1   Peutz–Jeghers' polyp. The surface is slightly lobulated and there is a broad pedicle at the base. 10 mm scale

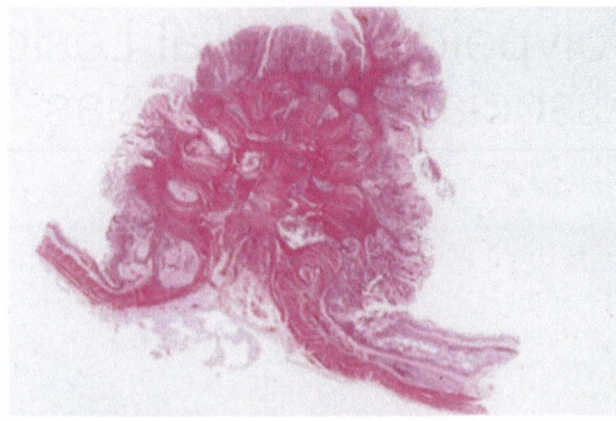

Figure 19.2   Peutz–Jeghers' polyp. The hyperplasia of the muscularis is well shown, clothed in normal large bowel mucosa. Islands of epithelium are buried in the muscularis. Whole mount section.   H & E × 4

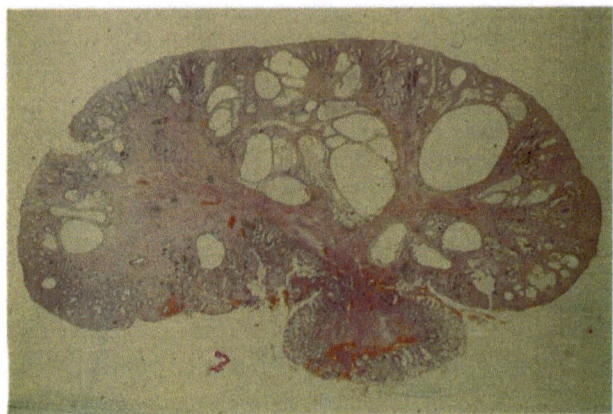

Figure 19.3   Juvenile polyp. The cut surface shows large cystic spaces which contain mucin and a narrow pedicle. Whole mount section.   H & E × 8

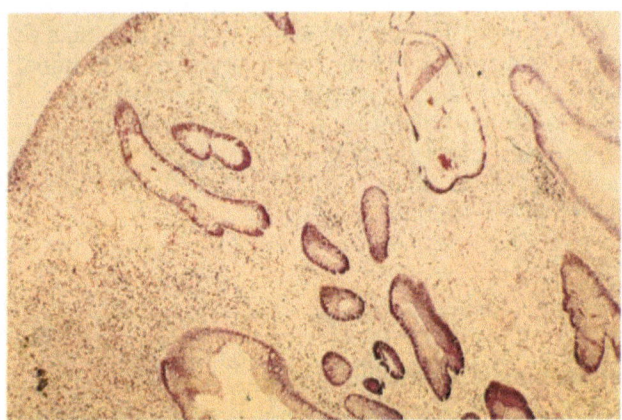

Figure 19.4   Juvenile polyp. The dilated spaces are lined by cubical or flattened columnar epithelium and there is an increase in the volume of lamina propria which is oedematous and has a mononuclear cell infiltrate.   H & E × 125

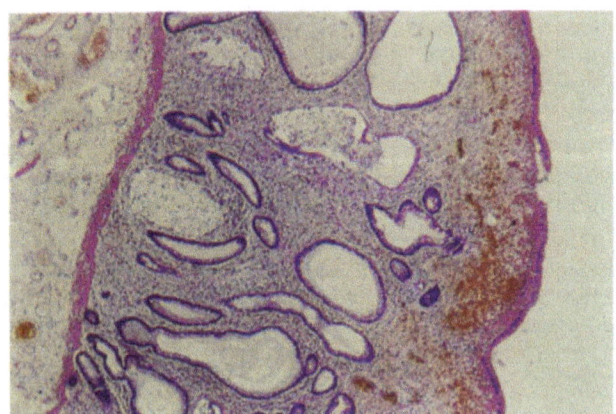

Figure 19.5   Cronkhite–Canada syndrome. There is marked cystic dilatation of glands with destruction of the epithelial lining and polymorphs within the cysts, forming a type of crypt abscess. The lamina propria contains an increased number of inflammatory cells.   H & E × 100

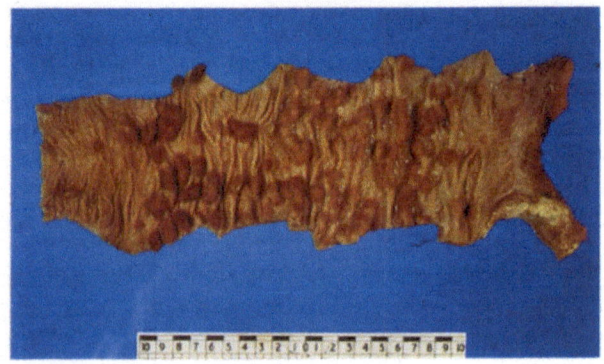

Figure 19.6   Metaplastic polyps. A resected rectum with numerous metaplastic polyps, with a maximum length of 10 mm and either sessile or having only a short and broad pedicle

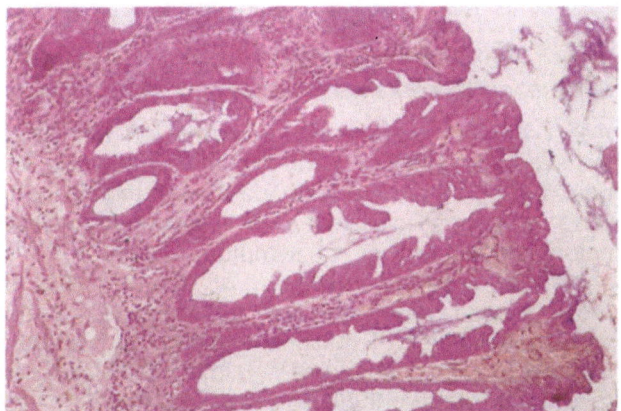

Figure 19.7 Metaplastic polyp. This section shows well the crypt lengthening and dilatation and the inward projection of papillary processes, with an increase in size of absorptive cells.   H & E × 125

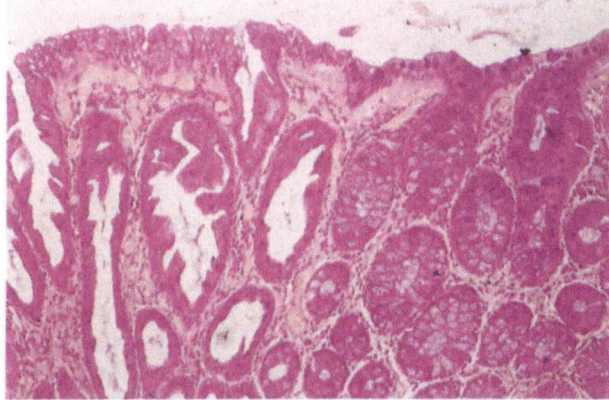

Figure 19.8 Metaplastic polyp. This incidental finding in a rectal biopsy shows the edge of an early metaplastic polyp which has not as yet projected from the surface.   H & E × 125

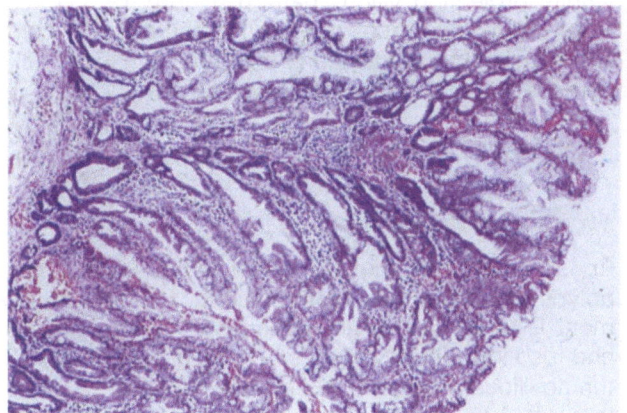

Figure 19.9 Metaplastic polyp with tubular adenomatous change. Both patterns can clearly be seen.   H & E × 125

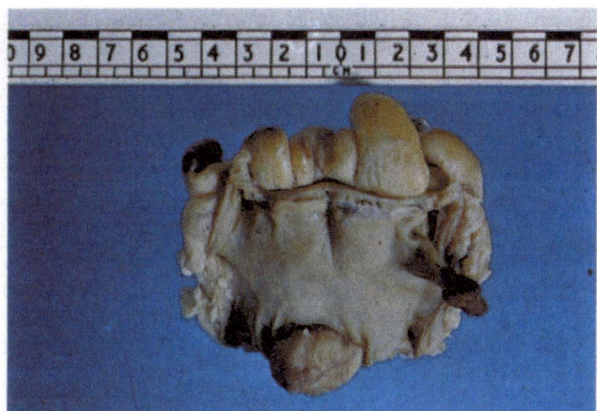

Figure 19.10 Adenoma. This resected specimen shows both a moderate sized sessile adenoma (left bottom) and a smaller pedunculated adenoma (right), both with a tubular pattern

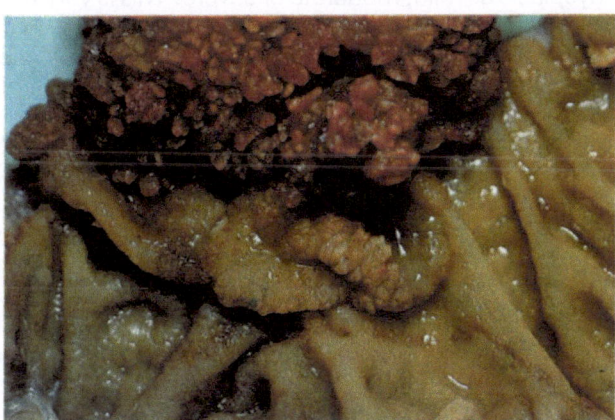

Figure 19.11 Villous adenoma. Resected specimen. Small projecting villous processes are clearly visible

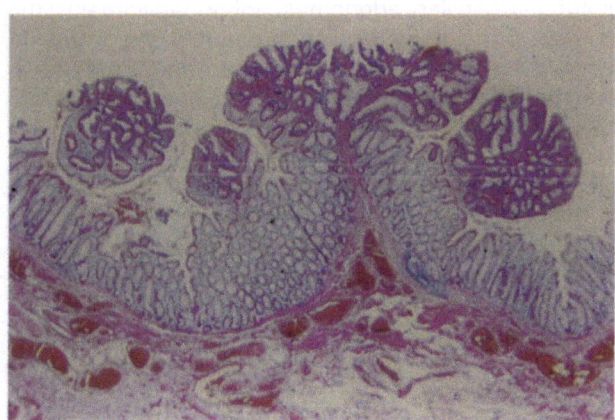

Figure 19.12 Tubular adenoma. It consists entirely of well-formed glandular elements.   H & E × 65

recognize them. They are more common in men than women and begin to appear around the age of 50, becoming more common as age advances. They are usually less than 10 mm in diameter, single and sessile, though multiple forms do occur (Figure 19.6) and some of the large polyps can develop a pedicle and show tubular or tubulovillous zones[5,6]. Endoscopically they have a smooth surface and it has been suggested that they can be distinguished from adenomas after resection by painting their surface with 1% trypan blue and examining them under a dissecting microscope[7]. I have no experience of this recently described technique. Microscopically there seems to be a delay in the normal upward migration of cells from the crypt zone, so that more mature cells are found at a lower level. This produces a characteristic appearance of crypt lengthening with dilatation and sometimes inward projection of papillary processes into the dilated crypt and an increase in size and number of absorptive cells. There is also fragmentation of the muscularis mucosae and an increased round cell infiltrate in the lamina propria (Figure 19.7). Sometimes a rectal biopsy in an elderly patient includes the edge of an early metaplastic lesion which has not yet projected as a polyp (Figure 19.8).

The epithelium does not usually show any hyperplastic changes or suggest a premalignant condition; studies which attempt to relate metaplastic polyps to carcinoma because of similarity of site have largely proved negative[8]. Nevertheless, in the larger polyps, particularly those over 10 mm in diameter, and in multiple lesions, there is sometimes evidence of adenomatous change, usually tubular (Figure 19.9) but sometimes tubulovillous[7].

Adenomas and Associated Epithelial Dysplasia

Pathologists are now well familiar with the WHO classification of large intestinal adenomas into tubular (adenomas), villous (papillomas) and tubulovillous or villotubular (papillary adenomas, adenopapillomas)[9]; the previous terminology is given in parentheses. They are also familiar with the concept of an adenoma–carcinoma (polyp–cancer) sequence in which adenomas are liable to undergo malignant transformation over a period which averages about 10 years[10]. There is little doubt that most carcinomas arise from pre-existing adenomas but the frequency with which malignant change occurs in adenomas has not yet been reliably determined. All adenomas, whatever their histological pattern, are in fact examples of epithelial polypoid dysplasia of varying patterns and degrees of severity, which change with the period of time during which they have developed. Nonpolypoid hyperplasias and the typical dysplasias seen in ulcerative colitis, which can be polypoid on occasion, are discussed in Chapter 20.

Biopsies of adenomas may include the whole lesion, with stalk if it is pedunculated, or merely represent an endoscopic nibble from the edge of a lesion. To obtain the maximum information close cooperation between endoscopist and pathologist is essential.

Endoscopic Appearances

Adenomas are more common in the left than in the transverse or right colon and in men than women; they become more frequent with age though the size range does not appear to increase[11,12]. In patients coming to colonoscopy because of symptoms, about 50% of adenomas will have a diameter of 10 mm or less and most of these will be tubular or tubulovillous, a pattern with reduced risk of malignant change as compared with purely villous adenoma[12]. It is therefore important to know the size of the lesion biopsied. Recent studies have suggested that painting the lesion with 1% trypan blue and examining it under a dissecting microscope may also help to identify possible malignancy[7]; I have no personal experience.

Small tubular and tubulovillous adenomas have a smooth or sometimes a lobulated surface, rather like a raspberry, and can be sessile or pedunculated (Figure 19.10); villous adenomas are larger and have a more definite projecting villous pattern (Figure 19.11). The larger lesions are more common in the sigmoid colon and rectum, and as they carry the greatest risk of malignant change adequate biopsy is essential.

Microscopic Appearances

Considerable care must be given to the embedding of polyps to include any stalk present. The first requirement is to decide whether the lesion is adenomatous and if so into which category – tubular (Figure 19.12), tubulovillous (Figure 19.13) or villous (Figure 19.14) – it falls. It has been my experience that the more thoroughly an adenoma is examined the more often can it be shown to have a mixed tubulovillous pattern (Figure 19.15). I agree with others[13] that it is preferable to categorize adenomas as tubular or villous when they contain 80% or more of that pattern even when some mixture of patterns is present.

The next requirement is to grade the degree of dysplasia as mild, moderate or severe. This is very much a subjective matter and pathologists working in the same institution for the same clinicians should constantly compare and discuss their criteria. In general in mild dysplasia there is little glandular irregularity apart from an increase in branching of glands; nuclei are enlarged, the nuclear–cytoplasmic ratio is slightly increased, there may be some early stratification, but the gland arrangement remains regular, there is no conspicuous cellular pleomorphism and mitoses are either normal in number or only slightly increased (Figure 19.16). In severe dysplasis there is marked glandular irregularity with compression of gland elements which obliterates gland lumina and gives a 'back-to-back' appearance. The nuclear–cytoplasmic ratio is greatly increased, there is much cellular pleomorphism with loss of normal nuclear polarity and an increased number of mitoses. Mucin secretion is greatly decreased (Figure 19.17). Moderate dysplasia falls between these two categories. The degree of dysplasia in villous components is more difficult to assess; more attention must be given to cellular pleomorphism and mitotic figures than to reproduction of villous pattern (Figures 19.18 and 19.19). When adenomas are multiple there is a greater tendency to severe dysplasia in at least some of them.

Having assessed the degree of dysplasia a search must be made for evidence of invasion, either by an examination of the stalk if it is included or of the muscularis mucosae and submucosa if these are present (Figure 19.20). Care must be taken not to diagnose buried epithelium in a polyp stalk[14] as early invasion (Figure 19.21). This can usually be avoided by assessing the regularity of gland elements and looking for endocrine cells; often there is also recognizable lamina propria present.

When all these factors have been evaluated it can still be impossible to determine, on biopsy which includes mucosa only, whether a particular adenoma has undergone malignant change. Aside from breach of the muscularis mucosae the most helpful indications are size, pattern and degree of dysplasia; malignant change is rare in adenomas less than 10 mm in diameter, of tubular pattern and without severe dysplasia. A repeat biopsy in larger lesions can be a very helpful procedure.

Familial Adenomatosis

Familial adenomatosis is inherited as an autosomal dominant though mutations are not uncommon. Patients usually present in the second or third decades with many hundreds of developing adenomas; it has been suggested that a minimum of 100 polyps is necessary to distinguish the condition from that of multiple adenomas[15]. Individual adenomas do not differ histologically from the solitary non-inherited adenomas already descibed; there is some evidence that they begin as an infolding of adenomatous surface epithelium between normal pre-existing glands[16] and that this may represent a significant difference in genesis between tubular adenomas and upgrowing villous adenomas. Some of my own material supports a surface origin (Figures 19.22 and 19.23) but I have also seen tubulovillous patterns in this condition.

Adenomatous Polyps associated with Other Conditions

Colonic adenomatous polyps are found in Gardner's syndrome[17], Turcot's syndrome[18] and as a complication of ureterosigmoidostomy[19] in which latter the polyps can also be reactive or juvenile in pattern.

The polypoid pattern of dysplasia sometimes seen in long-standing ulcerative colitis is described in Chapter 20.

Figures 19.13–19.23 will be found overleaf.

References

1. Lipper, S., Kahn, L. B., Sandler, R. S. and Varma, V. (1981). Multiple juvenile polyposis. A study of the pathogenesis of juvenile polyps and their relationship with colonic adenomas. *Hum. Pathol.*, **12**, 804

2. Goodman, Z. D., Yardley, J. H. and Milligan, F. D. (1979), Pathogenesis of colonic polyps in multiple juvenile polyposis. Report of a case associated with gastric polyps and carcinoma of the rectum. *Cancer*, **43**, 1906

3. Kindblom, L., Angervall, L., Santesson, R. and Selander, S. (1977). Cronkhite Canada syndrome – case report. *Cancer*, **39**, 2651

4. Ruymann, F. B. (1969). Juvenile polyps with cachexia. Report of an infant and comparison with Cronkhite Canada syndrome in adults. *Gastroenterology*, **57**, 431

5. Williams, G. T., Arthur, J. F., Bussey, H. J. R. and Morson, B. C. (1980). Metaplastic polyps and polyposis of the colorectum. *Histopathology*, **4**, 155

6. Vatn, M. H. and Stalsberg, H. (1982). The prevalence of polyps of the large intestine in Oslo. An autopsy study. *Cancer*, **49**, 819

7. Thompson, J. J. and Enterline, H. T. (1981). The macroscopic appearance of colorectal polyps. *Cancer*, **48**, 151

8. Correa, P., Strong, J. P., Reif, A. and Johnson, W. D. (1977). The epidemiology of colorectal polyps; prevalence in New Orleans and international comparison. *Cancer*, **39**, 2258

9. Morson, B. C. and Sobin, L. H. (1976). *Histological Typing of Intestinal Tumours.* (Geneva: World Health Organization)

10. Morson, B. C. and Dawson, I. M. P. (1979). *Gastrointestinal Pathology*, 2nd edn. Chapter 38. (Oxford: Blackwell)

11. Rickert, R. R., Auerbach, O., Garfinkel, L., Hammond, E. C. and Frasca, J. M. (1979). Adenomatous lesions of the large bowel. An autopsy survey. *Cancer*, **43**, 1847

12. Gillespie, P. E., Chambers, T. J., Chan, K. W., Doronzo, F., Morson, B. C. and Williams, C. B. (1979). Colonic adenomas; a colonoscopic survey. *Gut*, **20**, 240

13. Konishi, F. and Morson, B. C. (1982). Pathology of colorectal adenomas; a colonoscopic survey. *J. Clin. Pathol.*, **35**, 830

14. Muto, T., Bussey, H. J. R. and Morson, B. C. (1973). Pseudocarcinomatous invasion in adenomatous polyps of the colon and rectum. *J. Clin. Pathol.*, **26**, 25

15. Bussey, H. J. R. (1975). *Familial Polyposis Coli.* (Baltimore: Johns Hopkins University Press)

16. Maskens, A. P. (1979). Histogenesis of adenomatous polyps in the human large intestine. *Gastroenterology*, **77**, 1245

17. Danes, B. S. (1976). Increased tetraploidy: cell specific for the Gardner gene in the cultured cell. *Cancer*, **38**, 1983

18. Itoh, H., Ohsato, K., Yao, T., Iida, M. and Watanabe, H. (1979). Turcot's syndrome and its mode of inheritance. *Gut*, **20**, 414

19. Ansell, I. D. and Vellacott, K. D. (1980). Colonic polyps complicating ureterosigmoidostomy. *Histopathology*, **4**, 429

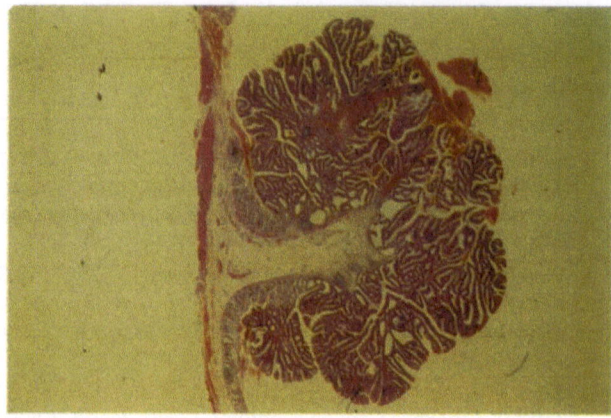

Figure 19.13 Tubulovillous adenoma. There is a mixed tubular and villous pattern. H & E × 32

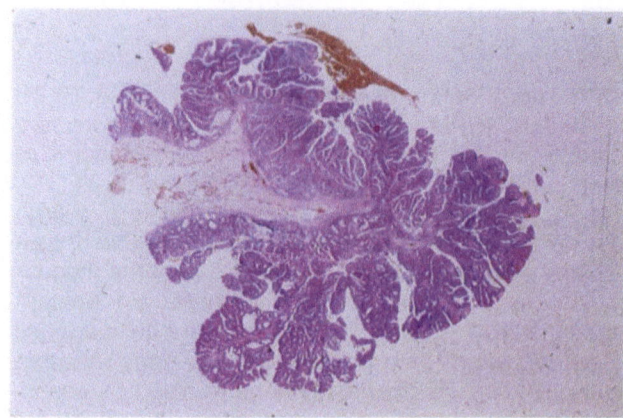

Figure 19.14 Villous adenoma. Although a few recognizable tubular elements are present, over 80% of the adenoma has a villous pattern. H & E × 25

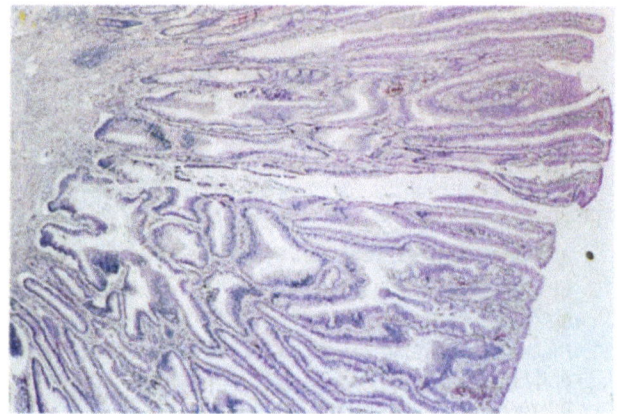

Figure 19.15 Tubulovillous adenoma. This adenoma appeared on first examination to be purely villous. A detailed search of many sections revealed zones of glandular pattern which, when added up, came to more than 20% of the total area sampled. The tumour was therefore classified as tubulovillous. H & E × 125

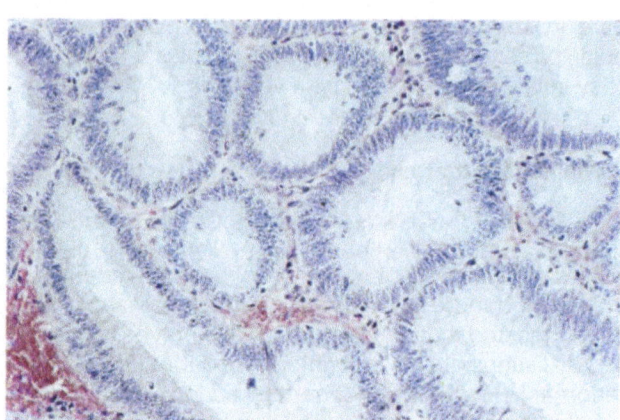

Figure 19.16 Tubular adenoma, mild dysplasia. Gland elements are regular, there is no conspicuous cellular pleomorphism and very few mitoses. H & E × 320

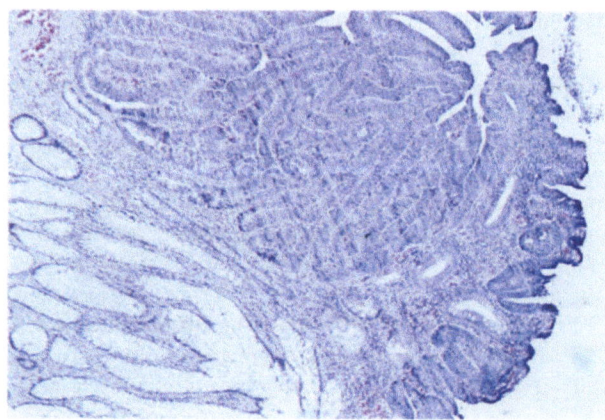

Figure 19.17 Tubular adenoma, severe dysplasia. There is marked glandular irregularity, cellular pleomorphism and an increased number of mitoses. In a biopsy without muscularis, this could not be distinguished from carcinoma. H & E × 100

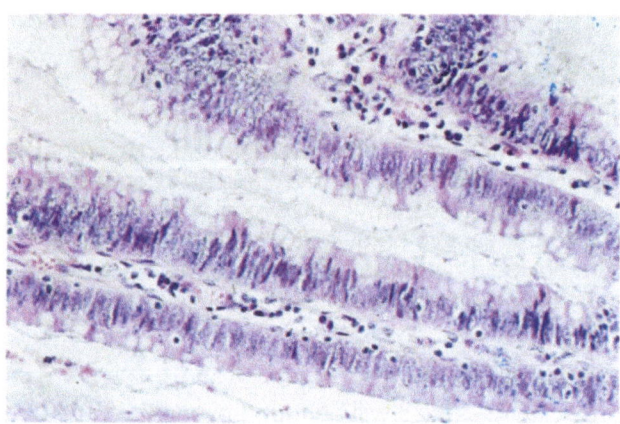

Figure 19.18 Villous adenoma. The villous pattern is retained but there is considerable cellular pleomorphism; this biopsy fits into the moderate dysplasias. H & E × 320

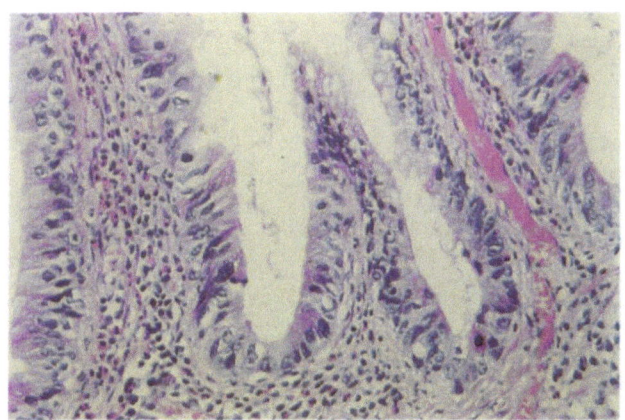

Figure 19.19 Villous adenoma. Same specimen as Figure 19.18 showing the increased cellular pleomorphism. H & E × 320

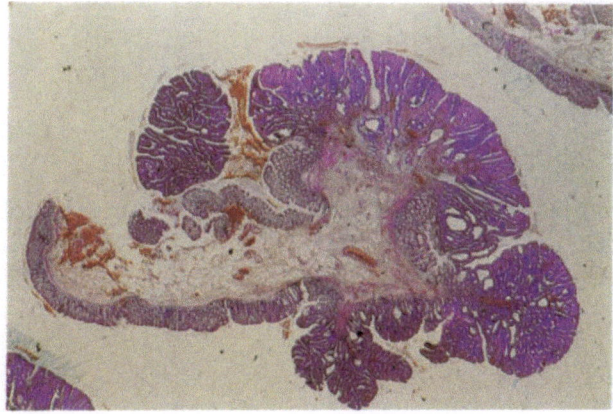

Figure 19.20 Tubulovillous adenoma showing early carcinomatous change with invasion of the muscularis mucosae. H & E × 32

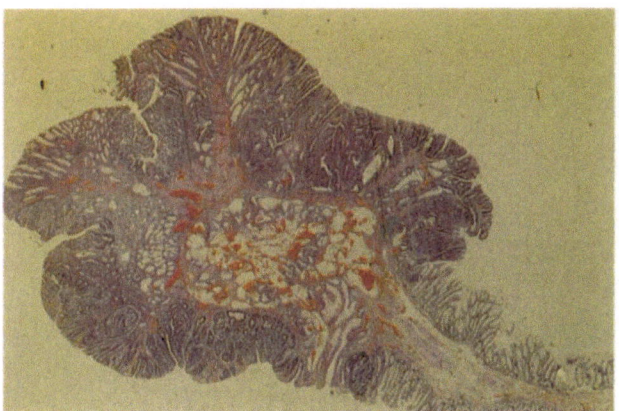

Figure 19.21 Tubulovillous adenoma with buried epithelium in the stalk. The epithelial elements are regular, though some glands are distended with mucus, and there is no cellular pleomorphism. H & E × 25

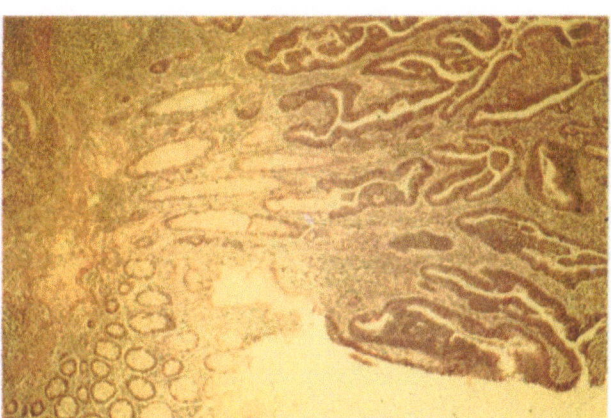

Figure 19.22 Familial adenomatosis. An adenoma is arising from the superficial mucosa with the deeper parts of the glands still remaining normal. H & E × 125

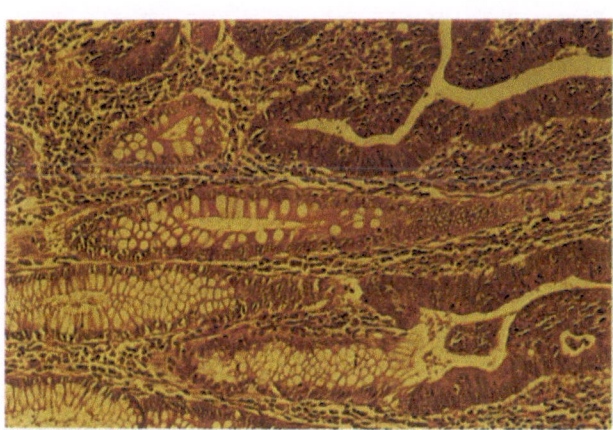

Figure 19.23 Higher-power view of Figure 19.22 to show the abrupt origin of the adenomatous change. H & E × 250

20

Large Intestine and Anal Canal: Dysplasias and Malignant Neoplasms

Precancerous Epithelial Changes

Most, if not all, large bowel adenocarcinomas unassociated with other disorders arise from pre-existing adenomas; the development in these of dysplasia prior to carcinomatous change has been discussed in Chapter 19. There are, however, a group of cancers arising in association with chronic inflammatory bowel disease in which dysplasia is an important feature and it is also necessary to discuss the recently described 'transitional' change in large bowel epithelium adjacent to neoplasms.

Dysplasia in Inflammatory Bowel Disease

It is well recognized that in long-standing chronic or quiescent ulcerative colitis there is a risk of carcinoma developing which increases with the duration of the colitis[1]. In patients who have had resections of large bowel with ileorectal anastomoses it is current practice to biopsy the rectal stump at regular intervals to look for precancerous dysplastic changes. Regular colonoscopy with multiple biopsies is also often offered to patients with colitis of more than 10 years standing who have not had a resection. It is thus important to be able to recognize dysplastic epithelium in a biopsy, to grade the dysplasia and to separate it from the chronic hyperplastic change sometimes seen in active ulcerative colitis.

Dysplastic changes are most common in the sigmoid colon and rectum. They may have an adenomatous or a flat mucosal appearance. Those which are adenomatous endoscopically can appear nodular or velvety; peduncle formation is rare. More than one such zone may be present. Microscopically there are two patterns. The adenomatous may resemble sessile tubular adenomas as already described (Figure 20.1) or may have a more tubulovillous pattern and extend over a wide area of mucosa (Figure 20.2). The flat pattern, which is not always visible endoscopically, arises in an atrophic mucosa and shows gland irregularities, nuclear pleomorphism, hyperchromatism and often an absence of goblet cells (Figure 20.3), and there may be abnormal cell proliferation throughout elongated crypts (Figures 20.4 and 20.5). More extensive sampling may show both patterns (Figure 20.6), and early invasion may be present in the submucosa (Figure 20.7). The differentiation from inflammatory hyperplasia can be difficult, particularly when dysplasia is mild, but this is less

significant than it may seem, for there is evidence that only severe dysplasia is likely to progress to carcinoma[2-4] . There is also some evidence that when dysplasia is associated with polypoid or plaque-like lesions the risk of neoplasia is greater[5] but this observation needs confirmation. To summarize, rectal biopsy in long-standing colitis is of value in detecting dysplasia which, when severe, is likely to presage carcinomatous change either at the site of biopsy or elsewhere in the colon. Because dysplastic changes are patchy a negative biopsy may represent a sampling error and more accurate reports are likely if regular colonoscopic survey and multiple biopsies are available[6,7].

Dysplastic and malignant changes in the large bowel in association with long-standing Crohn's disease are much less common but are well recognized[8,9]; appearances are similar to those seen in ulcerative colitis but the cancer risk is much less.

Transitional Mucosa

Although dysplastic precancerous changes are described as developing within existing adenomas and in the epithelium in chronic inflammatory bowel disease, they are not normally seen in the epithelium adjacent to the edge of a developing carcinoma or adenoma. In the belief that a sharp transition from completely normal to neoplastic mucosa without an intermediate phase was inherently unlikely, a number of workers have studied the epithelium within 5–10 mm of the edge of adenomas and carcinomas in the hope of detecting changes which, though less florid than dysplasia, could be characterized as pre-neoplastic[10-12]. Certain histological changes have been found, of which the most significant are elongation of crypts with branching and distension and an increase in goblet cell numbers without evidence of hyperplasia (Figure 20.8). A more detailed study of mucins and enzyme systems within this epithelium[10,11,13,14] showed that changes were present which paralleled the histological findings; the most significant were the mucin studies, which revealed a relative absence of the normal sulphomucin content and an increase in sialomucins (Figures 20.9 and 20.10). Ultrastructural studies, which included scanning and transmission electron micrographs, have also supported the presence of mucosal abnormalities[15]; the choice of the term 'transitional' to describe them is unfortunate since it is purely descriptive and

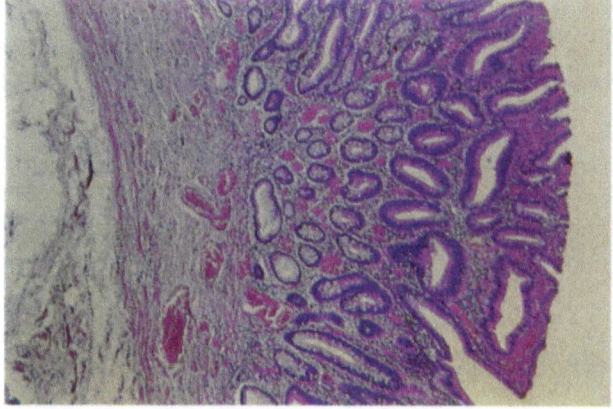

Figure 20.1 Dysplasia in ulcerative colitis (U.C.). Localized adenomatous dysplasia in the superficial mucosa. H & E × 100

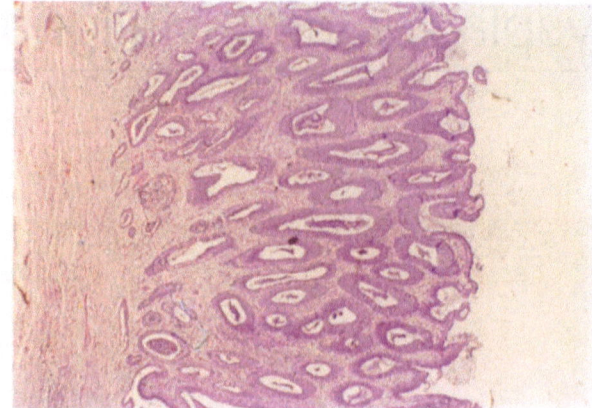

Figure 20.2 Dysplasia in U.C. More diffuse tubulovillous pattern of dysplasia. H & E × 100

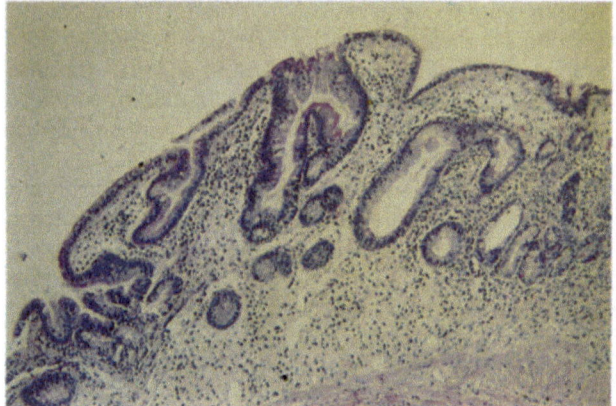

Figure 20.3 Dysplasia in U.C. This shows a moderate dysplasia in a flat mucosa; there is no suggestion here of an adenomatous type pattern. H & E × 100

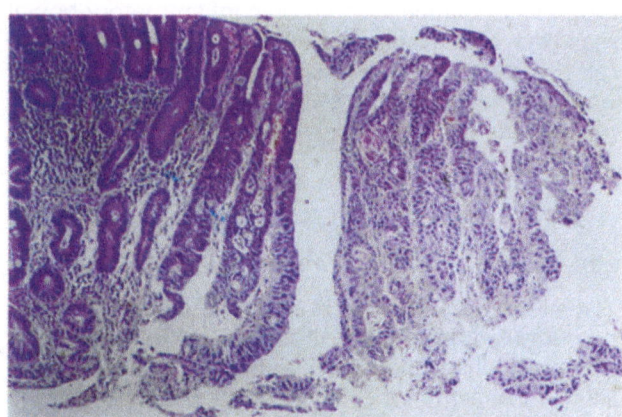

Figure 20.4 Dysplasia in U.C. This biopsy shows severe dysplasia in a flat mucosa. The dysplasia extends throughout the elongated crypts. H & E × 125

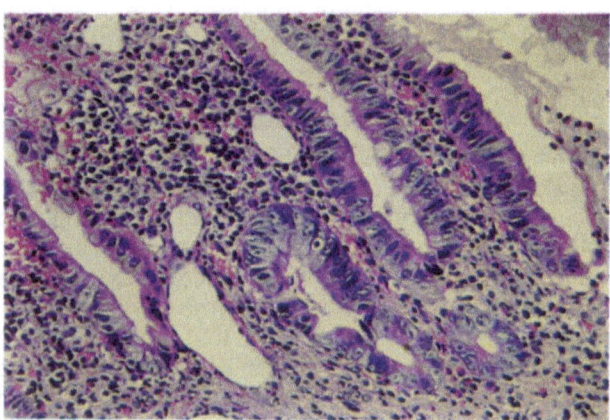

Figure 20.5 Dysplasia in U.C. A higher-power view from the same biopsy as Figure 20.4, showing the nuclear pleomorphism and absence of goblet cells. H & E × 320

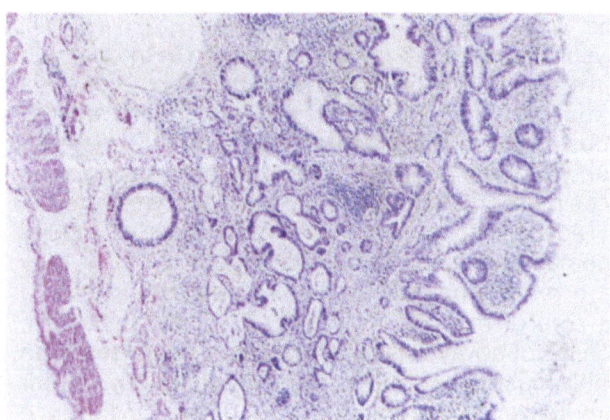

Figure 20.6 Dysplasia in U.C. A mixed type of pattern showing adenomatous-type hyperplasia superficially and a more severe glandular pattern of dysplasia in the deeper mucosa. H & E × 125

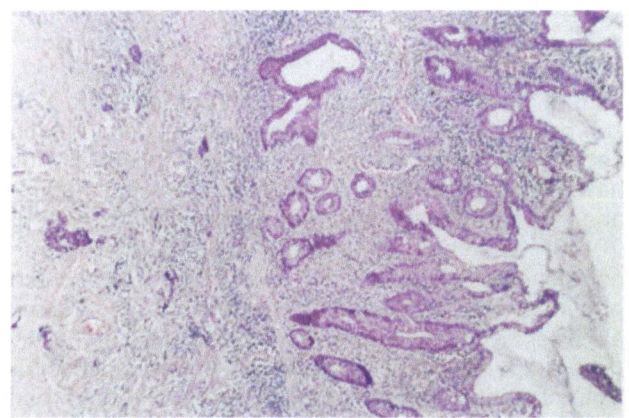

Figure 20.7 Early carcinoma in U.C. The epithelium shows severe dysplasia and there is invasion into the submucosa indicating carcinomatous change. H & E × 80

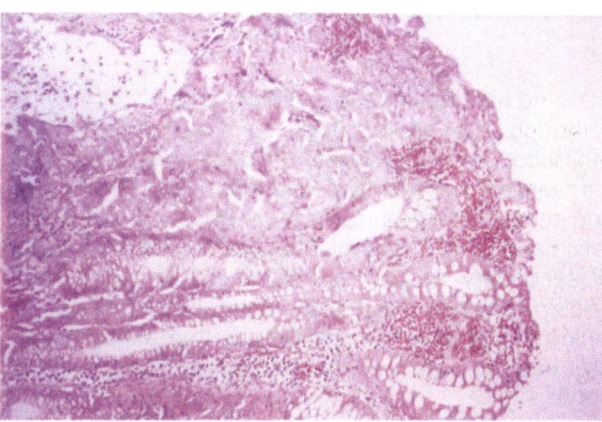

Figure 20.8 Transitional mucosa. This biopsy shows carcinoma (upper half) and adjacent transitional mucosa (lower half). Note the elongated crypts and increase in goblet cell numbers and the lack of any hyperplasia. H & E × 125

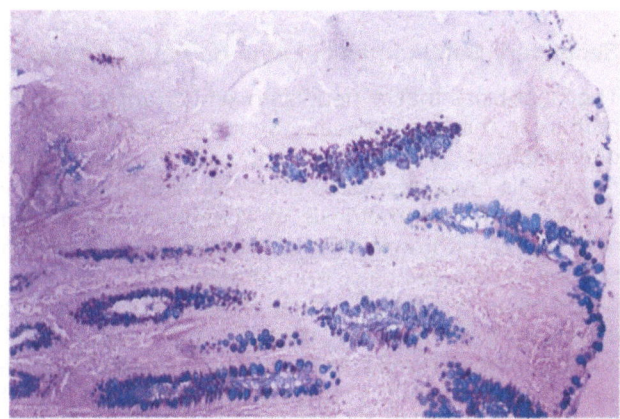

Figure 20.9 Transitional mucosa. Step section to Figure 20.8. The carcinoma (top) contains no mucin; the transitional mucosa below is secreting sialomucins (blue) but little or no sulphomucin (brown). High iron diamine (HID) technique × 125

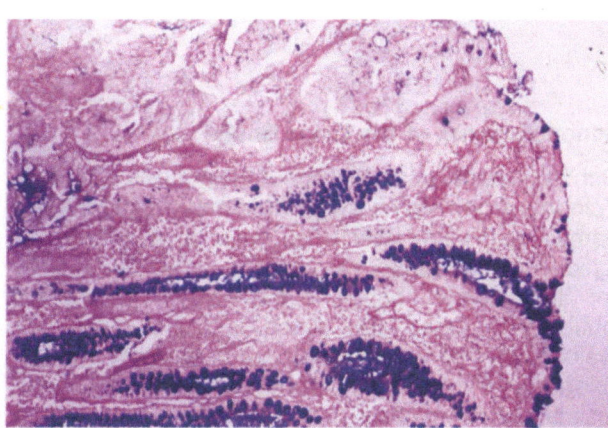

Figure 20.10 Transitional mucosa. A similar picture to Figure 20.9 using a PAS Alcian blue (pH 2.5) technique × 125

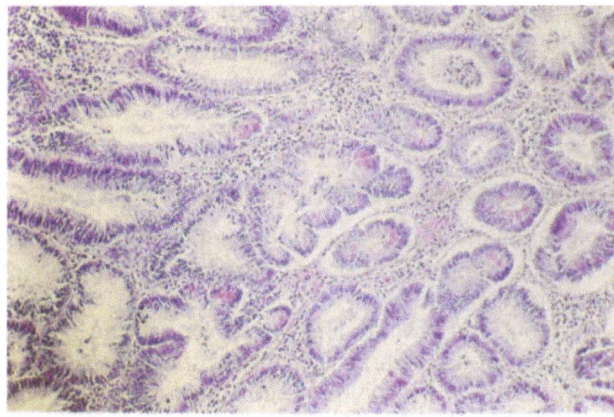

Figure 20.11 Adenocarcinoma with Paneth cells. The cells are clearly a part of the neoplastic epithelium and not included normal cells. H & E × 320

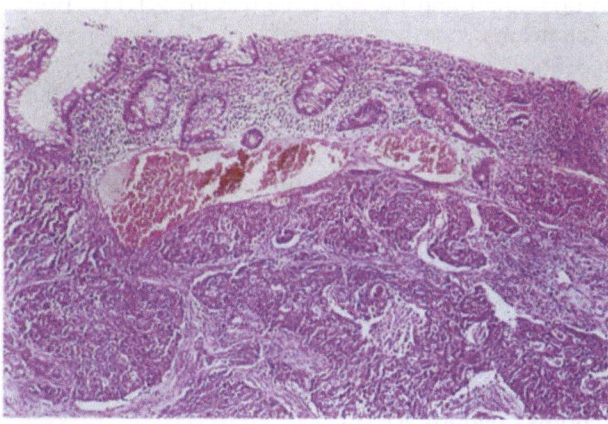

Figure 20.12 Adenocarcinoma of sigmoid colon showing squamous metaplasia. Some growths of this pattern appear to be purely squamous, others have a mixed pattern. H & E × 100

there is no resemblance to urothelium.

Although the presence of such a zone is now established, the usefulness of detecting it remains controversial, since similar changes are described in association with other neoplasms and with non-neoplastic conditions[16], and the changes may be equally as well secondary as primary. My own fairly extensive studies[17] convince me that the changes described are genuine in that they can regularly be found if searched for, but are not yet of any proven value in diagnosis or prognosis.

Anal Canal Dysplasias

Squamous metaplasia occurs not uncommonly in the epithelium covering prolapsed haemorrhoids, but is not, in that situation, premalignant.

Adenocarcinoma of the Large Bowel

Much has already been said about the genesis of adenocarcinoma from pre-existing adenomas or chronically inflamed epithelium which has become severely dysplastic. Whether adenocarcinomas arise *de novo* or after 'transitional' change in the epithelium, though probable, is uncertain. Once a carcinoma has developed its diagnosis is not usually a problem, though in biopsies which consist of mucosa only it may be impossible to differentiate invasive carcinoma from severe dysplasia within an adenoma (see Figure 19.17). It seems pointless to illustrate in detail changes which have already been shown in adenomas with dysplasia and are well known to all pathologists and I have not done so, preferring to illustrate and comment on some of the peculiarities which can be observed.

Specialized cells can be incorporated into large bowel carcinomas and are occasionally seen in biopsies. I have seen endocrine and Paneth cells (Figure 20.11); both appear to be component parts of the carcinoma, suggesting that a stem cell can differentiate in different ways under a single carcinogenic stimulus. Squamous metaplasia, though rare, is also well recorded in adenocarcinomas and adenomas[18], distanced too far from the anal canal for direct extension to be possible (Figure 20.12). Rarely a primary large bowel carcinoma can have a signet ring pattern reminiscent of intra-epithelial gastric carcinoma[19] (Figures 20.13 and 20.14); care needs to be taken in diagnosis here, since carcinomas of stomach and pancreas can spread intramucosally right down to the rectum (see Figure 20.20). Malakoplakia is also described[20] in association with adenomas and carcinomas (Figure 20.15).

Endocrine Cell Tumours

Endocrine cell tumours are uncommon in the large bowel and when present are usually sited in caecum or rectum, either as small nodules often lying more in the submucosa than in the mucosa or as larger ulcerating and sometimes polypoid growths. Microscopically they have either a characteristic type 1(A) carcinoid pattern and are argyrophil but rarely argentaffin[21] (Figure 20.16), or a type 2(B) ribbon pattern in which the component cells are smaller than the corresponding pattern seen in the pancreas[22] (Figure 20.17), and may also be argyrophilic and lead haematoxylin positive (Figure 20.18). Most are apparently non-functional but a number of different hormone secretions have been described in them[23]. Mixed patterns are not uncommon and more than one pattern can appear in a single biopsy. It is always worthwhile to use argentaffin, argyrophil and lead haematoxylin techniques on suspected endocrine cell tumours.

Secondary Carcinomas in Large Bowel and Anus

The possibility that a neoplasm which appears to be primary in the large bowel may in fact result from the direct spread of an adjacent primary tumour or be a metastasis must always be borne in mind, as must the possibility of endometriosis in a female. I have seen direct spread from prostate and cervix into the rectum and secondary deposits from breast, lung, ovary and pancreas in the large bowel (Figure 20.19). Points especially to look for are the site of the tumour cells within the bowel wall and the tumour pattern. Deposits are more common in submucosa than mucosa though they can ulcerate through to reach the lumen, and if mucosal, often consist of scattered malignant cells rather than formed glandular elements (Figure 20.20). Carcinomas of stomach and pancreas often produce a diffuse intramural spread of malignant cells throughout the gastrointestinal tract (Figure 20.20). Secondary deposits may produce their own characteristic patterns such as the 'indian file' appearance of carcinoma of breast, and histochemical techniques for mucins and enzymes can sometimes help in their differentiation.

Malignant Melanomas of Rectum and Anal Canal

The epithelium of the anal canal contains melanocytes and it is therefore not surprising that malignant melanomas occasionally occur. Proctoscopically they arise above the dentate line, are polypoid and usually pigmented and can be mistaken for thrombosed piles (Figure 20.21); the pigmentation itself can look like altered blood. They tend to spread upwards and primary anal growths can appear to be of rectal origin. Histologically there may or may not be junctional change at the lower anal edge; I have only once seen it. The growths have a characteristic melanomatous appearance, sometimes with whorling, and cells containing pigment can usually be found if carefully searched for (Figure 20.22). Because of the likelihood of coincidental traumatic haemorrhage in this situation stains for both iron and melanin should always be used. Cellular pleomorphism and the presence of tumour giant cells are also common and can be helpful in the distinction of melanoma from other anaplastic tumours.

The diagnosis of malignant melanoma does not necessarily indicate a primary lesion and a careful search should always be made for a possible primary lesion elsewhere.

Primary Neoplasms in the Anal Canal

Neoplasms arising in the lower anal canal and at the anal margin are squamous or very rarely basal cell carcinomas such as are found in the skin, and are not discussed here. Those which arise at or above the dentate line have a variable pattern in keeping with the epithelium from which they arise.

Basaloid (Cloacogenic) Carcinoma

This pattern accounts for 50–70% of all anal canal carcinomas, which are usually found high up in the anal canal above the embryological site where the cloaca fuses with the solid ectodermal anal plug. A number of histological patterns are possible, including basaloid (the most common), squamous, transitional and muco-epidermoid, and more than one of these patterns is commonly present in any one tumour[24] (Figures 20.23 and 20.24). There is an interesting variant with a much poorer prognosis, presenting usually as painful rectal stricture with or without fissuring (Figure 20.25), in which small islands of anaplastic glandular epithelium surrounded by reactive fibrosis are scattered sparsely throughout the deeper tissues and muscle without obvious surface mucosal involvement (Figure 20.26). The example in Figures 20.25 and 20.26 required three separate biopsies, all serially sectioned, before carcinoma cells were found in the submucosa just beneath the muscularis; even in retrospect they could not be detected in the first two (adequate) biopsies. Some neoplasms are so anaplastic that no real pattern can be determined (Figure 20.27) and their nature remains uncertain until resection.

Carcinomas of Anal Glands and Ducts

These are extremely rare and have to be differentiated from carcinomas arising in anorectal fistulae. Since many of these fistulae which are not inflammatory result from embryological malformations of duplication type, in which channels are present which are lined by rectal type mucosa and are similar to normal anal glands, differentiation between the two types of carcinoma can be impossible. Both types show the development of an adenocarcinoma from lining epithelium of a tract or duct (Figure 20.28); claims have been made that they can be

distinguished by histochemical examination of the mucins they secrete[25] but I have no personal experience.

Paget's Disease of the Perianal Region

Strictly speaking this condition, which occurs in perianal skin, is outside the scope of this atlas. I include it because it can be associated with anal carcinomas, particularly of apocrine type, and can be confused with spread of tumour from an anaplastic carcinoma of rectum or anal canal. It resembles Paget's disease elsewhere. Cells which contain Alcian blue (pH 2.5) and PAS-positive material are found in the epidermis and in the ducts of apocrine glands (Figures 20.29 and 20.30).

Lymphoid Tumours and Tumour-like Lesions

There are three ways in which lymphoid hyperplasias or neoplasms can present in the large bowel and it can be difficult to distinguish them on biopsy.

Benign Lymphoid Polyps

These are usualy single, sessile and occur in adults in the submucosa of the lower half of the rectum. Microscopically they resemble a normal lymph node without sinuses; the follicles are hyperplastic and can or need not contain well-defined germinal centres (Figure 20.31). Infiltration of the muscle coats is uncommon but the overlying mucosa is sometimes ulcerated. They are not liable to lymphomatous change, though occasional examples have been reported. In children they can rarely be multiple throughout the large bowel and probably then represent a heightened physiological response to antigenic material[26], though they are also seen in immunodeficiency states.

Malignant Lymphomatous Polyposis

This condition occurs in adults and may represent a form of chronic lymphatic leukaemia[27,28]. Endoscopically there may be either raised sessile whitish nodules (Figure 20.32) or a more diffuse brain-like thickening not unlike that seen in the stomach in Menetrier's disease (Figure 20.33). There is often splenomegaly and bone marrow involvement. Histologically the nodules consist of lymphocytes without follicular pattern but not showing pleomorphism or increased or abnormal mitoses. Biopsy interpretation can be difficult (Figure 20.34); in the patient illustrated in Figures 20.32 and 20.34 the initial diagnosis was undifferentiated endocrine cell tumour and a knowledge of the endoscopic appearances would greatly have assisted the pathologist.

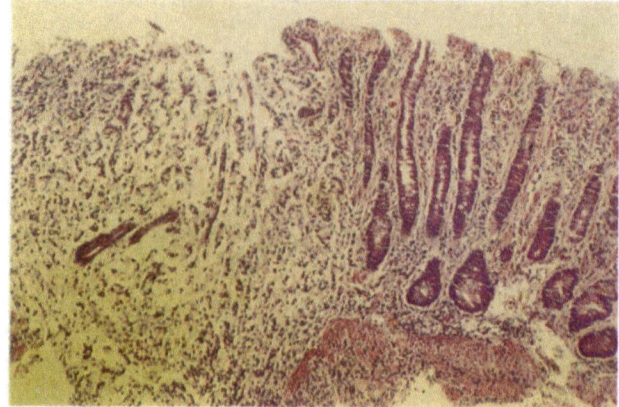

Figure 20.13 Adenocarcinoma, signet ring pattern. This resembles intra-epithelial carcinoma of stomach, but subsequent resection showed a widely invasive carcinoma with some poorly formed gland structures. H & E × 100

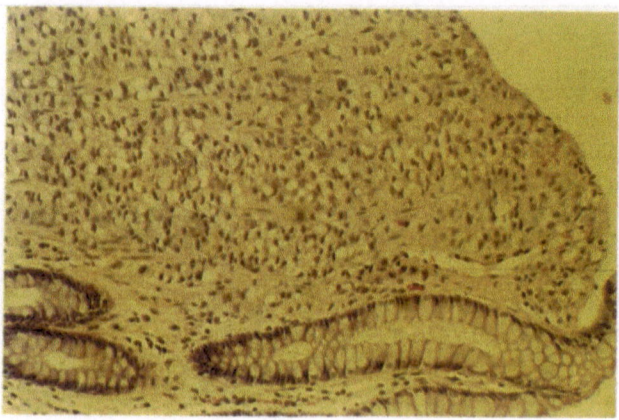

Figure 20.14 Higher-power view of a similar growth to that in Figure 20.13. The signet ring pattern is obvious. H & E × 250

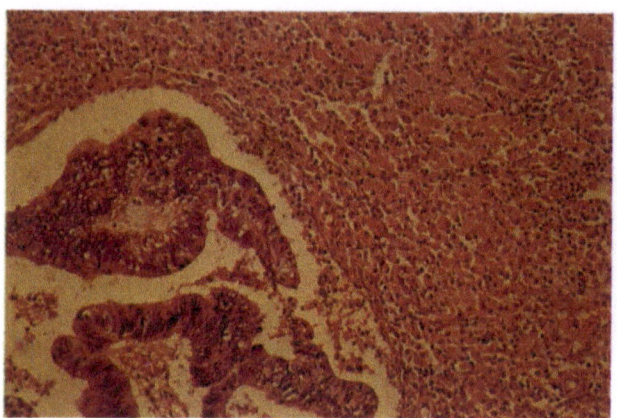

Figure 20.15 Adenocarcinoma of rectum with malakoplakia. H & E × 250

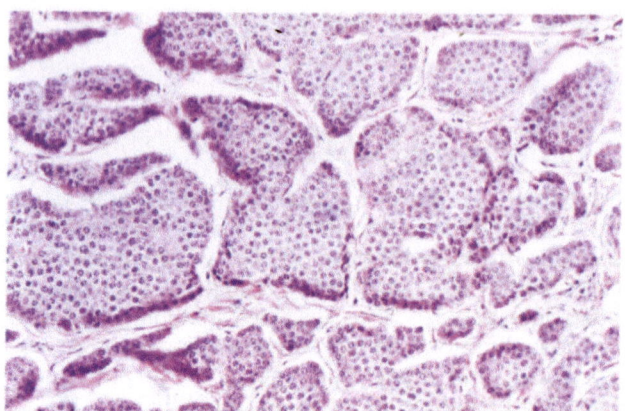

Figure 20.16 Endocrine cell tumour of 'carcinoid' type 1(A) pattern. This particular tumour was argentaffin-negative but argyrophil and lead haema-toxylin-positive. H & E × 125

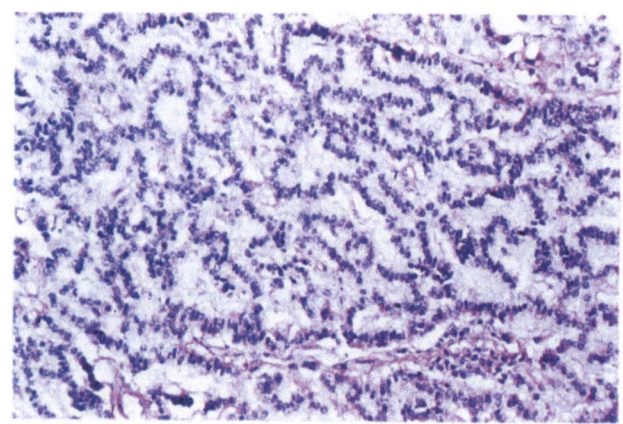

Figure 20.17 Endocrine cell tumour of ribbon type 2(B) pattern. Constituent cells are smaller than those of corresponding pancreatic tumours. H & E × 125

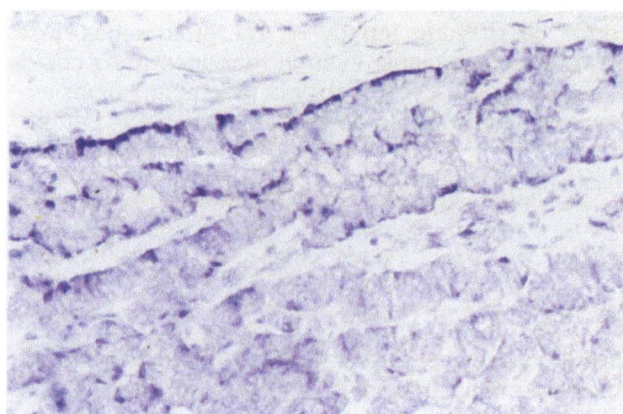

Figure 20.18 Endocrine cell tumour, ribbon pattern. Many granules stain with lead haematoxylin. × 320

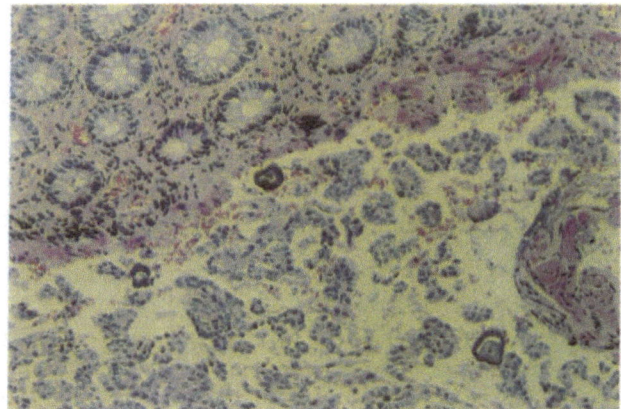

Figure 20.19 Secondary carcinoma of ovary in a rectal biopsy. The carcinoma cells lie in the superficial submucosa and the poorly formed gland elements are smaller than one would expect in a large bowel carcinoma; but differentiation can be impossible.   H & E × 250

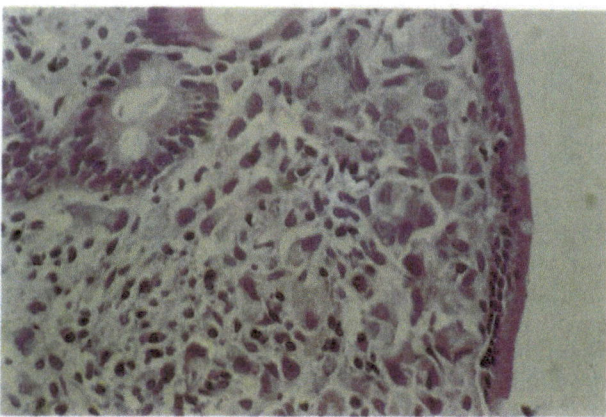

Figure 20.20 Secondary carcinoma of pancreas, intramucosal spread. This has to be distinguished from intraepithelial primary carcinoma, but the cells here are larger and more pleomorphic, and none are of signet ring pattern. H & E × 320

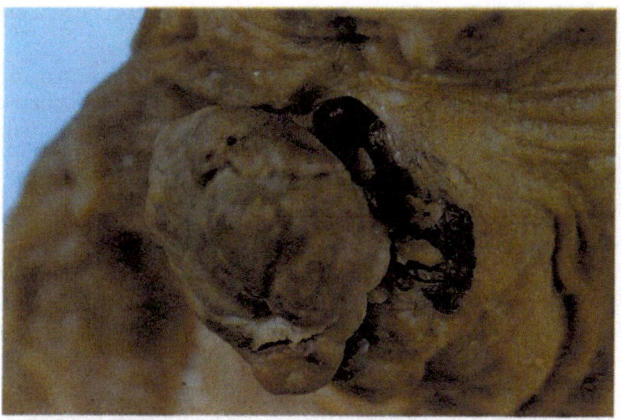

Figure 20.21 Primary malignant melanoma just above the dentate line. The tumour is polypoid and the black zone to the right could be melanin pigmentation or due to altered blood; it was in fact the former

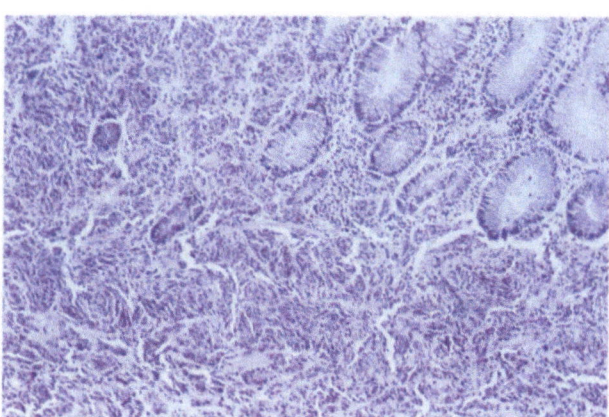

Figure 20.22 Primary malignant melanoma. There is a whorled pattern with little pigment in this section, though other sections showed large amounts. H & E × 125

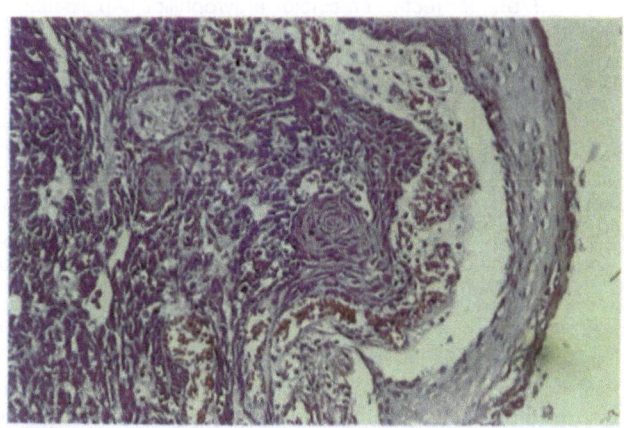

Figure 20.23 Anal canal carcinoma. Predominantly basal cell pattern with some squamous elements and one or two ill-formed cell nests.   H & E × 125

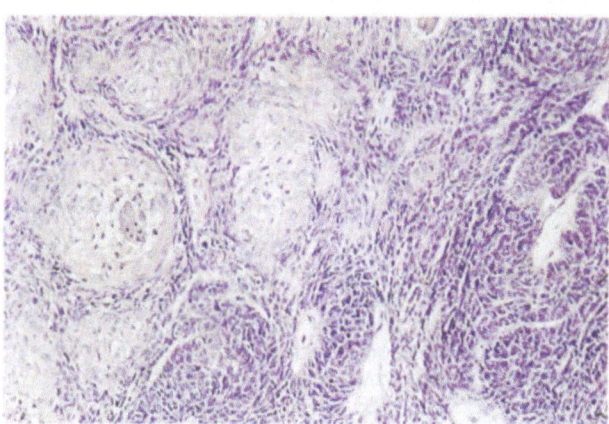

Figure 20.24 Anal canal carcinoma. A further example of a mixed basal cell and squamous pattern.   H & E × 250

Malignant Lymphoma

Malignant lymphomas in the large bowel can be primary or secondary. Secondary infiltration may present as a single or as multiple infiltrating masses which later ulcerate through the mucosa, or as a plaque, indicating more diffuse infiltration. Primary lymphoid tumours can be annular and constricting or polypoid and projecting. On biopsy, any histological pattern of lymphoma can be present, though those primary lymphomas which at one time were thought to be Hodgkin's disease are now considered to be immunoblastic or histiocytic. They can be associated with gluten-induced enteropathy, ulcerative colitis[29] and disturbances of immune competence. Their histological appearances do not differ from those of lymphomas elsewhere.

Tumours of Smooth Muscle

Smooth muscle tumours are rare in the large bowel and have the features of leiomyomas elsewhere in the gut. Secondary ulceration with bleeding is not uncommon. Histologically it can be virtually impossible to distinguish benign from malignant, and the size of the tumour is still a good criterion for assessment. The dispassionate observer may like to study Figures 20.35 and 20.36 without reading the relevant captions (both are biopsies from tumours of approximately equal size at subsequent resection) and decide which patient died a year later from multiple metastases and which was alive and well 6 years later.

References

1. Morson, B. C. and Dawson, I. M. P. (1979). *Gastrointestinal Pathology*. 2nd edn., Chapter 33. (Oxford: Blackwell)

2. Morson, B. C. and Pang, L. (1967). Rectal biopsy as an aid to cancer control in ulcerative colitis. *Gut*, **8**, 423

3. Riddell, R. H. (1976). The precarcinomatous phase of ulcerative colitis. *Curr. Top. Pathol.*, **63**, 179

4. Lennard-Jones, J. E., Morson, B. C., Ritchie, J. K., Shove, D. C. and Williams, C. B. (1977). Cancer in colitis : assessment of the individual risk by clinical and histological criteria. *Gastroenterology*, **73**, 1280

5. Blackstone, M. O., Riddell, R. H., Rogers, B. H. G and Levin, B. (1981). Dysplasia-associated lesion or mass (DALM) detected by colonoscopy in longstanding ulcerative colitis; an indication for colectomy. *Gastroenterology*, **80**, 366

6. Riddell, R. H. and Morson, B. C. (1979). Value of sigmoidoscopy and biopsy in detection of carcinoma and premalignant change in ulcerative colitis. *Gut*, **20**, 575

7. Butt, J. H. and Morson, B. C. (1981). Dysplasia and cancer in inflammatory bowel disease. *Gastroenterology*, **80**, 865

8. Greenstein, A. J., Sachar, D. B., Smith, H., Janowitz, H. D. and Aufses, A. H. J. (1980). Patterns of neoplasia in Crohn's disease and ulcerative colitis. *Cancer*, **46**, 403

9. Craft, C. F., Mendelsohn, G., Cooper, H. S. and Yardley, J. H. (1981). Colonic 'precancer' in Crohn's disease. *Gastroenterology*, **80**, 578

10. Filipe, M. I. and Branfoot, A. C. (1974). Abnormal patterns of mucus secretion in apparently normal mucosa of large intestine with carcinoma. *Cancer*, **34**, 282

11. Filipe, M. I. and Branfoot, A. C. (1976). Mucus histochemistry of the colon. *Curr. Top. Pathol.*, **63**, 143

12. Saffos, R. O. and Rhatigan, R. M. (1977). Benign (nonpolypoidal) mucosal changes adjacent to carcinoma of colon. A light microscopic study of 20 cases. *Hum. Pathol.*, **8**, 441

13. Culling, C. F. A., Reid, P. A., Worth, A. J. and Dunn, W. L. (1977). A new histochemical technique of use in the interpretation and diagnosis of adenocarcinoma and villous lesions in the large intestine. *J. Clin. Pathol.*, **30**, 1056

14. Marsden, J. R. and Dawson, I. M. P. (1974). An investigation into the enzyme histochemistry of adenocarcinomas of human large intestine and of the transitional epithelium immediately adjacent to them. *Gut*, **15**, 783

15. Riddell, R. H. and Levin, B. (1977). Ultrastructure of the 'transitional' mucosa adjacent to large bowel carcinoma. *Cancer*, **40**, 2509

16. Isaacson, P. and Atwood, P. R. A. (1979). Failure to demonstrate specificity of the morphological and histochemical changes in mucosa adjacent to colonic carcinoma (transitional mucosa). *J. Clin. Pathol.*, **32**, 214

17. Dawson, I. M. P. (1981). The value of histochemistry in the diagnosis and prognosis of gastrointestinal diseases. In Stoward, P. J. and Polak, J. M. (eds.). *Histochemistry, the Widening Horizons.* Chapter 9, pp. 127–162. (Chichester: John Wiley & Sons)

18. Williams, G. T., Blackshaw, A. J. and Morson, B. C. (1979). Squamous carcinoma of the colorectum and its genesis. *J. Pathol.*, **129**, 139

19. Amorn, Y. and Knight, W. A. Jr (1978). Primary linitis plastica of the colon. Report of two cases and review of the literature. *Cancer*, **41**, 2420

20. Chaudry, A. P., Saigal, K. P., Intengan, M. and Nickerson, P. A. (1979). Malakoplakia of the large intestine found incidentally at necropsy. Light and electron microscopic features. *Dis. Col. Rectum*, **22**, 73

21. Husoda, S., Kito, H., Nogaki, M., Masumori, S. and Ito, S. (1975). Is rectal carcinoid argyrophilic? Application of Grimelius' silver nitrate stain in four cases. *Dis. Col. Rectum*, **18**, 386

22. Jones, R. A., and Dawson, I. M. P. (1977). Morphology and staining patterns of endocrine cell tumours in the gut, pancreas and bronchus and their possible significance. *Histopathology*, **1**, 137

23. Alumets, J., Alm, P., Falkmer, S., Hakanson, R., Ljundberg, O., Martensson, H. *et al.* (1981). Immunohistochemical evidence of polypeptide hormones in endocrine cell tumours of the rectum. *Cancer*, **48**, 2409

24. Pang, L. S. C. and Morson, B. C. (1967). Basaloid carcinoma of the anal canal. *J. Clin. Pathol.*, **20**, 28

25. Fenger, C. and Filipe, M. I. (1977). Pathology of the anal glands with special reference to their mucin histochemistry. *Acta Pathol. Microbiol. Scand.*, **85A**, 273

26. Louw, J. H. (1968). Polypoid lesions of the large bowel in children with particular reference to benign polyposis. *Pediatr. Surg.*, **3**, 195

27. Sheahan, D. G., Martin, F., Baginsky, S., Mallory, G. K. and Zamcheck, N. (1971). Multiple lymphomatous polyposis of the gastrointestinal tract. *Cancer*, **28**, 408

28. Fromke, V. L. and Weber, L. W. (1974). Extensive leukaemic infiltration of the gastrointestinal tract in chronic lympho-sarcoma cell leukaemia. *Am. J. Med.*, **56**, 879

29. Wagonfeld, J. B., Platz, C. E., Fishman, F. L., Sibley, R. K. and Kirsner, J. B. (1977). Multicentric colonic lymphoma complicating ulcerative colitis. *Am. J. Dig. Dis.*, **22**, 502

Figures 20.25–20.36 will be found overleaf.

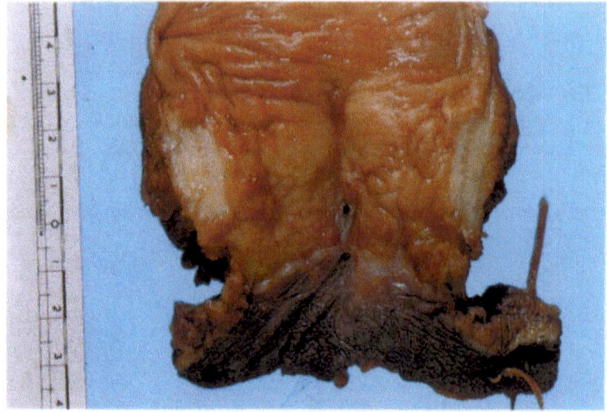

Figure 20.25 Anal canal carcinoma; anaplastic adenocarcinoma pattern. The patient presented with pain on defaecation and was found to have a stricture with fissuring. Carcinoma was only found on the third biopsy

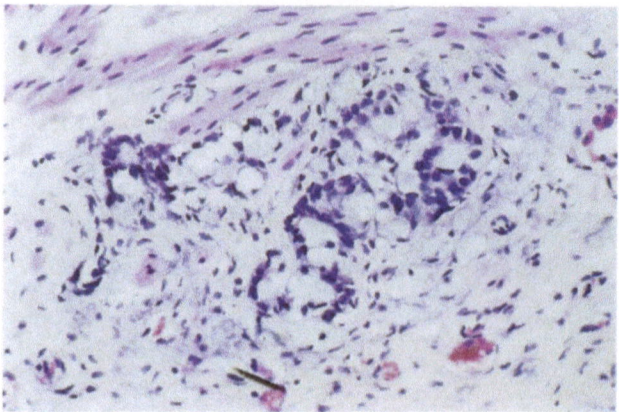

Figure 20.26 Biopsy from anal canal as shown in Figure 20.25. Anaplastic signet ring carcinoma, see text.   H & E × 320

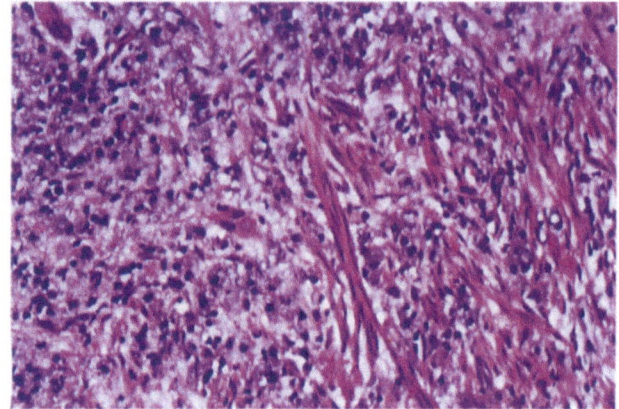

Figure 20.27 Another example of an anaplastic adenocarcinoma of anal canal; a PAS stain was helpful here in demonstrating mucin in occasional cells.   H & E × 250

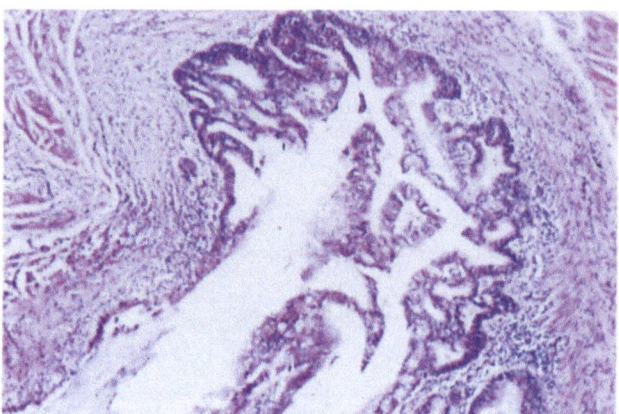

Figure 20.28 Carcinoma of anal ducts. This growth is developing in the deeper part of a duct and can really only be diagnosed as ductal by knowing its position   H & E × 125

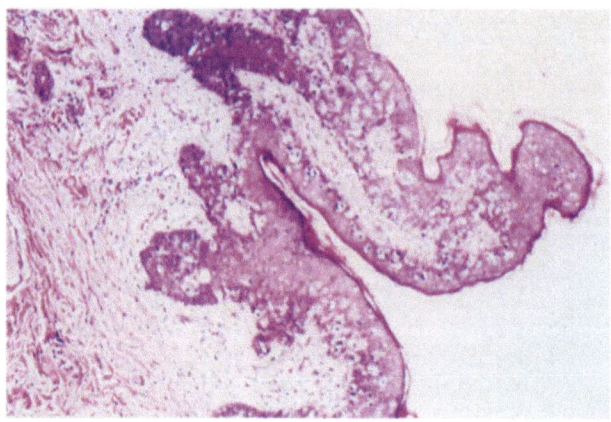

Figure 20.29 Paget's disease of perianal region. The Paget cells are clearly visible in the epidermis.   H & E × 100

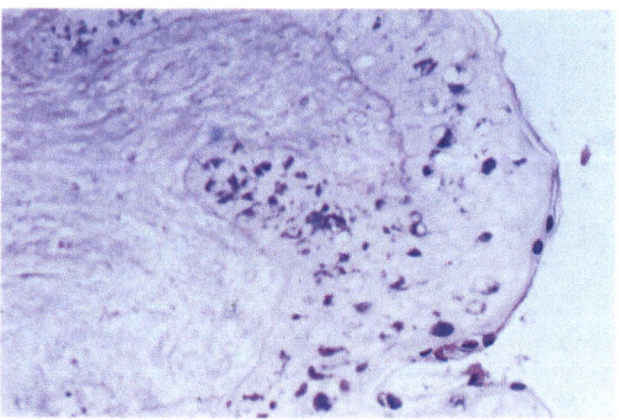

Figure 20.30 Paget's disease. A combined Alcian blue (pH 2.5) and PAS technique shows mucin in the cells. × 320

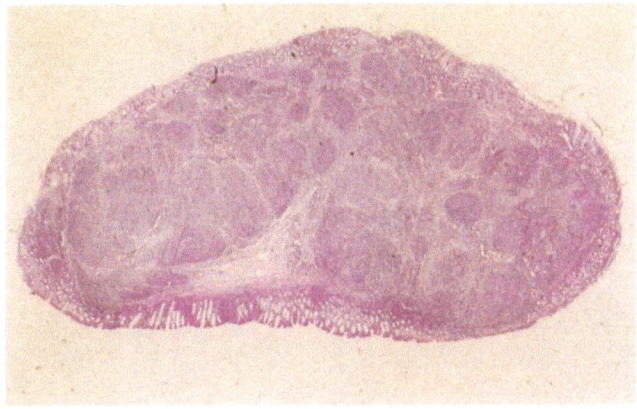

Figure 20.31 Benign lymphoid polyp in lower rectum. Follicles are hyperplastic but there are few obvious germinal centres. Whole mount section, H & E × 8

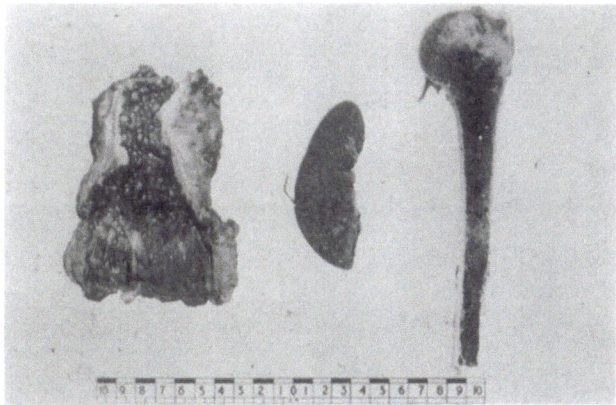

Figure 20.32 Malignant lymphomatous polyposis. These postmortem specimens show the lymphoid nodules in the lower rectum, a slightly enlarged spleen (600 g) and bone marrow involvement

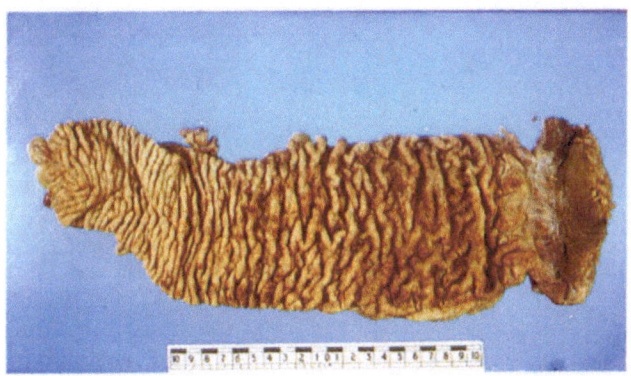

Figure 20.33 Malignant lymphomatous polyposis. This resected specimen of rectum and anus shows the brain-like thickening which can sometimes be seen

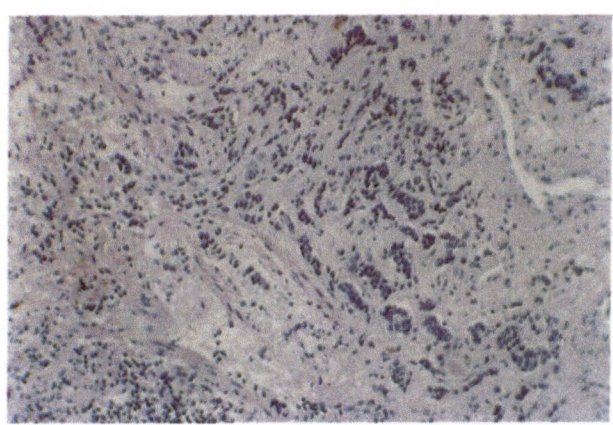

Figure 20.34 Malignant lymphomatous polyposis. This biopsy, from the specimen illustrated in Figure 20.32, was first diagnosed as an anaplastic endocrine cell tumour. Its true nature might have been appreciated more readily had a knowledge of the endoscopic appearances been available to the pathologist. H & E × 125

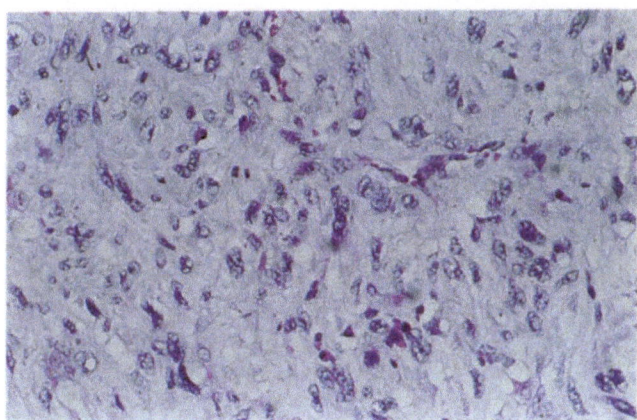

Figure 20.35 Smooth muscle tumour. There is some cellular pleomorphism and in places an 'epithelioid' pattern like that described in smooth muscle tumours in the stomach. Mucin stains, however, were negative. This patient died a year later from multiple metastases. H & E × 250

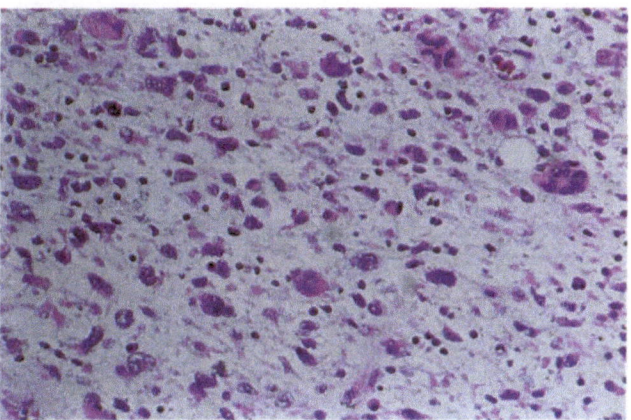

Figure 20.36 Smooth muscle tumour. The cellular pleomorphism is more marked in this biopsy and there are some tumour giant cells and a few abnormal mitoses. Nevertheless, this patient was alive and well 6 years later. H & E × 250

The advent of colonoscopy and the ease of sigmoidoscopy and proctoscopy virtually means that any visible lesion in the large intestine can be biopsied. Once the main disease categories have been described a number of unrelated lesions remain which, for ease, are discussed in alphabetical order below.

Amyloid

The large bowel is commonly involved in systemic amyloidosis and rectal biopsy is an accepted technique for its diagnosis. Amyloid is found extracellularly in submucosal arterioles and is also occasionally seen in the vessels supplying lymphoid aggregates in the mucosa and muscularis mucosae (Figure 21.1). Its presence should be confirmed by staining with Congo or Sirius red and subsequent examination using polarized light (Figure 21.2).

Brown Bowel Syndrome

This condition, already described on page 87, is occasionally seen in the muscularis mucosae of the large bowel in patients with long-standing malabsorption. Pigment granules which are autofluorescent and stain positively with PAS and Sudan black are readily recognizable (Figures 21.3 and 21.4; see also Figures 14.10, 14.11).

Cathartic Colon

Cathartic colon results from the long-continued use of purgatives, especially those of the anthraquinone group, and is therefore usually accompanied by melanosis coli (see below). Anthraquinones appear to act as neurotoxins, first stimulating and later destroying ganglion cells with loss of myenteric ganglia followed by Schwann cell proliferation[1]. Secondary changes which are most commonly recognizable are the presence of melanosis, the presence of adipose tissue in the submucosa and atrophy of the muscularis propria sometimes with hypertrophy of muscularis mucosae (Figure 21.5).

Cysts in Colonic Epithelium

There are, in the literature, three unrelated cystic conditions which are often confused and which merit separate discussion.

Colitis Cystica Profunda

This is the presence of mucin-containing cysts in the submucosa of the colon following bacillary dysentery, and presumably the result of displacement of epithelium at the time of the acute infection[2]. The cysts can attain a large size and may have a recognizable epithelial lining at least in part (Figure 21.6); if they rupture an inflammatory granulomatous reaction with muciphages can often be seen.

Colitis Cystica Superficialis

This describes a condition found in infants and young children who are malnourished and in adults with pellagra or debilitating diseases; it is especially common after kwashiorkor[3]. It is not specifically related to infection. Cysts containing gas are present in the mucosa and submucosa of small and large intestine (Figure 11.24) and the glands are usually reduced in number and irregular in pattern (Figure 21.7). There may be a surrounding inflammatory reaction with giant cells but this is less common than in gas cysts of the colon in adults.

Gas Cysts of the Colon (Pneumatosis Coli)

In this condition, which occurs mainly in adults and usually in association with chronic lung disease, numerous gas-filled cysts are present in the submucosa or serosa of the small and/or large intestine[4]. The endoscopic appearances of dilated submucosal cysts are dis-

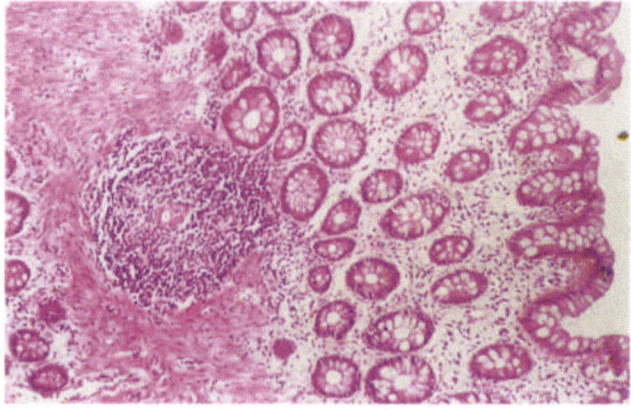

Figure 21.1 Amyloid. Deposits are present in the walls of an arteriole in the centre of a lymphoid aggregate. H & E × 125

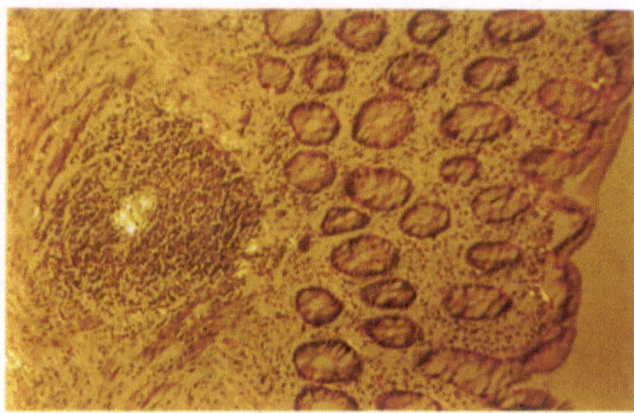

Figure 21.2 Amyloid. Serial section to Figure 21.1, stained with Sirius red and examined under crossed prisms. × 125

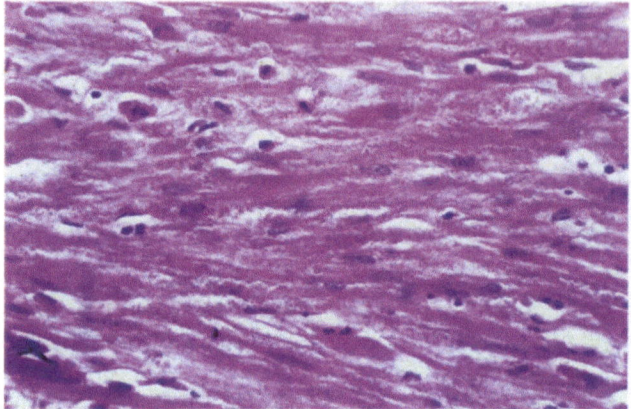

Figure 21.3 Brown bowel syndrome. Pigment granules are visible within muscle fibres in the muscularis mucosae. H & E × 400

Figure 21.4 Brown bowel syndrome, showing the autofluorescence of the granular material. Unstained section, ultra-violet excitation. × 400

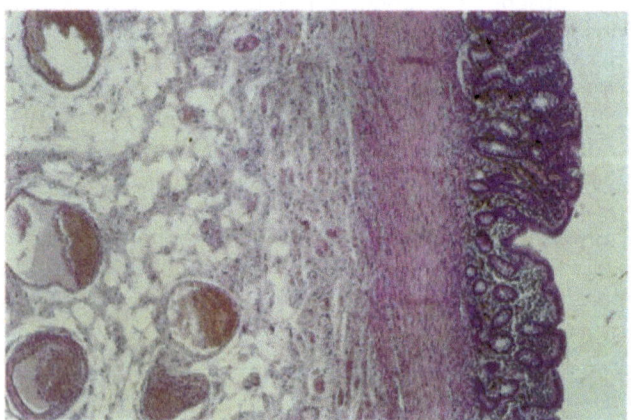

Figure 21.5 Cathartic colon. The muscularis mucosae is hypertrophic and there is a marked increase in adipose tissue in the submucosa. Melanosis coli was also present but cannot be seen at this magnification. H & E × 65

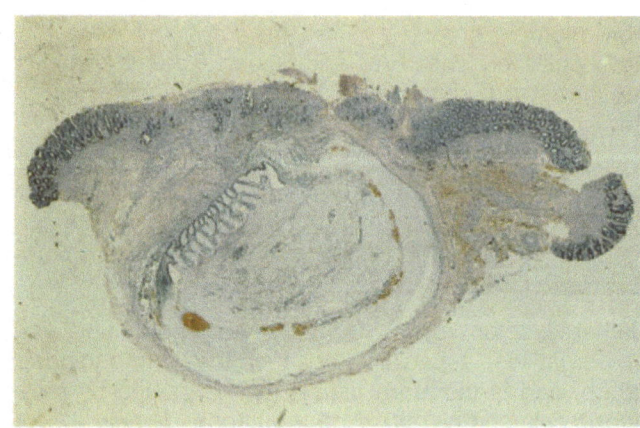

Figure 21.6 Colitis cystica profunda. A large cyst with an epithelial lining in part and containing inspissated mucin is distending the submucosa. H & E × 25

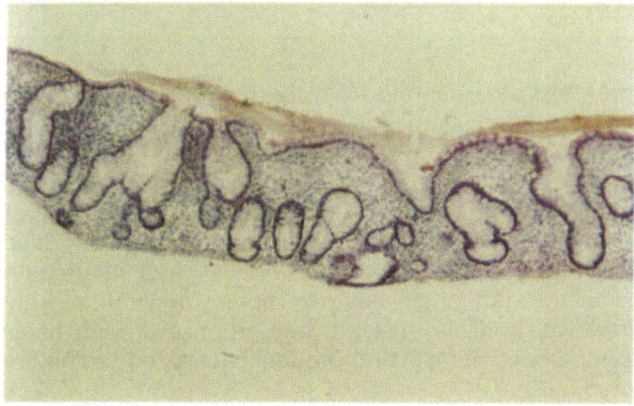

Figure 21.7 Colitis cystica superficialis. The gland pattern is irregular and glands are reduced in number. No cyst included in this biopsy.   H & E × 80

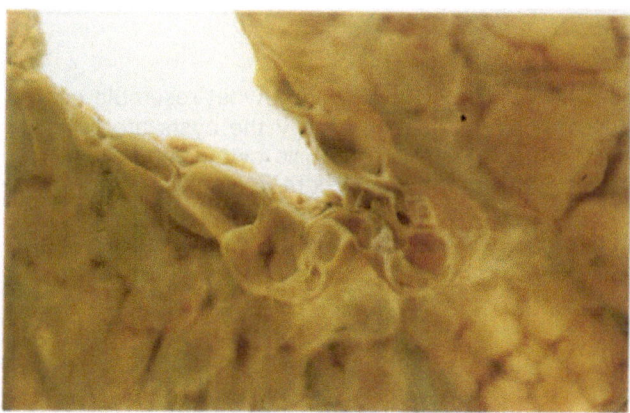

Figure 21.8 Gas cysts of colon. A resected specimen which shows multiple gas-filled cysts in the submucosa

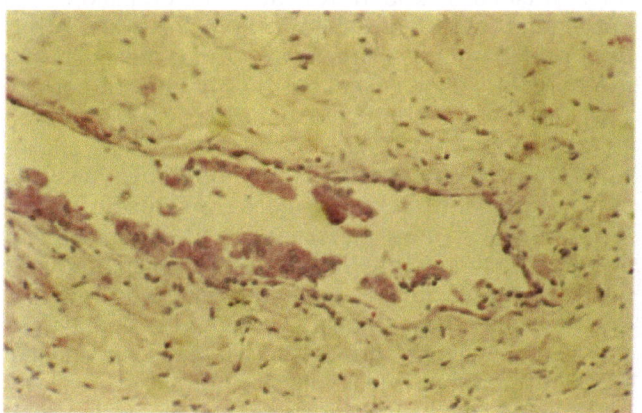

Figure 21.9 Gas cysts of colon. The cyst has an endothelial-type lining with macrophages present.   H & E × 250

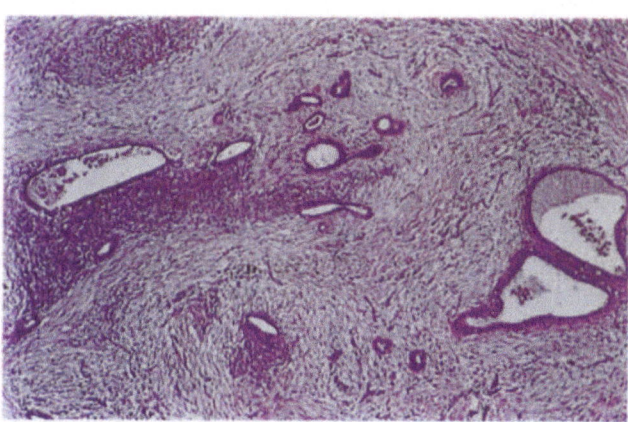

Figure 21.10 Endometriosis. The glands are non-specific but the stroma is characteristic of endometrium.   H & E × 100

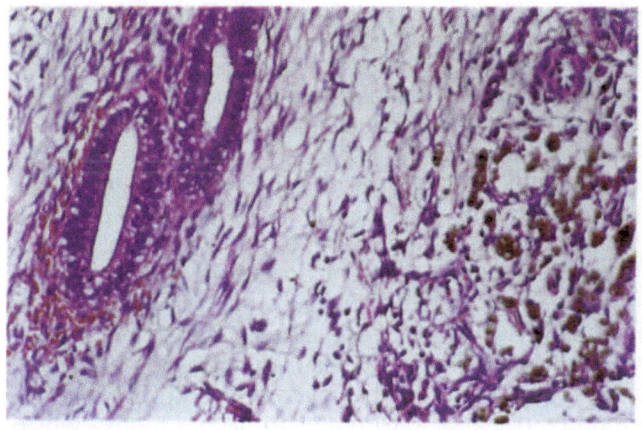

Figure 21.11 Endometriosis. Glands show recognizable early secretory changes as subnuclear vacuolation and there is iron pigment on the right. H & E × 250

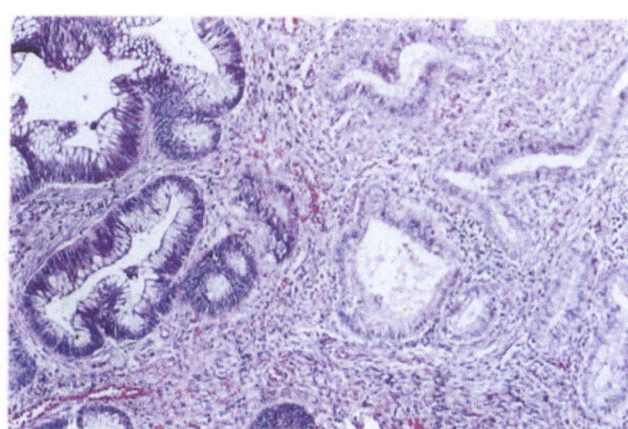

Figure 21.12 Endometriosis. This could easily be missed on a cursory inspection. There are large intestinal glands on the left, endometrial glands on the right.   H & E × 125

tinctive (Figure 21.8) and somewhat resemble coarse cobblestoning. Microscopically the cysts are lined by macrophages with eosinophilic cytoplasm which may fuse to form giant cells. There is sometimes an endothelial pattern of lining (Figure 21.9) but there is no inflammatory response and no muciphages are present. The overlying mucosa may or need not be thinned.

Diverticular Disease

This common condition constricts the descending and sigmoid colons and may be biopsied to exclude carcinoma as a cause of stricture. Mucosal biopsies taken from the mouths of diverticula or from the intervening mucosa may contain an increased number of lymphoid follicles and aggregates, but are essentially normal.

Endometriosis

Involvement of the large intestine and the perianal region by endometriosis is not uncommon[5,6] and must always be considered and rejected (as must spread of prostatic carcinoma in men) before a biopsy diagnosis of rectal or anal canal carcinoma is made in a woman. Macroscopically lesions are usually poorly defined and firm or hard to the touch, and may project into the lumen as polypoid lesions. They are not usually difficult to diagnose on biopsy provided that they are borne in mind. The gland elements are regular; though not always readily recognizable as of endometrial origin they may show subnuclear vacuoles or other secretory changes. There is usually detectable surrounding endometrial-type stroma and often numerous macrophages containing haemosiderin and surrounded by reactive fibroblastic tissue (Figures 21.10–21.12).

Heterotopias

Heterotopic tissue is rare in the large bowel; when present it is virtually always gastric epithelium in rectal mucosa[7]. I have seen a single example.

Hirschsprung's Disease

In the developing normal large bowel it is thought that preganglionic parasympathetic fibres first grow down from the vagus and out from the presacral parasympathetic system to reach the submucosa and muscle coats. These fibres are non-argyrophilic and cholinergic. There follows an outgrowth of sympathetic fibres which are argyrophilic and adrenergic. Still later

ganglion cells migrate from the neural crest along the course of parasympathetic fibres and aggregate to form submucosal and myenteric plexuses (see Figures 15.9 and 15.10). The efferent nerve supply to the muscle coats arises from them and appears to be entirely of parasympathetic origin. Ganglion cells probably also migrate along sympathetic nerves and aggregate similarly, but their effector fibres do not directly innervate muscle; instead they arborize around parasympathetic ganglia and probably act as co-ordinators of impulses[8].

In Hirschsprung's disease there is an absence of ganglion cells in the lower part of the rectum, which extends upwards for a variable distance to a so-called 'transitional zone' in which ganglion cells begin to appear in both plexuses and so to a normally innervated bowel. Short-segment Hirschsprung's disease, in which the aganglionic region extends only over the terminal 10–20 mm of the rectum, comprises about 40% of all cases and in over 90% the condition does not extend more than 400 mm from the anus. It has been said that there are never skip zones present, but a recent report suggests that this may not be correct[9].

Linked with the absence of ganglion cells is a marked increase in and thickening of non-argyrophilic cholinesterase-containing nerve fibres, both between the muscle coats and in the submucosa, and recent studies have shown that small nerve fibres in the lamina propria may also be more numerous and thicker than normal[10]. Clinically the rectum is markedly narrowed and the muscle is apparently unable to relax in the aganglionic segment; the bowel proximally becomes secondarily greatly dilated, but is histologically normal.

The material which reaches the pathologist is varied and must be a matter for discussion between him and the clinician. For diagnostic purposes it was usual to send a full-thickness biopsy from the narrowed segment so that both plexuses were available for study. This was serially sectioned and the pathologist looked for the presence or absence of ganglion cells and thickened nerve trunks, which were more easily seen in the myenteric plexus (Figure 21.13). With the development of histochemical techniques for esterases the recognition of ganglion cells became easier and some pathologists were happy to rely on biopsies which included the submucosal plexus only (Figure 21.14). More recently still some workers[10] have claimed that a punch biopsy consisting of mucosa and muscularis mucosae only is sufficient; they rely on the demonstration of an increased number of thickened nerve fibres using a cholinesterase technique (Figure 21.15). While these can sometimes be present and unmistakable, I have now seen a number of biopsies in which it has been difficult to decide whether the appearance of the nerves was outside the normal limits (Figure 21.16), but which have proved on further biopsy to be examples of Hirschsprung's disease. I still prefer to have a biopsy which includes the submucosal plexus, but I always use cholinesterase techniques.

Biopsies may also be sent for rapid section when the surgeon is performing a 'pull-through' type of operation and wishes to know that he or she is clear of the aganglionic segment. These biopsies can be of full thickness and do not usually present any problem. I use a rapid non-specific esterase' technique (usually indoxyl esterase) which delineates ganglion cells. With experience a report can be given within 10–12 min of receiving the biopsy.

Immune-type Transplant Reactions

Rectal biopsies have been used to assess graft versus host reactions in patients undergoing allogeneic bone marrow transplants[11]. In patients who clinically showed graft v. host reactions there were focal abnormalities, particularly crypt dilatation and crypt cell degeneration (Figure 21.17) which are attributable to a possible immunological mechanism. I have insufficient personal experience to assess the value of biopsy in this situation.

Irradiational Changes

Changes in the bowel can follow irradiation to the abdomen or pelvis and at one time were not uncommon in women treated for cervical carcinoma. The damage takes two forms. In one there is acute mucosal damage with erosion and ulceration, followed by repair in which irregular mucosal hyperplasia is conspicuous and can be indistinguishable from dysplasia or intraepithelial carcinoma (Figure 21.18), though a careful study sometimes shows that irregularities in gland shape are greater than changes in the nuclear–cytoplasmic ratio in individual cells (Figure 21.19) and there is sometimes conspicuous lamina proprial fibrosis with the presence of bizarre fibroblasts. In the second, which occurs later in time, there is intimal arteriolar proliferation and endarteritis obliterans in the submucosa (Figure 21.20) with fibrosis and stricture formation and often mucosal atrophy.

Malakoplakia

A number of examples of malakoplakia of the large intestine are now reported[12]. The condition is probably related to an abnormal response by macrophages to a Gram-negative micro-organism, and therefore has aetiological and pathological similarities to Whipple's disease. Macroscopically there may be one or several projecting polypoid lesions caused by aggregates of macrophages with distended eosinophilic cytoplasm (Figure 21.21) containing PAS-positive material and sometimes calcified micro-spherules. Malakoplakia can also be associated with adenomas and carcinomas of large bowel (see Figure 20.15).

Melanosis Coli

This condition results from the long-continued use of purgatives, particularly those of the anthracene group which also give rise to cathartic colon. It is less common now than formerly. The pigment may be sufficient to give a brown colour to the bowel, visible with the naked eye, but it is usually seen as an incidental finding in colonic carcinoma. Macrophages containing pigment are found in the lamina propria and sometimes in the submucosa (Figure 21.22). Despite its name, the pigment is not melanin, but a lipofuscin which probably results from damage to intracellular organelles by the purgative, followed by their ingestion by macrophages. It gives the usual histochemical reactions for lipofuscins and is autofluorescent.

Muciphages

Muciphages are macrophages which have phagocytosed mucin particles; they are found in the lamina propria, and stain readily with PAS and usually also with Alcian blue at pH 2.5 (Figure 21.23). They are an indication of non-specific mucosal damage with destruction of gland elements and for some reason are particularly common in long-standing Hirschsprung's disease. They must not be mistaken, as they have been, for the macrophages of Whipple's disease.

Mucoviscidosis

My own (unreported) studies on rectal biopsies taken with informed consent from the parents of children with this condition, who must be carriers of the abnormal gene, showed some goblet cells larger than normal and more distended with mucin (Figure 21.24), but on precise measurements the differences were not statistically significant. Histochemical studies on these parents, and on biopsies from patients with the condition, have shown no differences in the distribution of sialo- or sulphomucins. Organ culture studies[13] suggest that surface columnar cells may contain lipid droplets, but I have not found these in studies on my own material.

Neutropenias

Biopsy appearances are described in chronic granulomatous disease and in so-called neutropenic enterocolitis[14] which is a consequence of antimitotic drug therapy. In both there is patchy loss of gland elements with or without surface mucosal erosion or ulceration. The lamina propria is heavily infiltrated with lymphocytes and plasma cells, often with some eosinophils and a granulomatous pattern is often recognizable (Figure

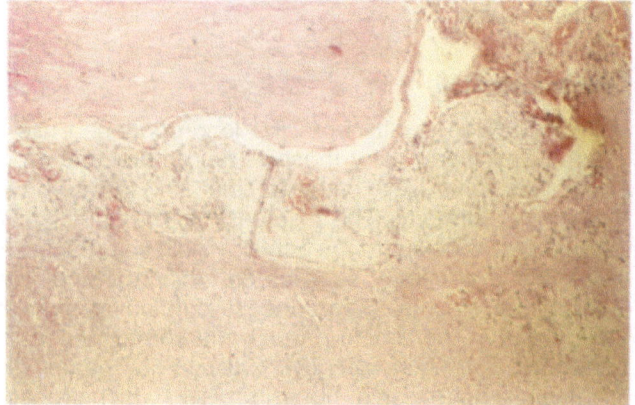

Figure 21.13 Hirschsprung's disease. Absence of ganglion cells and presence of thickened nerve trunks in the myenteric plexus.   H & E × 100

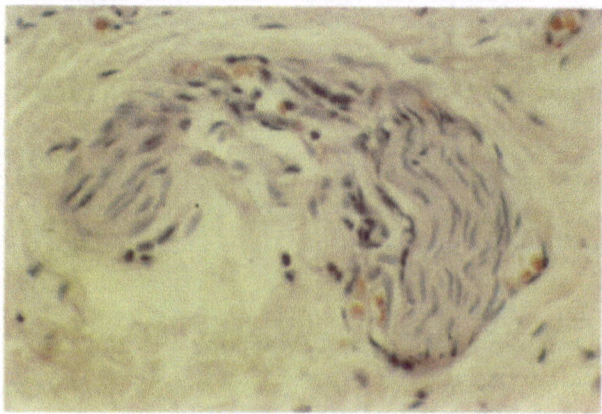

Figure 21.14 Hirschsprung's disease. Thickened nerve trunk in the submucosal plexus.   H & E × 320

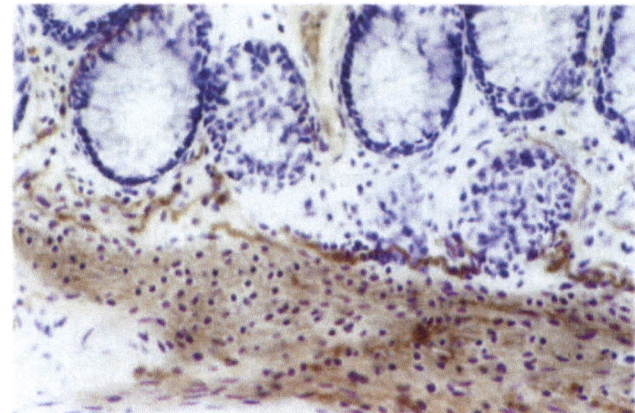

Figure 21.15 Hirschsprung's disease. Small thickened nerve fibres in the muscularis mucosae and lamina propria.   Acetylcholinesterase (AChE) technique × 320

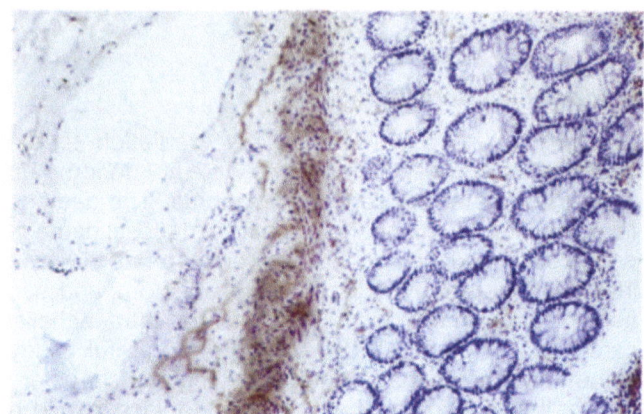

Figure 21.16 Hirschsprung's disease. A doubtful positive biopsy. There are a few thickened fibres in the submucosa, but none in the lamina propria. This boy did in fact have the disease.   AChE technique × 125

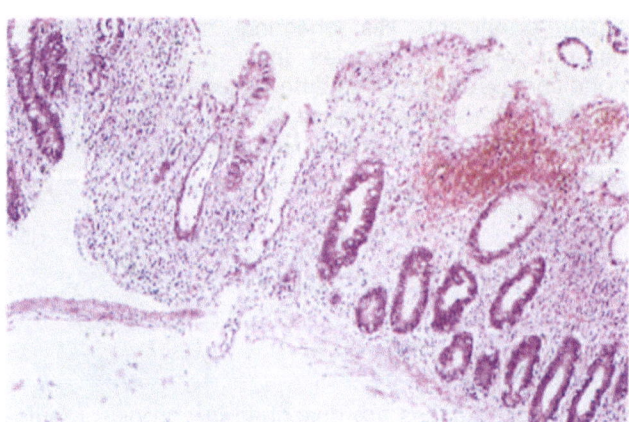

Figure 21.17 Immune-type transplant reaction. There is crypt cell degeneration and dilatation of crypts with surface erosion. The changes themselves are non-specific, but are a guide to an immune reaction in a patient without other evidence of large bowel disease.   H & E × 100

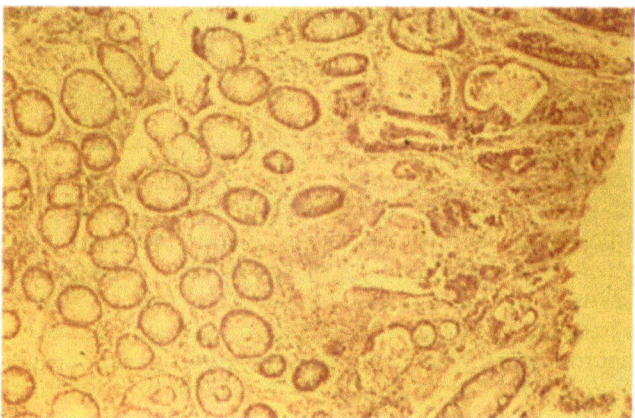

Figure 21.18 Irradiational change. The superficial mucosa has been eroded and replaced by an irregular hyperplastic epithelium indistinguishable from dysplasia. No lamina proprial fibrosis is present here.   H & E × 125

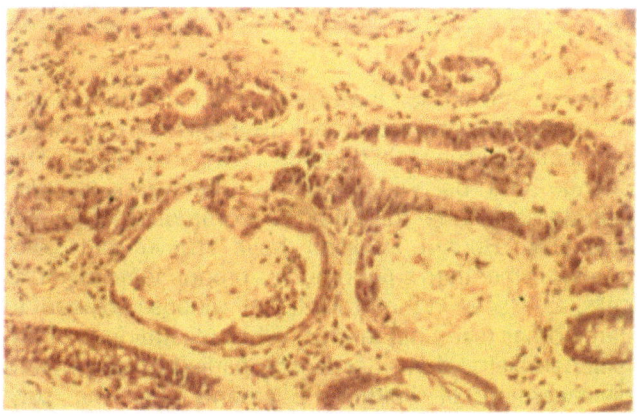

Figure 21.19 Irradiational change. A higher-power view of Figure 21.18. The glandular irregularity is marked but individual cells do not show a great deal of hyperchromasia or alteration in nuclear-cytoplasmic ratio, and there is no increase in mitotic figures. H & E × 320

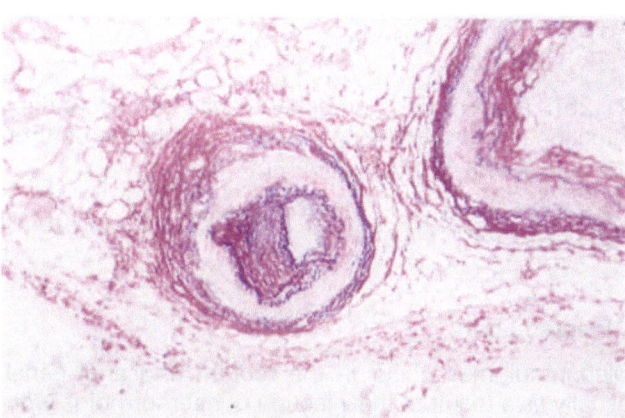

Figure 21.20 Irradiational change. There is marked endarteritis obliterans in small submucosal arteries, with, in this biopsy, a marked increase in adipose tissue. Elastic–Van Gieson stain × 125

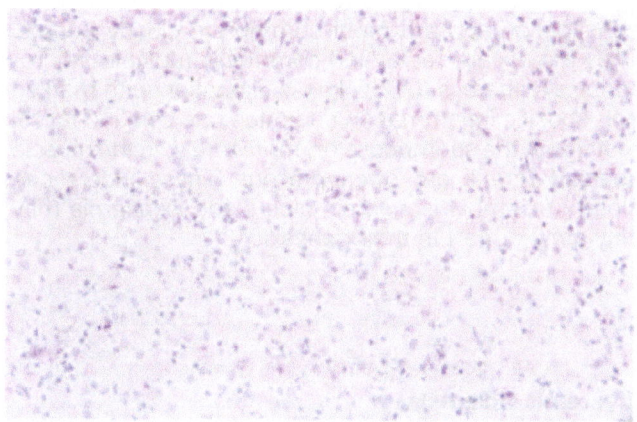

Figure 21.21 Malakoplakia. The macrophage cytoplasm has a characteristic eosinophilic appearance but calcified microspherules are not conspicuous. H & E × 250

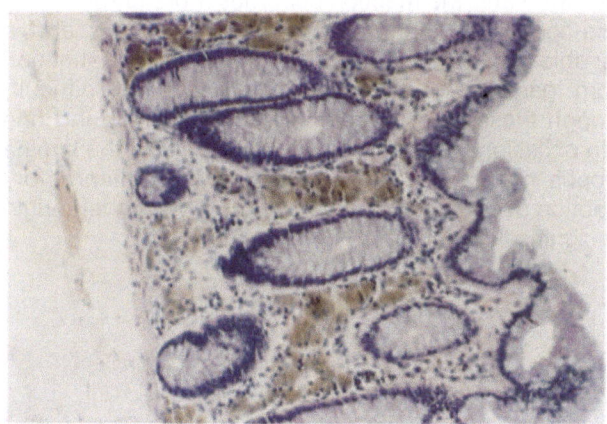

Figure 21.22 Melanosis coli. The pigment is present in aggregates of macrophages within the lamina propria. H & E × 125

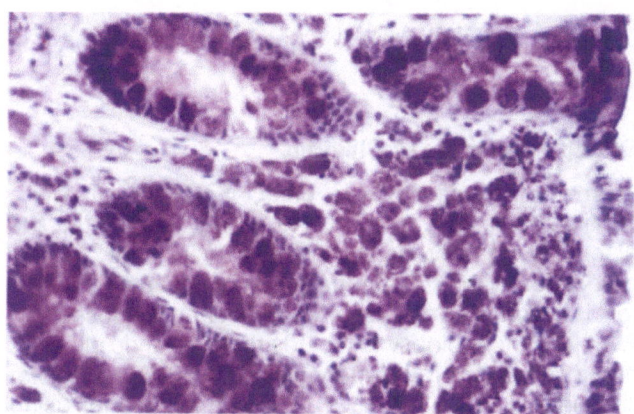

Figure 21.23 Muciphages in rectal mucosa. Macrophages are distended with mucin which has the same tinctorial properties as the mucin within adjacent goblet cells. PAS × 250

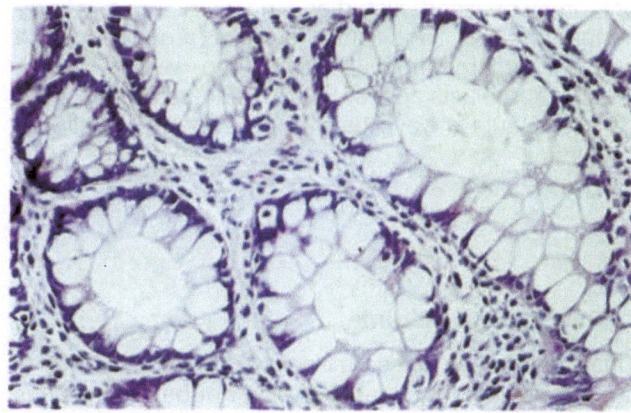

Figure 21.24 Mucoviscidosis, carrier state. The glands in this biopsy, which came from the parent of a child with mucoviscidosis, show a normal appearance, except that individual cells are perhaps slightly more distended with mucin than normal H & E × 250

21.25). These lesions probably result from secondary infection rather than being primarily due to the neutropenia or to the antimitotic therapy.

Oleogranuloma

Oleogranulomas occur in the rectum and anal canal usually as a result of the injection of haemorrhoids with sclerosing fluids in an oily suspension; vegetable oils cause the least, mineral oils the greatest reaction. They present as submucosal swellings which can ulcerate and fibrose and can mimic anal canal or low rectal carcinoma.

Microscopically there is first an acute inflammatory response, in which eosinophils are common, surrounding roughly circular spaces in which oil has been present. Later the reaction becomes more chronic with lipid-containing macrophages and giant cells and a variable degree of fibrosis (Figure 21.26). Distinction from gas-filled cysts can occasionally be difficult, though these must be rare in the anal canal, and one can occasionally see lipid-containing cells in the lamina propria in the absence of any surrounding inflammatory reaction (Figure 21.27). I do not know what their origin or significance is.

Self-induced Proctitis

There is some evidence that patients who are habitually constipated or have a psychological fear of constipation will use manual means to evacuate the bowel, and that traumatic ulceration can be caused in this way. Somewhat similar lesions may be seen in male homosexuals, but are usually masked by superadded infection. The lesion resembles that seen in solitary ulcer syndrome. There is fibrosis within the lamina propria with gland distortion and sometimes inflammatory change, and often surface erosion with a purulent inflammatory exudate into which lamina proprial fibroblasts appear to grow (Figure 21.28). This pattern should always prompt an appropriate clinical enquiry.

Solitary Ulcer Syndrome

This syndrome is indeed misnamed, since ulceration is not invariable and the lesions need not be solitary! It is also still poorly recognized and often misdiagnosed. The cause is probably mucosal prolapse with secondary ischaemia. Endoscopically there is a roughened red area confined to the anterior or anterolateral rectal wall, which may later ulcerate[15,16]. Microscopically there is some broadening of the lamina propria with tortuosity and sometimes dilatation of crypts. The muscularis mucosae is thickened and strands of muscle extend

upwards into the lamina propria in which there is also increased fibrosis, often best distinguished by using a connective tissue stain (Figures 21.29 and 21.30). This change can be widespread. Surface erosion with pseudomembrane formation is common though not invariable. Recent studies[16] have shown that sialomucins rather than sulphomucins predominate in goblet cells, as is seen in the 'transitional' mucosa adjacent to carcinomas (see Chapter 20). When ulceration occurs it is superficial and is often accompanied by downward displacement of epithelial elements into the submucosa.

Stercoral Ulceration

Stercoral ulcers are caused by the pressure of solid faecal matter on large bowel mucosa in long-standing constipation and are most common in elderly people. They are usually rectal and commonly multiple. Microscopically there is full-thickness ulceration with marked non-specific inflammation and often one can find faecal material in the submucosa or, more rarely, in the muscle coats. Bacteria are often present. These ulcers can closely resemble ischaemic ulcers and ischaemia may play a major part in their genesis.

Systemic Sclerosis

The large bowel is not uncommonly involved in systemic sclerosis, but the principal changes – which are fibrosis, elastosis and sclerosis in the muscle coats – are not seen on biopsy. There is often some non-specific patchy fibrosis in the submucosa and there can be a non-specific mucosal atrophy; arterial changes in the submucosa are rare. A definitive diagnosis on biopsy is probably impossible.

Storage Disorders in Children

In specialized paediatatric units, including our own, considerable use is made of rectal biopsy in the diagnosis of storage disorders, which are usually associated with mental retardation, such as the various forms of Batten's disease and other gangliosidoses[17,18]. A full-thickness biopsy to include the myenteric plexus is essential, and this is quenched unfixed and cryostat sectioned. I follow Lake[17] in including techniques using PAS with and without diastase, Sudan black, Oil red O, Luxol fast blue, Feyrter's thionin method and a technique for acid phosphatase, as well as an unstained section for autofluorescence[18]. Interpretation needs time and care but is not essentially difficult provided that the biopsy is adequate. Full details are available in Brett and Lake's excellent paper[17].

References

1. Smith, B. (1972). Pathology of cathartic colon. *Proc. R. Soc. Med.*, **65,** 288

2. Goodall, H. B. and Sinclair, I. S. R. (1957). Colitis cystica profunda. *J. Pathol. Bacteriol.*, **73**, 33

3. Barbezat, G. O., Bowie, M. D. and Kaschula, R. O. C. (1967). Studies on the small intestinal mucosa of children with protein calorie malnutrition. *S. Afr. Med. J.*, **41**, 1031

4. Ecker, J. A., Williams, R. G. and Clay, K. L. (1971). Pneumatosis cystoides intestinalis – bullous emphysema of the intestine. A review of the literature. *Am. J. Gastroenterol.*, **56**, 125

5. Spjut, H. J. and Perkins, D. E. (1969). Endometriosis of the sigmoid colon and rectum. *Am. J. Roentgenol.*, **82**, 1070

6. Gordon, P. H., Schottler, J. L., Balcos, E. G. and Goldberg, S. M. (1976). Perianal endometrioma. Report of five cases. *Dis Col. Rectum*, **19**, 260

7. Wolf, M. (1971). Heterotopic gastric epithelium in the rectum. *Am. J. Clin. Pathol.*, **55**, 604

8. Meier-Ruge, W. (1974). Hirschsprung's disease: its aetiology, pathogenesis and differential diagnosis. *Curr. Top. Pathol.*, **59**, 131

9. MacMahon, R. A., Moore, C. C. M. and Cussen, L. J. (1981). Hirschsprung-like syndrome in patients with normal ganglion cells on suction rectal biopsy. *J. Pediatr. Surg.*, **16**, 835

10. Patrick, W. J. A., Besley, G. T. N. and Smith, I. I. (1980). Histochemical diagnosis of Hirschsprung's disease and a comparison of the histochemical and biochemical activity of acetylcholinesterase in rectal mucosal biopsies. *J. Clin. Pathol.*, **33**, 336

11. Epstein, R. J., McDonald, G. B., Sale, G. E., Shulman, H. M. and Thomas, E. D. (1980). The diagnostic accuracy of the rectal biopsy in acute graft-versus-host disease; a prospective study of 13 patients. *Gastoenterology*, **78**, 764

12. Chaudhry, A. P., Satchidanand, S. K., Anthone, R. Baumler, R. A. and Gaeta, J. F. (1980). An unusual case of supraclavicular and colonic malakoplakia – a light and ultrastructural study. *J. Pathol.*, **131**, 193

13. Neutra, M. R. and Trier, J. S. (1978). Rectal mucosa in cystic fibrosis. Morphological features before and after short term organ culture. *Gastroenterology,* **75**, 701

14. Kies, M. S., Luedka, D. W., Boyd, J. F. and McCue, M. J. (1979). Neutropenic enterocolitis. Two case reports of long term survival following surgery. *Cancer*, **43**, 730

15. Rutter, K. R. P. and Riddell, R. H. (1975). The solitary ulcer syndrome of the rectum. *Clin. Gastroenterol.*, **4**, 505

16. Franzin, G., Scarpa, A., Dina, A. and Novelli, P. (1981). 'Transitional' and hyperplastic–metaplastic mucosa occurring in solitary ulcer of the rectum. *Histopathology,* **5**, 527

17. Brett, E. M. and Lake, B. D. (1975). Reassessment of rectal approach to neuropathology in childhood. Review of 307 biopsies over 11 years. *Arch. Dis. Child.*, **50**, 753

18. Dawson, I. M. P. (1981). The value of histochemistry in the diagnosis and prognosis of gastrointestinal diseases. In Stoward, P. J. and Polak, J. M. (eds.). *Histochemistry. The Widening Horizons.* Chapter 9 (Chichester: John Wiley & Sons)

Figures 21.25–21.30 will be found overleaf.

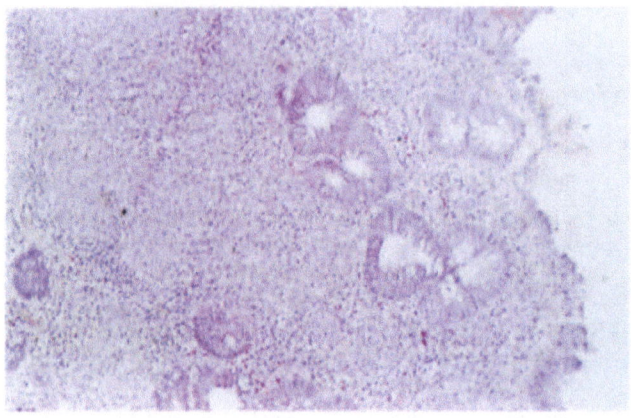

Figure 21.25 Chronic granulomatous disease. There is patchy loss of gland elements, a heavy inflammatory cell infiltrate in the lamina propria and a definite granulomatous reaction. H & E × 125

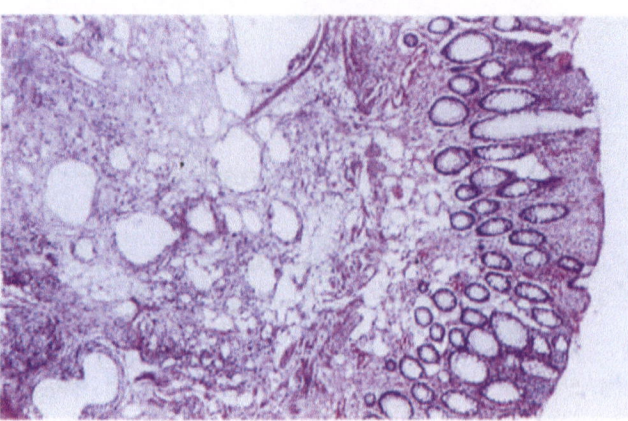

Figure 21.26 Oleogranuloma. There are numerous roughly spherical spaces where oil has escaped into the tissues; these are surrounded by macrophages and giant cells but there is little fibrosis in this biopsy. H & E × 65

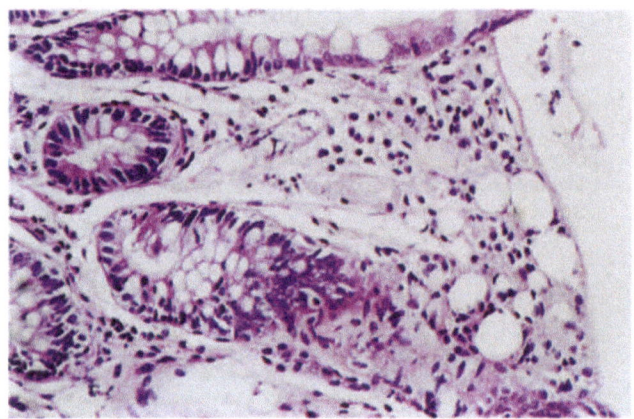

Figure 21.27 Lipid-containing cells in lamina propria. It is difficult to say what these represent. They may be small deposits of oil used as a lubricant, or may be genuine adipose tissue cells. There is little or no accompanying inflammatory reaction. H & E × 250

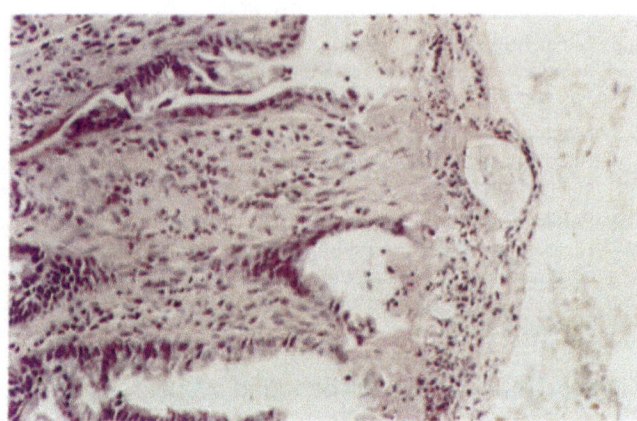

Figure 21.28 Self-induced proctitis. There is surface mucosal erosion with an inflammatory exudate, and a fibroblastic reaction in the lamina propria which is growing outwards into the exudate. From a woman who habitually used a fingerstall to aid faecal evacuation. H & E × 250

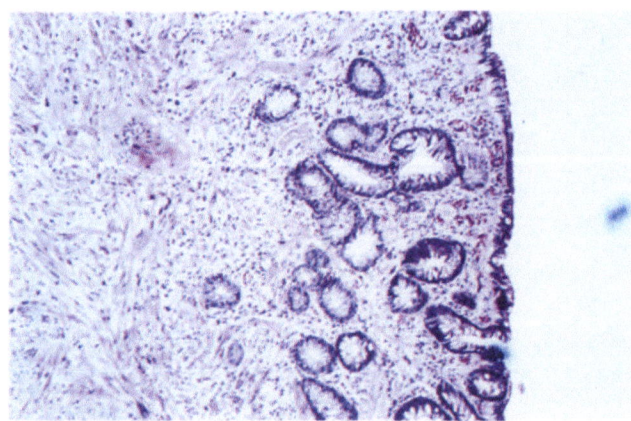

Figure 21.29 Solitary ulcer syndrome. There is gland drop-out with some glandular irregularity, but the main features are fibrosis in the lamina propria and upgrowth of muscularis mucosae into it. H & E × 100

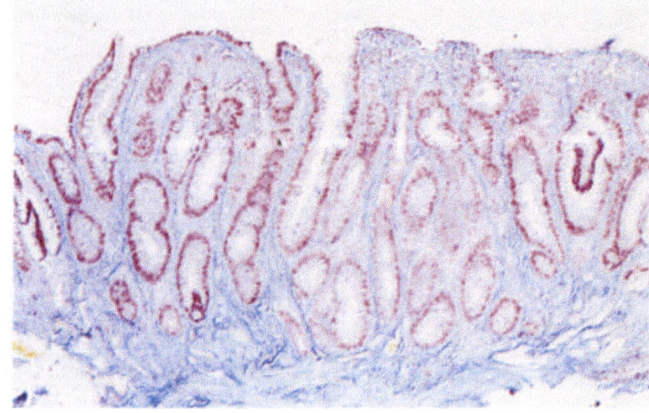

Figure 21.30 Solitary ulcer syndrome. Trichrome stain to show the extent of fibrous tissue proliferation. × 80

Index